Practical Neurology of the Elderly
Volume I

Edited by

Jacob I. Sage, MD

Professor, Department of Neurology
Director, Division of Movement Disorders
University of Medicine and Dentistry of New Jersey
Robert Wood Johnson Medical School, New Brunswick, New Jersey

and

Margery H. Mark, MD

Associate Professor, Department of Neurology
University of Medicine and Dentistry of New Jersey
Robert Wood Johnson Medical School, New Brunswick, New Jersey

Brought to you by an educational grant from Cephalon, Inc., a neuroscience company dedicated to the discovery, development, and marketing of pharmaceutical products for the treatment of neurological disorders.

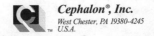
Cephalon®, Inc.
West Chester, PA 19380-4245
U.S.A.

ISBN: 0-8247-9694-2

The publisher offers discounts on this book when ordered in bulk quantities. For more information, write to Special Sales/ Professional Marketing at the address below.

This book is printed on acid-free paper.

MARCEL DEKKER, INC.

270 Madison Avenue, New York, New York 10016

Current printing (last digit):
10 9 8 7 6 5 4 3 2 1

PRINTED IN THE UNITED STATES OF AMERICA

Preface

Elderly people, a growing segment of our population, present special challenges in their medical management that are the *raison d'être* of this book. Although there are very few ailments that are exclusive to older patients, there are some that are predominantly diseases of older age groups (for example, Alzheimer's disease and other dementing disorders, parkinsonism, and stroke). Many problems are encountered more frequently in the elderly or are more difficult to diagnose correctly in older patients (e.g., confusional states, drug-induced movements, dizziness, fatigue, gait disorders, neurourological problems, infections, and symptoms in the border zone between neurology and psychiatry). Differential diagnosis and treatment may differ between older and younger patients in conditions such as myasthenia gravis, myopathies, neuropathies, sleep disorders, visual complaints, headaches, and seizures. Finally, the needs for legal protection, rehabilitation, and the proper interpretation of neurophysiologic tests are common to all ages but have special significance for quality-of-life issues in older patients. In this book, we have tried to address all these different topics in two convenient volumes.

To illustrate the differences between elderly and younger adults, let us take one with which the editors of this book are most familiar: the treatment of Parkinson's disease. Levodopa is the single most efficacious agent for the treatment of this disease. It can ameliorate many of the functional impairments associated with parkinsonism, and yet we use it differently in senior citizens than in those who are younger. A 55-year-old plumber with some right-arm bradykinesia interfering with the use of a wrench or screwdriver would probably get levodopa treatment. A 75-year-old retired plumber with bilateral hand tremor, generalized bradykinesia, mild fine motor incoordination, and a slow but stable gait would probably have treatment deferred. Not only has the very definition of functional impairment changed with the 20-year difference in age, but the increased fear of debilitating side effects such as psychotoxicity has altered our perception of the risk–benefit ratio in the aged. A middle-aged lawyer with right-hand tremor appearing only in the courtroom might legitimately be started on an anticholinergic, yet that same drug would be carefully avoided if he were 75. Knowledge of these distinctions reflects the quality of medical care and is essential to any physician who treats elderly patients.

This book is aimed at anyone who sees elderly patients: family physicians, internists, geriatricians, psychiatrists, and neurologists. Most of the neurological disorders and related issues that affect the elderly are covered. Most chapters are oriented around a specific subject or constellation of signs and symptoms (confusional states; hyperkinetic and drug-induced movement disorders; the borderline of psychiatry and neurology; gait disturbances and spinal cord diseases; myopathic disorders; neuropathic disorders; stroke; dizziness; fatigue; sleep disorders; visual disorders; pain, headaches, and neuralgias; seizures; neurourology; and infections). Some chapters cover a single disease or a group of related diseases of special importance in elderly patients (e.g., myasthenia gravis, Alzheimer's disease, non-Alzheimer dementing disorders, Parkinson's disease, diffuse Lewy body disease, and atypical parkinsonisms). The final two chapters of Volume I and the final chapter of Volume II are of general significance to those treating the elderly: neurorehabilitation, how to interpret neurophysiological tests in an elderly patient, and legal and ethical issues. Notably, we have chosen to exclude certain neurological conditions such as brain tumors and multiple sclerosis, as these disorders affect young and old similarly and there is nothing peculiar to the treatment of these diseases when they occur in the aged.

We believe that this approach provides an up-to-date and practical book that will be of use to physicians treating an ever-increasing segment of the population.

Jacob I. Sage
Margery H. Mark

Contents

3. Acute Confusion and Delirium   115
David S. Geldmacher

4. Gait Disturbances and Cervical Spondylosis   145
Rodger J. Elble

6. Myopathic Disorders

237

David Lacomis and David A. Chad

Volume II

Contributors

David N. Alexander, M.D.   Associate Clinical Professor, Department of Neurology, University of California at Los Angeles School of Medicine; and Director of Stroke Rehabilitation, Daniel Freeman Hospitals, Los Angeles, California

Anthony A. Amato, M.D.   Assistant Clinical Professor of Medicine (Neurology), Department of Neurology, Wilford Hall Medical Center; and University of Texas Health Science Center at San Antonio, San Antonio, Texas

Richard J. Barohn, M.D.   Associate Professor, Department of Neurology, University of Texas Southwestern Medical Center at Dallas, Dallas, Texas

H. Richard Beresford, M.D., J.D.   Professor, Department of Neurology, University of Rochester School of Medicine, Rochester; and Cornell Law School, Ithaca, New York

Susan E. Boruchoff, M.D.   Assistant Professor, Department of Medicine, Division of Allergy, Immunology, and Infectious Diseases, University of Medicine and Dentistry of New Jersey–Robert Wood Johnson Medical School, New Brunswick, New Jersey

David A. Chad, M.D.   Professor, Department of Neurology and Pathology, University of Massachusetts Medical Center, Worcester, Massachusetts

Sudhansu Chokroverty, M.D.   Chief, Neurology Service, Veterans Administration Medical Center, Lyons, New Jersey; Associate Chairman of Neurology and Chief of Neurophysiology, St. Vincent's Hospital and Medical Center, New York,

New York; Professor, Department of Neurology, University of Medicine and Dentistry of New Jersey–Robert Wood Johnson Medical School, New Brunswick, New Jersey; and Adjunct Professor of Neurology, New York Medical College, New York, New York

Cynthia L. Comella, M.D. Associate Professor, Department of Neurological Sciences, Rush-Presbyterian-St. Luke's Medical Center, Chicago, Illinois

P. K. Coyle, M.D. Department of Neurology, State University of New York at Stony Brook School of Medicine, Stony Brook, New York

Andrew C. Coyne, Ph.D. Assistant Professor of Clinical Pshchiatry, Division of Geriatric Psychiatry, Department of Psychiatry, University of Medicine and Dentistry of New Jersey–Robert Wood Johnson Medical School, Piscataway, New Jersey

Rodger J. Elble, M.D., Ph.D. Associate Professor and Interim Chairman, Department of Neurology; and Director of the Center for Alzheimer Disease and Related Disorders, Southern Illinois University School of Medicine, Springfield, Illinois

Nancy Forman, M.D. Assistant Professor, Department of Psychiatry, University of Medicine and Dentistry of New Jersey–Robert Wood Johnson Medical School, New Brunswick, New Jersey

Joseph H. Friedman, M.D. Professor, Department of Clinical Neurosciences, Brown University School of Medicine; Director, Brown University Parkinson's Disease and Movement Disorders Unit; Chief, Division of Neurology, Roger Williams Medical Center; and Adjunct Clinical Professor, School of Pharmacy, University of Rhode Island, Providence, Rhode Island

David S. Geldmacher, M.D. Assistant Professor, Department of Neurology, Case Western Reserve University School of Medicine; and Clinical Director, University Alzheimer Center, University Hospitals of Cleveland, Cleveland, Ohio

Stephen M. Gollomp, M.D.   Clinical Professor, Department of Neurology, University of Pennsylvania School of Medicine; and Parkinson's Disease and Movement Disorders Center, Graduate Hospital, Philadelphia, Pennsylvania

Timothy C. Hain, M.D.   Associate Professor, Departments of Otolaryngology and Psychology, Univesity of Miami School of Medicine, Miami, Florida

Susan J. Herdman, Ph.D., P.T.   Departments of Neurology and Otolaryngology, Northwestern University School of Medicine, Chicago, Illinois

James F. Howard, Jr., M.D.   Professor, Department of Neurology, The University of North Carolina at Chapel Hill, Chapel Hill, North Carolina

Timothy R. Kelliher, M.D.   Clinical Instructor in Neurology, Boston University School of Medicine; and Staff Neurologist, Neurological Unit, Boston City Hospital, Boston, Massachusetts

Janice E. Knoefel, M.D.   Assistant Professor, Department of Neurology, Boston University School of Medicine; and Chief, Geriatric Evaluation and Management Unit, Veterans Administration Medical Center, Boston, Massachusetts

Kenji Kosaka, M.D.   Professor and Chairman, Department of Psychiatry, Yokohama City University School of Medicine, Yokohama, Japan

Lauren B. Krupp, M.D.   Associate Professor, Department of Neurology, State University of New York at Stony Brook School of Medicine, Stony Brook, New York

David Lacomis, M.D.   Assistant Professor, Departments of Neurology and Pathology, University of Pittsburgh School of Medicine, Pittsburgh, Pennsylvania

Margery H. Mark, M.D. Associate Professor, Department of Neurology, University of Medicine and Dentistry of New Jersey–Robert Wood Johnson Medical School, New Brunswick, New Jersey

Matthew A. Menza, M.D. Associate Professor, Departments of Psychiatry and Neurology, University of Medicine and Dentistry of New Jersey–Robert Wood Johnson Medical School, New Brunswick, New Jersey

Brian E. Mondell, M.D. Assistant Professor, Department of Neurology, The Johns Hopkins University School of Medicine, Baltimore; and Medical Director, Baltimore Headache Institute, Lutherville, Maryland

Brian R. Ott, M.D. Assistant Professor, Department of Clinical Neurosciences, Brown University School of Medicine; and Director, Alzheimer's Disease and Memory Disorders Unit, Roger Williams Medical Center, Providence, Rhode Island

Russell C. Packard, M.D. Director, Headache Management and Neurology; and Adjunct Professor, University of West Florida, Pensacola, Florida

William E. Reichman, M.D. Division of Geriatric Psychiatry, Department of Psychiatry, University of Medicine and Dentistry of New Jersey–Robert Wood Johnson Medical School, Piscataway, New Jersey

David E. Riley, M.D. Assistant Professor, Department of Neurology, Case Western Reserve University School of Medicine; and Director, Movement Disorders Center, Mt. Sinai Medical Center, Cleveland, Ohio

Thomas D. Sabin, M.D. Professor, Departments of Neurology and Psychiatry, Boston University School of Medicine, and Director, Neurological Unit, Boston City Hospital, Boston, Massachusetts

Ralph L. Sacco, M.D.   Assistant Professor of Neurology and Public Health (Epidemiology) in the Sergievsky Center, Columbia University College of Physicians and Surgeons; and Director, Northern Manhattan Stroke Study, Neurological Institute of New York, New York, New York

Jacob I. Sage, M.D.   Professor, Department of Neurology, and Director, Division of Movement Disorders, University of Medicine and Dentistry of New Jersey–Robert Wood Johnson Medical School, New Brunswick, New Jersey

Mark L. Scheuer, M.D.   Assistant Professor, Department of Neurology, Columbia University College of Physicians and Surgeons; and Comprehensive Epilepsy Center, Neurological Institute, New York, New York

Martin Sliwinski, Ph.D.   Department of Neurology, State University of New York at Stony Brook School of Medicine, Stony Brook, New York

Matthew B. Stern, M.D.   Associate Professor, Department of Neurology, University of Pennsylvania School of Medicine; and Director, Parkinson's Disease and Movement Disorders Center, Graduate Hospital, Philadelphia, Pennsylvania

Thaddeus S. Walczak, M.D.   Assistant Professor, Department of Neurology, Columbia University College of Physicians and Surgeons; and Comprehensive Epilepsy Center, Neurological Institute, New York, New York

Melvin P. Weinstein, M.D.   Professor, Department of Medicine, Division of Allergy, Immunology and Infectious Diseases, University of Medicine and Dentistry of New Jersey–Robert Wood Johnson Medical School, New Brunswick, New Jersey

M. Cristina Zamanillo, M.P.H., M.D.   Research Staff Associate, Department of Neurology, Columbia University College of Physicians and Surgeons; and Neurological Institute of New York, New York, New York

1

Alzheimer's Disease

William E. Reichman and Andrew C. Coyne
University of Medicine and Dentistry of New Jersey
Robert Wood Johnson Medical School
Piscataway, New Jersey

I. INTRODUCTION

Alzheimer's disease (AD) is the most common irreversible and progressive cause of dementia. It is the fourth leading cause of death in developed nations, after heart disease, cancer, and stroke. In the past few years, the disorder has come to the forefront of public attention. Improvements in the diagnosis, management, and treatment of dementia (1), coupled with demographic shifts in the population of the United States (2,3), have vastly increased the resources devoted to Alzheimer's disease (4).

The fundamental clinical consequence of AD is dementia, a syndrome characterized by acquired and persistent impairments in memory, cognition (problem solving, calculation, abstraction), language, and visuospatial abilities (5–7). Generally, accompanying these deficits is some alteration in behavior and mood. In all causes of dementia, including AD, intellectual decline leads to progressive functional impairment. The affected individual is eventually unable to fulfill some of the most essential roles of his or her life. The capacities to work, manage household affairs, parent a child, or support and comfort a spouse or friend are irretrievably lost.

II. HISTORICAL BACKGROUND

Clinical descriptions of disorders resembling dementia date back perhaps as much as 2500 years, with the term *dementia* itself first being used by the Roman medical writer Aurelius Cornelius Celsus during the first century A.D. More recent centuries saw the introduction of the terms *senile dementia* by Esquirol in 1838, as well as *presenile dementia* by Binswanger in 1898 (8). Furthermore, the clinical and neuropathological observations of Alzheimer (9), (i.e., cerebral atrophy, senile or neuritic plaques, and neurofibrillary tangles), coupled with related findings by Blocq and Marinesco (10) and Simchowicz (11), eventually led to widespread use of the label *Alzheimer's disease* as the designation for the most common form of dementia.

III. EPIDEMIOLOGY

Previous investigations into the prevalence of clinically diagnosed AD have provided estimates ranging from less than 2% of the 65 and older population to more than 10% (12–18). A comprehensive review of descriptive epidemiologic studies dealing with AD has been provided by Rocca and colleagues (19). Two recent studies serve to illustrate the range of estimates of the prevalence of AD in the community that have been reported. In one study, Folstein and colleagues (14) conducted a three-stage survey of community-residing adults in Baltimore, Maryland. The first stage involved screening interviews with 3481 adults; the second stage involved a standardized clinical psychiatric examination of 810 individuals seen during the first stage; and the third, or differential diagnosis, stage collected additional data for 32 individuals through a neurological examination, laboratory tests, review of previous medical records, and interviews with informants. Findings indicated that 4.5% of the over-65 population suffered from some form of dementia. More specifically, among those 65 and older, 2% suffered from AD; 2% had multi-infarct dementia (MID); and 0.5% had mixed dementia (AD and MID). As shown in Table 1, the prevalence of dementia

Table 1 Estimated Age Specific Prevalence of DSM-III Dementing Disorders Among 31,200 Eastern Baltimoreans over Age 65

Diagnosis	Ages 65–74			Ages 75–84			Ages 85+		
	N	%	(SE)	N	%	(SE)	N	%	(SE)
Alzheimer's disease	1	0.3	(0.3)	7	3.7	(1.3)	4	8.2	(3.4)
Multi-infarct dementia	3	0.7	(0.4)	2	1.0	(0.7)	2	15.5	(13.2)
Mixed dementia	1	0.2	(0.2)	1	0.6	(0.6)	1	1.9	(1.9)
All dementia	5	1.2	(0.6)	10	5.3	(1.5)	7	25.6	(13.5)

Source: Ref. 14.

was found to rise with age; for AD in particular, Folstein and coworkers reported a rate of 0.3% among 65- to 74-year-olds; 3.7% among 75- to 84-year-olds; and 8.2% among those 85 and older.

In a similar investigation, Evans and associates (13) examined the cognitive functioning of 3623 community-residing adults above the age of 65 in East Boston, Massachusetts. Individuals were initially screened with a brief test of cognitive functioning and classified into three memory performance groups (i.e., good, intermediate, and poor). A stratified sample of 467 individuals selected from these three groups then underwent a comprehensive clinical evaluation designed to diagnose Alzheimer's disease, other dementias, and other medical conditions that may have produced cognitive impairment.

The application of National Institute of Neurological and Communicative Disorders and Stroke (NINCDS)–Alzheimer's Disease and Related Disorders Association (ADRDA) (20) diagnostic criteria for probable AD, as well as modified DSM-III-R (21) criteria for primary degenerative dementia, resulted in an overall estimated prevalence rate of 10.3% for those 65 years of age and older. Prevalence of dementia was found to vary by age; among 65- to 74-year-olds, the prevalence was 3.0%; among 75- to 84-year-olds, 18.7%; and among those 85 and older, 47.2%.

Clearly, wide interstudy variation in prevalence estimates—making for difficulty in interpreting and comparing results of previous investigations—is not uncommon. Such variation may reflect methodological differences, as well as a lack of agreement regarding diagnostic criteria for specific dementias (19,22). At least some improved comparability across future studies, however, should have resulted from the adoption of uniform diagnostic criteria over the last decade (20,23).

A. Risk Factors

In addition to prevalence data, another important issue from an epidemiological standpoint is that of risk factors for the development of Alzheimer's disease. Perhaps the largest single risk factor is age. Katzman and Saitoh (24) point out that "AD is the epitome of an age-dependent disorder . . . its age-specific prevalence increases logarithmically with age" (Figure 1).

Gender may represent another risk factor for AD. For example, recent data from Folstein and colleagues (14) indicated that the prevalence of AD was higher for females than males. This echoes earlier findings of Kay (25), who observed a higher prevalence of senile dementia among females than males. Still other phenomena that have been implicated (although not necessarily confirmed) as risk factors for the de-

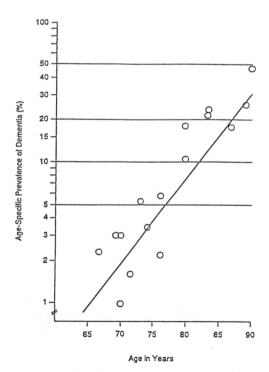

Figure 1 Age-specific prevalence of dementia.

velopment of AD include the following: a family history of affected members (26–28). the presence of Down's syndrome in the individual with suspected dementia (29–31), and Down's syndrome among family members of the individual (32,33). Additional factors that have been considered are exposure to environmental toxins such as aluminum or organic solvents (34,35), head trauma (36), and surgical anesthesia (36,37). Finally, low educational level has been related to a greater prevalence of dementia (38,39) and to greater severity of dementia (40).

IV. CLINICAL FEATURES

A. Neuropsychological Features

In all patients affected with AD, dementia is an inevitable feature. Classically, dementia of the Alzheimer type has been described as having an insidious onset with gradual progression of severity. While relatively brief plateau phases are often noted in the clinical course of the disorder, the deleterious effects of AD on intellectual ability and functional performance in the activities of daily living are unremitting and ultimately catastrophic.

AD consists of impairment in several intellectual spheres including memory, language, visuospatial skill, and cognition (calculation, problem solving, abstraction). As the disease advances, intellectual impairment is accompanied by apraxia and agnosia. Early in the course of the disease, patients demonstrate impaired recent recall and mild word-finding difficulties. The typical language output of such patients has been described as circumlocutory. There is a vague or empty quality to the individual's discourse, reflecting the presence of anomia. As the fluent language disturbance progresses, patients begin to demonstrate difficulties with language comprehension; repetition ability, however, is relatively well preserved (transcortical sensory aphasia). Many patients will demonstrate paraphasic errors (substitutions of words or phonemes) and manifest difficulty in writing and reading comprehension. The ability to read aloud, despite impaired reading comprehension, is a common finding in the middle stages of the disease. Reiterative language disturbances such as logoclonia and palilalia are also notable. In the later stages of AD, language output becomes less fluent, comprehension is severely impaired, and repetition ability is lost. Patients are unable to read or write. In the terminal stage of AD, the patient may be mute (41).

With progression of language deficits, memory impairment becomes more striking. Patients become unable to learn new information and have difficulty with remote recall. Orientation to the date and surroundings is impaired. Memory for recent and remote historical events, personal history, and fund of information becomes severely restricted.

Disruptions in visuospatial ability result in navigational difficulties as many patients wander or get easily lost. The abilities to manipulate numbers and solve problems become increasingly disturbed.

B. Neurological Features

In classic, early AD, the neurological examination is strikingly unremarkable. Most commonly, there are no notable sensorimotor, cerebellar, extrapyramidal, or other pathological signs. Across stages of disease severity, the prevalence of extrapyramidal signs (EPS) has been reported to vary between 9% and 67% (42–44). Most such series note that tremor uncommonly accompanies bradykinesia and rigidity in these patients. A recent study (45) reported that extrapyramidal signs appeared in 17% of early-onset AD patients compared with 26% of late-onset patients. Taken as a group, most of these studies report an increasing prevalence of EPS with disease progression. Throughout all stages of dementia severity, bradykinesia, rigidity, ataxia, and postural abnormalities are more common in AD patients than in age-matched, healthy controls (46). The pathogenesis of EPS in AD is still unresolved. In some postmortem studies, the pathological changes of AD and Parkinson's disease accompany each other (47–49). Morris and coworkers (44), however, have reported the relative absence of striatonigral pathology in AD patients with parkinsonism.

In addition to EPS, a variety of other neurologic signs have been documented in AD. Paulson and Gottlieb (50) described the reemergence of primitive reflexes and gegenhalten in patients with senile dementia. As AD advances, many patients demonstrate grasping, sucking, and snout reflexes. Urinary and fecal incontinence are also frequently observed. In late-stage AD, disturbed gait is often noted along with pyramidal signs such as the extensor plantar response and hyperactive jaw jerk reflex (46). Although seizures may be encountered in the early stages of AD, they are more often seen as the patient enters the later stages of the disorder (51). The prevalence of myoclonus in AD also seems to increase with disease progression (51,52). Dysarthria is notably rare in AD until the later stages are reached.

C. Psychiatric Features

In addition to the disability resulting from intellectual deterioration, approximately 60% of afflicted patients demonstrate clinically significant psychiatric and behavioral symptoms (53). Many patients become increasingly irritable, rigid, and coarse in their display of emotions (54). Additionally, several patients with AD appear apathetic, aloof, or withdrawn. With increasing passivity, initiative and interest may be deficient; many such patients appear to lack empathy for others and are notably self-centered (55). These common changes in demeanor may be accompanied by disinhibition and perseverative tendencies. Many patients become increasingly fretful and are afraid to be left alone; they may shadow the caregiver (viscosity) or pace throughout the home. Ill-defined anxiety and restlessness are also common findings. At times, many patients will demonstrate sudden severe spells of anxiety (catastrophic reactions) in response to minor stresses such as a change in routine.

Frank delusions occur in nearly half of AD patients and take several forms. Most commonly, delusional thoughts have paranoid themes, but are poorly elaborated. Delusions of theft, abandonment, and infidelity are often seen in routine clinical practice. Patients may also inexplicably insist on leaving their own house in order to "go home." Many of these patients falsely believe that they must leave to care for their children or go to work. Commonly, affected individuals argue that "others" have been milling about the house (phantom boarder delusion) or that the spouse or caregiver is an imposter (Capgras delusion) (53).

Hallucinations and illusions are not uncommon in AD, but are rarely as florid as in delirious states or psychiatric conditions such as schizophrenia or bipolar disorder. Occasionally, patients may hear voices or see things that are not there. Tactile or olfactory hallucinations are notably rare and should prompt an inquiry into other potential causes apart from AD.

Many patients with AD demonstrate verbal and physical aggression. Later-stage patients may engage in repetitive behaviors such as tray- and head-banging or self-mutilation.

Although major depression is unusual in AD, milder symptoms of dysphoria are relatively common (56). Alterations in the sleep/wake cycle and diet are also often noted in both depressed and nondepressed AD patients.

Despite the full spectrum of behavioral and intellectual changes in the disorder, the characteristic patient with AD remains relatively unconcerned. While many patients may be aware that they suffer from impaired memory, such individuals are typically not as concerned as one might expect. As a result, insight is felt to be impaired in the disorder (54).

As the broad range of neuropsychological deficits and psychiatric symptoms accumulate, the individual's functional abilities deteriorate. The vast majority of patients eventually experience great difficulty completing their work, managing household tasks, and attending adequately to grooming, hygiene and toileting. With progression of such impairments, the individual's vocational, social, and familial roles are abandoned.

D.   Psychosocial Features

A large number of previous investigations have provided evidence that Alzheimer's disease has a significant impact on the functioning of family-member caregivers (57–60). Although the exact consequences of providing daily care for cognitively impaired older adults on family-member caregivers are still in question (61), a number of potential outcomes have been identified. These include high levels of psychological stress and burden (58); a high incidence of clinical depression (62); compromised physical health (63–65); and an increased probability of physical abuse within the caregiving relationship (66).

E.   Clinical Course

The clinical course of AD is characterized by gradual progression of intellectual deficits. Over time, these deficits are accompanied by increasing functional and physical disability and psychiatric symptomatology (Table 2). Death generally results within 15 years of the diagnosis having been established. The rate of disease progression, however, is variable. This finding has historically prompted a search for clusters of clinical variables or AD subtypes that may predict a particular clinical course such as age of onset, gender, degree of aphasia, or the presence of myoclonus, apraxia, agnosia, or extrapyramidal features (67–69). Drachman and colleagues (70) have argued that only those measures that assess disease severity best predict the subsequent course of AD. To date, it remains unresolved as to whether in fact there are AD subtypes that give rise to a particularly rapid or slow course.

Table 2 Principal Clinical Findings in Each Stage of DAT

Stage I (duration of disease 1–3 years)
  Memory: new learning defective, remote recall mildly impaired
  Visuospatial skills: topographic disorientation, poor complex constructions
  Language: poor wordlist generation, anomia
  Personality: indifference, occasional irritability
  Psychiatric features: sadness or delusions in some
  Motor system: normal
  EEG: normal
  CT/MRI: normal
  PET/SPECT: bilateral posterior parietal hypometabolism/hypoperfusion

Stage II (duration of disease 2–10 years)
  Memory: recent and remote recall more severely impaired
  Visuospatial skills: poor construction, spatial disorientation
  Language: fluent aphasia
  Calculation: acalculia
  Praxis: ideomotor apraxia
  Personality: indifference or irritability
  Psychiatric features: delusions in some
  Motor system: restlessness, pacing
  EEG: slowing or background rhythm
  CT/MRI: normal or ventricular dilation and sulcal enlargement
  PET/SPECT: bilateral parietal and frontal hypometabolism/hypoperfusion

Stage III (duration of disease 8–12 years)
  Intellectual functions: severely deteriorated
  Motor: limb rigidity and flexion posture
  Sphincter control: urinary and fecal incontinence
  EEG: diffusely slow
  CT/MRI: ventricular dilatation and sulcal enlargement
  PET/SPECT: bilateral parietal and frontal hypometabolism/hypoperfusion

Source: Ref. 41.

V.   NEUROPATHOLOGICAL FEATURES

Upon gross inspection, the affected brain in AD is marked by diffuse cortical atrophy that is most prominent in the parietal, temporal, and anterior frontal areas. The primary motor area, somatosensory region, and occipital lobe are largely spared (71).

The hallmark microscopic histological findings of AD consist of neuronal loss, neuritic plaques, neurofibrillary tangles, and granulovacuolar degeneration. This is accompanied by astrocytic gliosis and neuronal lipofuscin deposition (72). The central core of the neuritic plaque consists of the glycoprotein amyloid. Surrounding this central core are fragments of degenerated neuronal processes. Within the plaque, synapses are significantly reduced in number. Presumably, this invariably leads to disrupted communication between neighboring neurons and subsequent functional loss (41). Amyloid is also noted to accumulate abnormally within the walls of the intracerebral vasculature (amyloid angiography) (73).

Neurofibrillary tangles (NFTs) are intraneuronal proteinaceous structures composed of pairs of twisted neurofilaments called paired helical filaments (PHFs). An abnormally phosphorylated form of the microtubule associated protein, tau, appears to be an important constituent of the PHFs (74). As neurons undergo neurofibrillary changes, PHFs become increasingly densely packed within the cellular cytoplasm (75). It remains unknown to what extent this hastens neuronal death. Bundles of PHF are also found within the neuritic plaque.

The predominant cortical sites of pathologic change in AD include the posterior temporoparieto-occipital junction, frontal association areas, and posterior cingulate. The hippocampus, amygdala, and entorhinal regions are also significantly involved (72).

The septal nucleus basalis of Meynert, the main origination site of cholinergic projections to the cortex, demonstrates significant neuronal loss, granulovacuolar degeneration, and neurofibrillary tangles (76). The brainstem nuclei locus ceruleus (noradrenergic) and median raphe (serotonergic) also show considerable neuronal loss (77).

VI. NEUROCHEMICAL FEATURES

The primary neurotransmitter deficit of AD is depletion of acetylcholine. This reflects the significant disruption of cholinergic projections emanating from the nucleus basalis that is consistently noted in the disease. Choline acetyltransferase, the enzyme responsible for acetylcholine synthesis, is especially diminished in the frontal and parietal regions, as well as the hippocampus. It is largely assumed that the disruption in cholinergic function noted in AD reflects presynaptic pathology; postsynaptic receptor numbers are only mildly reduced or normal (78).

Several other neurotransmitters have also been found to be deficient in AD, including norepinephrine, serotonin, and gamma-aminobutyric acid (72). Neuropeptides such as somatostatin, corticotropin-releasing factor, substance P, and vasopressin are also preferentially depleted in the disorder (79–81).

VII. PATHOGENESIS

Despite the consistent finding of neuritic plaques and neurofibrillary tangles in AD, the pathogenesis of the disorder remains a subject of considerable controversy. The lack of a suitable animal model in which to study AD has contributed to the uncertainty about which specific cellular processes lead to the clinical expression of the disorder. Some investigators point to the abnormally abundant extracellular accumulation of beta-amyloid as the hallmark event in the pathogenesis of AD (82). Apparently, the deposition of beta-amyloid is the consequence of its cleavage from amyloid precursor protein (APP), a glycosylated protein that extends the width of the cell membrane. There are two potential metabolic pathways that are responsible for the cleavage of APP into its constituent parts. The secretase pathway avoids the formation of amyloid-ogenic (plaque-forming) APP fragments (83). However, the lysosomal pathway, because of its particular site of cleavage of APP, leads to the cellular extrusion of potentially amyloid-ogenic fragments (84). Although data remain incomplete, act-ivation of muscarinic acetylcholine receptors has been dem-onstrated to stimulate release of APP fragments in cultured human cell lines (83). This finding provides preliminary evi-dence that there may be an important link between cholinergic neurotransmission and abnormal APP processing.

A. Genetic Factors

Over the past several years, the molecular genetics of AD has undergone intensive study. For early-onset AD, a familial gene has been mapped to chromosomes 14 (85) and 21 (28, 86). This latter finding was initially of particular interest as the gene coding for amyloid precursor protein (APP) was localized to the same chromosomal region (87–89). Although subject to continued debate, it appears that mutations within the APP gene may account for the expression of the disease in a subgroup of families with a relatively early disease on-set (late 40s and 50s) (90–93). Perhaps in additional families, other genetic mutations may be responsible for disruptions in cellular amyloid processing leading to the onset of the disease.

In late-onset AD, attention has been focused on the apo-lipoprotein E (ApoE) type 4 allele on chromosome 19 (94,95). Although data remain preliminary, available evidence suggests that the presence of the ApoE type 4 allele increases the risk of developing the disorder while the number of alleles influ-ences the age of disease onset (94).

Despite these important findings, most cases of AD do not appear to be familial. Although the first-degree relatives of AD patients have an increased risk of contracting the dis-order, the extent of the risk remains unknown (87). In fami-lies in which the disorder clusters, it often appears to dem-onstrate a pattern of autosomal dominant inheritance with full penetrance (87).

VIII. CLINICAL DIAGNOSIS

Clinical criteria for the diagnosis of AD have been well-established (20) (Table 3). The diagnosis relies on the presence of impaired memory accompanied by other intellectual deficits. Patients must be between the ages of 40 and 90 years. Documentation of progression of impairment over the course of one year must also be evident. The clinical diagnosis of "probable AD" requires that other potential causes of dementia such as stroke, metabolic abnormalities, infectious diseases, head trauma, or cerebral mass lesions have been excluded. If, in fact, such abnormalities are uncovered, but not considered to be etiologically related to the observed dementia, then the patient is given the diagnosis of "possible AD." This diagnosis is also applied if the clinical course deviates from the expected insidious onset and gradual progression of the disorder or the patient demonstrates an atypical constellation of deficits. A diagnosis of "definite AD" requires histopathological confirmation by brain biopsy or, more commonly, by postmortem examination. Using these clinical criteria, diagnostic accuracy approaches 90% (96).

The standard clinical evaluation of AD requires a set of established procedures that attempts to exclude all other causes of dementia and to identify the classic clinical features of the disorder. The evaluation initially consists of the taking of a thorough history, physical examination, neurological examination, and mental status assessment (Table 4).

Once the chief complaint is identified, the history must include questions that attempt to uncover the full breadth of neuropsychological and functional impairments (e.g., in activities of daily living). Additional queries are directed toward identifying the timing of dementia onset, its course, and whether or not there have been any associated medical, neurological, or psychiatric features.

A commonly used structured mental-status instrument is the Folstein Mini-Mental State Exam (MMSE) (Table 5) (97). The scale's items assess memory, language, visuoconstruct-

Table 3   Criteria for Clinical Diagnosis of Alzheimer's Disease

1. The criteria for the clinical diagnosis of *probable* Alzheimer's
    disease include:
    Dementia established by clinical examination and documented
       by the Mini-Mental Exam, Blessed Dementia Scale, or some
       similar examination and confirmed by neuropsychological
       tests
    Deficits in two or more areas of cognition
    Progressive worsening of memory and other cognitive functions
    No disturbance of consciousness
    Onset between ages 40 and 90, most often after age 65
    Absence of systemic disorders or other brain diseases that in and
       of themselves could account for the progressive deficits in
       memory and cognition
2. The diagnosis of *probable* Alzheimer's disease is supported by:
    Progressive deterioration of specific cognitive functions such as
       language (aphasia), motor skills (apraxia), and perception
       (agnosia)
    Impaired activities of daily living and altered patterns of behav-
       ior
    Family history of similar disorders, particularly if confirmed
       neuropathologically
    Laboratory results of:
       Normal lumbar puncture as evaluated by standard tech-
       niques
       Normal pattern of nonspecific changes in EEG, such as in-
       creased slow-wave activity, and evidence of cerebral atrophy
       on CT with progression documented by serial observation
3. Other clinical features consistent with the diagnosis of *probable*
    Alzheimer's disease, after exclusion of causes of dementia other
    than Alzheimer's disease, include:
    Plateaus in the course of progression of the illness
    Associated symptoms of depression, insomnia, incontinence,
       delusions, illusions, hallucinations, catastrophic verbal, emo-
       tional, or physical outbursts, sexual disorders, and weight loss
    Other neurologic abnormalities in some patients, especially with
       more advanced disease and including motor signs such as
       increased muscle tone, myoclonus, or gait disorder
    Seizures in advanced disease
    CT normal for age

Table 3 Continued

4. Features that make the diagnosis of *probable* Alzheimer's disease uncertain or unlikely include:

    Sudden, apoplectic onset

    Focal neurologic findings such as hemiparesis, sensory loss, visual field deficits, and incoordination early in the course of the illness

    Seizures or gait disturbances at the onset or very early in the course of the illness

5. Clinical diagnosis of *possible* Alzheimer's disease:

    May be made on the basis of the dementia syndrome, in the absence of other neurologic, psychiatric, or systemic disorders sufficient to cause dementia, and in the presence of variations in the onset, in the presentation, or in the clinical course

    May be made in the presence of a second systemic or brain disorder sufficient to produce dementia, which is not considered to be *the* cause of the dementia

    Should be used in research studies when a single, gradually progressive severe cognitive deficit is identified in the absence of other identifiable cause

6. Criteria for diagnosis of *definite* Alzheimer's disease are:

    The clinical criteria for probable Alzheimer's disease

    Histopathologic evidence obtained from a biopsy or autopsy.

7. Classification of Alzheimer's disease for research purposes should specify features that may differentiate subtypes of the disorder, such as:

    Familial occurrence

    Onset before age of 65

    Presence of trisomy-21

    Coexistence of other relevant conditions such as Parkinson's disease

Source: Ref. 20.

ional ability, calculation, and concentration. While scores below 24 are generally indicative of dementia, higher scores do not exclude the presence of acquired intellectual impairment. Additional scales that may be readily utilized to measure progression of such deficits over time include the Blessed

Table 4 Cornell Scale for Depression in Dementia. (Rating should be based on symptoms and signs occurring during the week prior to interview. No score should be given if symptoms result from physical disability or illness.)

	Mild/Absent 0	Intermittent 1	Severe 2	Unable to Evaluate 9
A. Mood-Related Signs				
1. Anxiety: anxious expression, ruminations, worrying	☐	☐	☐	☐
2. Sadness: sad expression, sad voice, tearfulness	☐	☐	☐	☐
3. Lack of reactivity to pleasant events	☐	☐	☐	☐
4. Irritability: easily annoyed, short tempered	☐	☐	☐	☐
B. Behavioral Disturbance				
5. Agitation: restlessness, handwringing, hairpulling	☐	☐	☐	☐
6. Retardation: slow movements, slow speech, slow reaction	☐	☐	☐	☐
7. Multiple physical complaints (score 0 if GI symptoms only)	☐	☐	☐	☐
8. Loss of interest: less involved in usual activities (score only if change occurred acutely, i.e., in less than 1 month)	☐	☐	☐	☐
C. Physical Signs				
9. Appetite loss: eating less than usual	☐	☐	☐	☐
10. Weight loss (score 2 if greater than 5 lb in 1 month)	☐	☐	☐	☐
11. Lack of energy: fatigues easily, unable to sustain activities (score only if change occurred acutely, i.e., in less than 1 month)	☐	☐	☐	☐

D. Cyclic Functions

   12. Diurnal variation of mood: symptoms worse in morning ☐ ☐ ☐ ☐

   13. Difficulty falling asleep: later than usual for this individual ☐ ☐ ☐

   14. Multiple awakenings during sleep ☐ ☐ ☐

   15. Early morning awakening: earlier than usual for this individual ☐ ☐ ☐

E. Ideational Disturbance

   16. Suicide: feels life is not worth living, has suicidal wishes, or makes suicide attempt ☐ ☐ ☐

   17. Poor self-esteem: self-blame, self-deprecation, feelings of failure ☐ ☐ ☐

   18. Pessimism: anticipation of the worst ☐ ☐ ☐

   19. Mood-congruent delusions: delusions of poverty, illness, or loss ☐ ☐ ☐

Totals

	×0		×1		×2		×0
=	_____	+	_____	+	_____	+	_____

Total Score: _____

Source: Alexopoulos GS, Abrams RC, Young RC, Shamoian CA. Cornell scale for depression in dementia. Biol Psychiatry 1988; 23: 271–284.

Table 5 Folstein Mini-Mental State Exam

Patient: _____ Date: _____

Administered By: _____

Maximum score	Score	
		ORIENTATION
5	( )	What is the (year) (season) (date) (month) (day of week)?
5	( )	Where are we (state) (county) (town) (hospital) (floor)?
		REGISTRATION
3	( )	Name 3 objects: 1 second to say each. Then ask the patient all 3 after you have said them. Give 1 point for each correct answer. Then repeat them until all 3 are learned. Count trials and record. No. of Trials_____
5	( )	Serial 7's. 1 point for each correct. Stop after 5 answers. Alternatively, spell "WORLD" backwards.
		RECALL
3	( )	Ask for 3 objects repeated above. Give 1 point for each correct.
		LANGUAGE
9	( )	Name a pencil and watch. (2 points)
	( )	Repeat the following "No ifs, ands, or buts." (1 point)
	( )	Follow 3-stage command: "Take a paper in your right hand, fold it in half, and put in on the floor." (3 points)
	( )	Read and obey the following: "Close your eyes." (1 point)
	( )	Write a sentence. (1 point)
	( )	Copy design. (1 point)
Total	_____	

Assess level of
consciousness _____
along a continuum. Alert   Drowsy   Stupor   Coma

Source: Ref. 97.

Dementia Scale (98) and the Clinical Dementia Rating Scale (99). The routine assessment of intellectual and memory function in AD may be enhanced by referral to a neuropsychologist. This may be especially important when a patient scores relatively well on a screening instrument such as the MMSE despite a clinical history of impairment. In so doing, more indepth exploration of the patient's neuropsychological functions is then available for discussion with the individual and his family.

Once it has been established that the patient is suffering from dementia, a full exploration of potential causes must be conducted. This typically consists of a screening laboratory battery to rule out the presence of other conditions that may cause or contribute to dementia. Such disorders include hematologic abnormalities, nutritional deficiencies (e.g., vitamin B_{12}, folic acid), endocrinopathies, infectious diseases (e.g., neurosyphilis, HIV infection), and hepatic, renal, or cardiopulmonary failure.

Generally, the search for any significant systemic illnesses is accompanied by neuroimaging to exclude the presence of stroke, tumor, or hydrocephalus (Table 6). In early AD, magnetic resonance imaging (MRI) or computed tomography (CT) of the brain is typically normal or demonstrates diffuse cortical atrophy that is consistent with the patient's age. As the disorder progresses, however, atrophy in excess of what would be expected for the patient's age is frequently noted; the degree of atrophy typically increases over time. The presence of periventricular lucencies on CT or increased signal intensity on T_2-weighted images on MRI does not exclude the diagnosis of AD.

Functional brain imaging such as single photon emission computed tomography (SPECT) is also becoming increasingly available for use as a clinical diagnostic tool. In AD, SPECT classically demonstrates symmetrically reduced cerebral blood flow to the temporoparietal regions. Bilateral frontal hypoperfusion may also be noted. There has been some debate

Table 6   The Clinical Evaluation of Dementia

History of present illness
Review of systems
Past medical history
Medication review
Family history
Physical examination
Neurologic examination
Psychiatric interview
Mental status examination (with rating of dementia severity)
Mandatory laboratory evaluation
   Complete blood count with differential
   Serum electrolytes, calcium, phosphorus, glucose
   Serum creatinine, blood urea nitrogen
   Urinalysis
   Liver function tests
   High-sensitivity thyroid stimulating hormone
   Syphilis serology
   Erythrocyte sedimentation rate
   Serum B_{12}, folic acid
Selective laboratory evaluation
   Lyme disease antibody titer
   Human immunodeficiency virus titer
   Rheumatologic studies (rheumatoid factor, antinuclear antibody
      titer, etc.)
   Endocrine studies (serum cortisol, parathyroid hormone, etc.)
   Arterial blood gas determination
Mandatory neuroimaging
   Computerized tomography or magnetic resonance imaging of the
      head
Selective neuroimaging
   Single photon emission computerized tomography
Additional studies
   Lumbar puncture
   Chest radiograph
   Electrocardiogram
   Electroencephalogram
   Neuropsychological evaluation

regarding the sensitivity of this method in early AD (100, 101). In some AD patients with relatively isolated language or visuospatial deficits, asymmetrically reduced blood flow has been noted in corresponding brain regions (102). In general, the classical AD finding on SPECT may be useful in fortifying a presumptive clinical diagnosis. However, a negative scan, or one that demonstrates focal or diffuse hypoperfusion, does not exclude the diagnosis of AD.

IX. NEUROPATHOLOGICAL DIAGNOSIS

The brains of nondemented elderly frequently show many of the pathological changes considered pathognomonic for AD. Upon histological examination, the essential difference between those individuals who are nondemented at the time of death and those who have AD appears to be the degree of neuropathologic change that is found. Most often, this is reported as a particular number of plaques and tangles per field of magnification ($200\times$) and whether this amount exceeds what is normally expected for the patient's age (103). Different pathological criteria for the diagnosis of AD have been established by a few notable groups, while no uniform criteria have been universally accepted (104).

X. TREATMENT

Contemporary strategies directed at the treatment of AD acknowledge the several biological, psychological, social, and economic facets of the disorder. Treatment is now available for memory and cognition enhancement and the management of the neuropsychiatric features of AD. Additionally, with a greater appreciation of the social and economic consequences of AD, psychosocial and legal services have become more responsive to the needs of afflicted individuals and their families.

A. Memory and Cognition Enhancement

Over the past several years, pharmacotherapy of impaired memory in AD has involved the use of many different classes of medications, with almost universally disappointing results (105). The most successful clinical approach to date involves the administration of agents whose primary functions are to restore deficient levels of acetylcholine in the brains of affected patients or to mimic the effects of acetylcholine on postsynaptic neurons (106). Three cholinergic approaches that have been extensively studied include acetylcholine precursor loading (choline and lecithin), cholinergic agonism (bethanechol, arecoline), and blockade of the degradation of acetylcholine by the use of acetylcholinesterase inhibitors (physostigmine, tacrine). Of these approaches, acetylcholinesterase inhibition with tacrine (tetrahydroaminoacridine) has been the most successful in placebo-controlled clinical trials (107–111). Studies vary significantly in the magnitude of clinical response that is detected; some trials have failed to demonstrate any significant clinical advantage over placebo (112,113). This has prompted considerable debate over whether the modest benefits of the drug outweigh its very significant dose-related side effects, which include hepatotoxicity and gastrointestinal disturbances (114). Despite these potentially difficult limitations, tacrine has been approved for clinical use in the United States under the trade name Cognex and has a clear role in the treatment of early to moderately advanced AD.

While the cholinergic approach to the treatment of AD may be limited by the observation that other neurotransmitters, in addition to acetylcholine, are depleted in the disorder, newer agents with effects on multiple transmitter systems are under investigation and are available to patients and their families through participation in experimental clinical drug trials. Other agents in development attempt to prevent further neuronal loss of function through restorative and protective means. Neurotrophic agents, such as nerve growth factor, and drugs that block oxidative damage to neurons, such as the selective monoamine oxidase B inhibitor deprenyl, may demonstrate promise in the future therapy of AD. On the horizon are treatment approaches that may interrupt the cascade of events leading to the accumulation of potentially neurotoxic amyloid (114).

B.   Psychiatric Management

Identification and management of the myriad psychiatric features of AD have a fundamental place in the contemporary treatment of the disorder. Once the target symptoms to be treated are noted through consultation with the patient's caregiver, a careful search for any triggers of disturbed behavior should be sought. Factors such as pain, the need to urinate, or other occult medical problems may cause or exacerbate such disruptive behaviors as restlessness, agitation, or sleep disturbances. Particular times of the day may also pose management difficulties for the caregiver. Many patients are particularly distressed around meal time, while bathing, or in the latter hours of the day. The appropriate uses of behavioral management techniques for dysfunctional behavior in AD have been well documented and generally consist of reassurance, distraction, and the timely provision of structured activity (115).

Multiple classes of psychotropic medications, including neuroleptics, sedative-hypnotics, anticonvulsants, serotonin-enhancement agents, and beta-adrenergic blockers, have been effectively employed for the treatment of dementia-associated behavioral problems (116–123) (Table 7). Although there are relatively few controlled clinical trials comparing the efficacy of different psychotropic agents in the treatment of dementia-associated behavioral problems, neuroleptics appear to be the drugs of first choice for clinically significant hallucinations, delusions, or aggressive behavior. No particular neuroleptic has advantage over any other in this regard. Choice of agent is therefore guided by the relative side effects of the available agents. High-potency neuroleptics such as haloperidol, fluph-

Table 7 Pharmacotherapy of Disturbed Behavior in Alzheimer's Disease

Antipsychotic agents

Agent	Starting daily dose	Relative side effects		
		Parkinsonism	anti-cholinergic/sedation	
Haloperidol	0.5–1 mg	High	Low	
Trifluoperazine	1 mg	Moderate	Moderate	
Thiothixene	1 mg	Moderate	Moderate	
Thioridazine	10 mg	Low	High	

Alternative agents for agitation/aggressiveness

Agent	Starting daily dose[a]	Side effects
Carbamazepine[b]	100 mg 2×/day	Sedation, ataxia, dysarthria, bone marrow suppression, hepatotoxicity
Trazodone	50 mg/day	Sedation, orthostasis, priapism (in males)
Buspirone	5 mg 2×/day	Dizziness, nausea, sedation
Clonazepam	0.5 mg 2×/day	Sedation, ataxia, dysarthria
Fluoxetine	10 mg/day	Restlessness, anxiety, insomnia
Propranolol[c]	10 mg 2×/day	Sedation, bradycardia, hypotension, depression, worsening of chronic obstructive pulmonary disease

Antidepressant agents

Agent	Dosing guidelines	Side effects
Nortriptyline, desipramine, doxepin	Initiate: i0 mg/day; increase dose by 10-mg increments/week until treatment response or side effects emerge	Confusion, sedation, anticholinergic effects, cardiac conduction delay
Trazodone	Initiate: 50 mg/day; increase dose by 50 mg/week until response or side effects emerge	Sedation, orthostasis, confusion, priapism (in males)
Fluoxetine, paroxetine	Initiate: 10 mg/day; increase dose to 20 mg/day after 1 week	Restlessness, insomnia, anxiety, anorexia, confusion
Sertraline	Initiate: 25 mg/day; increase dose to 50 mg/day after 1 week	Restlessness, insomnia, anxiety, anorexia, confusion
Bupropion	Initiate: 75 mg/day; increase dose after 4 days to 150 mg/day; maintain at 300 mg/day maximum	Insomnia, anxiety, confusion, seizures

[a]Dosing will need to be increased for all agents at weekly intervals until response or emergence of side effects.
[b]Monitor serum levels, complete blood count, and liver function.
[c]Monitor pulse and blood pressure closely.

enazine, and thiothixene (0.5–2 mg po qd) have a greater tendency to produce extrapyramidal side effects than lower-potency agents such as thioridazine and chlorpromazine (10–50 mg po qd) (124). However, these latter drugs are generally more sedating and cause more significant anticholinergic effects such as dry mouth, constipation, urinary retention, and exacerbation of narrow-angle glaucoma. Further, the lower-potency drugs often lead to more frequent cardiac conduction problems and orthostatic hypotension. As a result, neuroleptic agents need to be used with great care in elderly AD patients and in relatively low dosage ranges.

Relatively mild to moderately severe anxiety and restlessness may be treated with divided doses of benzodiazepines that have short elimination half-lives, such as oxazepam (10–30 mg po qd), lorazepam (0.5 to 2 mg po qd), or alprazolam (0.5–1 mg po qd). These medications, however, can lead to increased confusion, ataxia, sedation, and dysarthria (125). Buspirone may be an effective alternative for the treatment of anxiety or aggression in these patients (20–30 mg po qd) (126, 127). With this agent, therapeutic benefit may not become apparent for several weeks and may be complicated by gastrointestinal complaints.

For patients with aggressive behavior or agitation that is treatment resistant, anticonvulsant medications such as clonazepam (0.5–2 mg po qd), carbamazepine (400–1200 mg po qd), or valproic acid (250 mg po bid to qid) may be efficacious (128–130). With these latter two medications, serum levels, complete blood counts, and liver function tests must be carefully monitored at regular intervals such as once per week for the first month of treatment followed by once per month for the next few months. Frequently, the emergence of side effects such as gait ataxia, dysarthria, confusion, and excessive sedation limit the usefulness of these particular agents.

Trazodone may be an effective agent for the treatment of insomnia or aggressive behavior in dementia patients (131, 132). Treatment is generally initiated at 50 mg po hs and gradually increased until therapeutic benefits are noted or side effects emerge (e.g., hypotension, excess sedation, priapism in males). Improvement in agitation or aggression may not become evident for 6–10 weeks following the start of treatment. Chloral hydrate is also occasionally used for the treatment of insomnia in AD patients. Doses of 500–1500 mg po hs may be employed but can lead to increased confusion, lethargy, and ataxia. Beta-adrenergic blockers have also demonstrated efficacy for the treatment of disruptive behavior in dementia, but must be used cautiously in those elderly who may be particularly susceptible to bradycardia or chronic obstructive pulmonary disease (133,134).

No particular antidepressant agent has demonstrated special efficacy in the treatment of clinically-significant depressive symptoms in AD. Older agents such as amitriptyline or imipramine have prominent anticholinergic side effects and are best avoided in this patient population.

XI. MANAGEMENT OF CAREGIVER: SOCIAL AND ECONOMIC ISSUES

A variety of psychological and social interventions may provide assistance to family members caring for dementia patients (135–140). For example, much work has been directed toward reducing caregiver stress or burden (141), the measurement of which Brown, Potter, and Foster (142) have argued should become a routine part of geriatric assessment. The measurement of stress associated with caregiving for dementia patients may be accomplished through Zarit's "Burden Interview" (143–146), Kinney and Stephens' (147) "Hassles Scale," or other related scales (148,149).

Stress among caregivers of Alzheimer's disease patients may involve up to four domains (150) (Figure 2). These include 1) the background and context of stress (e.g., family composition, socioeconomic status, history of caregiving within the family); (2) stressors themselves (e.g., bathing/toileting the patient, financial demands); (3) mediators of stress (e.g.,

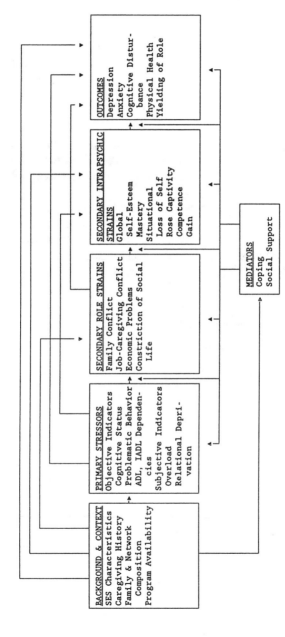

Figure 2 A conceptual model of stress among caregivers for Alzheimer's disease patients

social support, community services); and (4) outcomes (e.g., anxiety, depression, changes in physical health status).

Of these four domains, interventions tapping into mediators of stress such as community services have yielded mixed findings (141). While some studies have demonstrated that relatively straightforward psychosocial interventions result in significant reductions in phenomena such as caregiver stress and depression, others have found little if any impact on caregiver functioning.

In one study that attempted to reduce caregiver burden and depression, Kahan et al. (136) contrasted a time-limited, educational/social support group program with a waiting-list control. At the start of the 8-week intervention, all participants completed the Zarit Burden Interview (144), the Zung Self-Rating Depression Scale (SDS) (151), and a 13-item questionnaire covering knowledge about dementia. All measures were completed again at the end of the 8-week project. Experimental subjects (i.e., those in the support group) showed a significant decrease in burden, a decrease in Zung SDS scores, and an increase in knowledge about dementia. Control (i.e., waiting-list) subjects, on the other hand, displayed a significant increase in burden coupled with no changes in either depression or knowledge about dementia. Thus, time-limited caregiver groups offering "practical knowledge about dementia and the opportunity to discuss individual problems within a supportive environment" (136) represent one means of reducing the negative impact of caregiving.

In a related study, Zarit et al. (146) examined the effectiveness of two interventions commonly employed to reduce caregiver stress: family counseling and support group participation. These interventions were contrasted with a waiting-list control condition. Subjects (119 family-member caregivers for dementia patients) received either: (1) 8 weeks of family counseling that focused on understanding dementia, managing disruptive behavior, and accessing community resources; (2) 8 weeks of participation in a support group with a similar focus; or (3) an 8-week stay on a waiting list (followed by assignment to counseling or support groups). Outcome measures included the Zarit Burden Interview, the Brief Symptom Inventory (152), the Memory and Behavior Problems Checklist (153), and subjective ratings of adequacy of support received and efficacy of the study intervention.

Overall, results indicated that while both family therapy and support group interventions reduced burden and psychiatric symptoms in caregivers, the extent of change was no different from that seen among subjects who remained on a waiting list. Zarit and colleagues suggested that the failure to demonstrate differential improvement on the part of intervention subjects versus waiting list subjects may have been due to the selection of too short a treatment period and may have also involved a failure to control for alternative interventions sought out by waiting-list subjects. An additional hypothesis proposed was that the interventions tested may not have produced a stronger outcome as they did not significantly reduce the day-to-day demands placed on caregivers by dementia patients. Specifically, interventions such as day care or respite care may more effectively reduce stress as they directly limit the amount of time spent in caregiving.

In a similar study, Thompson et al. (154) examined the impact on caregiver burden of six different types of social support: "intimate interaction and confiding," "positive feedback," "advice," "material aid," "physical assistance," and "social participation." Results indicated that only "social participation" exerted a significant mitigating effect on caregiver burden. What Thompson and colleagues referred to as "pleasant social activities" may serve to distract caregivers from their difficult daily routine and may also be physiologically rewarding to caregivers. Thus, interventions designed to promote social activities with family and friends should have utility for alleviating caregiver burden.

The above findings related to stress and burden also highlight the need for specific interventions designed to provide short-term respite from caregiving activities. Perhaps the most important intervention in this respect is adult day care, which typically provides structured, therapeutic activity programming in a safe and secure environment. The goals of day care include (1) fostering orientation to person, place, and time; (2) cognitive stimulation through the use of familiar subjects, objects, and tasks; (3) socialization with peers; (4) physical exercise; and (5) education, case management, and social support for caregivers. Similarly, caregivers and patients alike may benefit from respite care, which is designed to provide "short-term, intermittent substitute care for impaired family members on behalf and in the absence of the family caregiver" (155). Respite care may be provided by a nursing home, hospital, day care center, or home health care agency. In each instance, caregiving responsibilities are temporarily assumed by others, allowing the primary caregiver to attend to personal needs, obtain medical care, or even take a long-overdue vacation.

Yet another intervention important for decreasing caregiver stress involves the use of home care services. These include visiting nurse associations (VNAs), home health aide/homemaker services, hospice programs, community outreach/case management programs, and home-delivered, "concrete" services (e.g., Meals-On-Wheels, chore services, home shopping) (156). Each of these community-based resources, which range from the provision of nonskilled assistance with activities of daily living to highly skilled nursing care (e.g., parenteral nutrition, chemotherapy), expands the range of care that may be provided in the home and has the potential for reducing stress and burden on family-member caregivers while improving the quality of life of dementia patients in the community. In addition, caregivers may also benefit from community-based self-help and advocacy groups, such as those run by the Alzheimer's Association; state or local telephone-based information and referral help lines (135); and the National Institute on Aging's Alzheimer's Disease Education and Referral Center (1-800-438-4380) and General Information Center (1-800-222-2225). Finally, caregivers may want to consider consultation with an attorney familiar with or specializing in "elder law" issues. Because legal steps such as durable power of attorney, financial trust agreements, conservatorship or guardianship, and advance directives for health care may be crucial to a family's continued ability to provide care for a relative with dementia, they must be discussed and put into place prior to the onset of cognitive impairment.

REFERENCES

1. Advisory Panel on Alzheimer's disease. Fourth Report of the Advisory Panel on Alzheimer's Disease, 1992. NIH Pub. No. 93-3520. Washington, DC: U.S. Government Printing Office, 1993

2. American Association of Retired Persons. A Profile of Older Americans. Washington, DC: AARP, 1993

3. U.S. Department of Commerce, Bureau of the Census. Statistical Abstract of the United States: 1990. Washington, DC: U.S. Government Printing Office

4. Fox P. From senility to Alzheimer's disease: The rise of the Alzheimer's disease movement. Milbank Q 1989; 67:58–102

5. Chui HC. Dementia: A review emphasizing clinicopathologic correlation and brain–behavior relationships. Arch Neurol 1989; 46:806–814

6. Cummings JL. Dementia syndromes: Neurobehavioral and neuropsychiatric features. J Clin Psychiatry 1987; 48:3–8

7. Weiner MF. The diagnosis of dementia. In Weiner MF, ed, The Dementias: Diagnosis and Management. Washington, DC: American Psychiatric Press, 1991:1–28

8. Cohen GD. Historical views and evolution of concepts. In Reisberg B, ed., Alzheimer's Disease: The Standard Reference. New York: The Free Press, 1983:29–33

9. Alzheimer A. "Uber eine eigenartige Erkrankung der Hirnrinde." Allegmeine Zeitschrift für Psychiatrie 1907; 64: 146–148

10. Blocq P, Marinesco G. "Sur les lésions et la pathogie de l'épilepsie dite essentielle." Sem Med (Paris) 1892; 12:445

11. Simchowicz T. "Histologische Studien über die senile Demenz." Hist Histopath Arb 1910; 4:267

12. Akesson, H. O. A population study of senile and arteriosclerotic psychoses. Human Heredity 1969; 19:546–566

13. Evans DA, Funkenstein HH, Albert MS, Scherr PA, Cook NR, Chown MJ, Hebert LE, Hennekens CH, Taylor JO. Prevalence of Alzheimer's disease in a community population of older persons: Higher than previously reported. J Amer Med Assn 1989; 262:2551–2556

14. Folstein MF, Bassett SS, Anthony JC, Romanoski AJ, Nestadt GR. Dementia: Case ascertainment in a community survey. J Gerontol: Medical Sciences 1991; 46:132–138

15. Katzman R. The prevalence and malignancy of Alzheimer's disease: a major killer. Arch Neurol 1976; 33:217–218

16. Kay DWK, Beamish P, Roth M. Old age mental disorders in Newcastle upon Tyne. Part I: A study of prevalence. Brit J Psychiatry 1964; 110:146–158

17. Schoenberg BS, Anderson DW, Haerer AR. Severe dementia. Prevalence and clinical features in a biracial U.S. population. Arch Neurol 1985; 42:740–743

18. Zhang M, Katzman R, Salmon D, Jin H, Cai G, Wang Z, Qu G, Grant I, Yu E, Levy P, Klauber MR, Liu WT. The prevalence of dementia and Alzheimer's disease in Shanghai, China: Impact of age, gender, and education. Ann Neurol 1990; 27:428–437

19. Rocca WA, Amaducci LA, Schoenberg BS. Epidemiology of clinically diagnosed Alzheimer's disease. Ann Neurol 1986; 19:415–424

20. McKhann G, Drachman D, Folstein M, Katzman R, Price D, Stadlan EM. Clinical diagnosis of Alzheimer's disease: Report of the NINCDS–ADRDA Work Group under the auspices of Department of Health and Human Services Task Force on Alzheimer's Disease. Neurology 1984; 34:939–944

21. American Psychiatric Association. Diagnostic and Statistical Manual of Mental Disorders, 3rd ed. revised. Washington, DC: APA, 1987

22. Larson EB. Alzheimer's disease in the community [editorial]. J Amer Med Assoc 1989; 262:2591–2592

23. Roman GC, Tatemichi TK, Erkinjuntti T, Cummings JL, Masdeu JC, Garcia JH, Amaducci L, Orgogozo JM, Brun A, Hofman A, Moody DM, O'Brien MD, Yamaguchi T, Grafman J, Drayer BP, Bennett DA, Fisher M, Ogata J, Kokmen E, Bermejo F, Wolf PA, Gorelick PB, Bick KL, Pajeau AK, Bell MA, DeCarli C, Culebras A, Korczyn AD, Bogousslavsky J, Hartmann A, Scheinberg P. Vascular dementia:

Diagnostic criteria for research studies. Report of the NINDS-AIREN International Workshop. Neurology 1993; 43: 250–260

24. Katzman R, Saitoh T. Advances in Alzheimer's disease. FASEB J 1991; 5:278–286

25. Kay DWK. Epidemiological aspects of organic brain disease in the aged. In: Gaitz CM, ed., Aging and the Brain. New York: Plenum, 1972:15–27

26. Heston LL, Mastri AR, Anderson VE, White J. Dementia of the Alzheimer type: Clinical genetics, natural history, and associated conditions. Arch Gen Psychiatry 1981; 38: 1085–1090

27. Nee LE, Eldridge R, Sunderland T, Thomas CB, Katz D, Thompson KE, Weingartner H, Weiss H, Julian C, Cohen R. Dementia of the Alzheimer type: Clinical and family study of 22 twin pairs. Neurology 1987; 37:359–363

28. St. George–Hyslop PH, Tanzi RE, Polinsky RJ, Haines JL, Nee L, Watkins PC, Myers RH, Feldman RG, Pollen D, Drachman D, Growdon J, Bruni A, Foncin JF, Salmon D, Frommelt P, Amaducci L, Sorbi S, Placentini S, Stewart GD, Hobbs WJ, Conneally PM, Gusella JF. The genetic defect causing familial Alzheimer's disease maps on chromosome 21. Science 1987; 235:885–890

29. Evenhuis HM. The natural history of dementia in Down's syndrome. Arch Neurol 1990; 47:263–267

30. Ropper AH, Williams RS. Relationship between plaques, tangles, and dementia in Down syndrome. Neurology 1980; 30(6):639–644

31. Wisniewski KE, Wisniewski HM, Wen GY. Occurrence of neuropathological changes and dementia of Alzheimer's disease in Down's syndrome. Ann Neurol 1985; 17:278–282

32. Heston LL. Alzheimer's disease, trisomy 21, and myeloproliferative disorders: Associations suggesting a genetic diathesis. Science 1976; 196:322–323

33. Heston LL, Mastri AR. The genetics of Alzheimer's disease: Associations with hematologic malignancy and Down's syndrome. Arch Gen Psychiatry 1977; 34:976–981

34. Crapper DR, Krishnan SS, Quittkat S. Aluminium, neurofibrillary degeneration and Alzheimer's disease. Brain 1976; 99(1):67–80

35. Perl DP. Pathologic association of aluminum in Alzheimer's disease. In: Reisberg B, ed., Alzheimer's Disease: The Standard Reference. New York: The Free Press, 1983:116–121

36. Paschalis C, Polychronopoulos P, Lekka NP, Harrison MJG, Papapetropoulos T. The role of head injury, surgical anesthesia and family history as anetiological factors in dementia of Alzheimer type. Dementia 1990; 1:52–55

37. Sotaineimi KA, Mononen H, Hokkanen TE. Long-term cerebral outcome after open-heart surgery. A 5-year neuropsychological follow-up study. Stroke 1986; 17:410–416

38. Fratiglioni L, Grut M, Forsell Y, Viitanen M, Grafstrom M, Holmen K, Ericsson K, Backman L, Ahlbom A, Winblad B. Prevalence of Alzheimer's disease and other dementias in an elderly urban population: Relationship with age, sex, and education. Neurology 1991; 41:1886–1892

39. Katzman R. Education and the prevalence of dementia and Alzheimer's disease. Neurology 1993; 43:13–20

40. Moritz DJ, Petitti DB. Association of education with reported age of onset and severity of Alzheimer's disease at presentation: Implications for the use of clinical samples. Am J Epidemiology 1993; 137:456–462

41. Cummings JL, Benson DF. Dementia: A Clinical Approach. 2nd ed. Boston: Butterworth-Heinemann, 1992

42. Koller WC, Wilson RS, Glatt SL, Fox JH. Motor signs are infrequent in dementia of the Alzheimer type. Ann Neurol 1984; 16(4):514–516

43. Mölsä PK, Marttila RJ, Rinne UK. Extrapyramidal signs in Alzheimer's disease. Neurology 1984; 34:1114–1116

44. Morris JC, Drazner M, Fulling K, Grant EA, Goldring J. Clinical and pathological aspects of parkinsonism in Alzheimer's disease. Arch Neurol 1989; 46:651–657

45. Wallin A, Blennow K. Neurologic motor signs in early and late onset Alzheimer's disease. Dementia 1992; 3(5-6):314–319

46. Franssen EH, Kluger A, Torossian CL, Reisberg MA. The neurologic syndrome of severe Alzheimer's disease. Arch Neurol 1993; 50:1029–1039

47. Leverenz J, Sumi M. Parkinson's disease in patients with Alzheimer's disease. Arch Neurol 1986; 43:662–664

48. Ditter DM, Mirra SS. Neuropathologic and clinical features

of Parkinson's disease in Alzheimer's disease patients. Neurology 1987; 37:754–760

49. Hansen LA, Masliah E, Terry RD, Mirra SS. A neuropathological subset of Alzheimer's disease with concomitant Lewy body disease and spongiform change. Acta Neuropathologica 1989; 78:194–201

50. Paulson G, Gottlieb G. Developmental reflexes: The reappearance of foetal and neonatal reflexes in aged patients. Brain 1968; 91:37–52

51. Hauser WA, Morris ML, Heston LL, Anderson VE. Seizures and myoclonus in patients with Alzheimer's disease. Neurology 1986; 36:1226–1230

52. Chen JY, Stern Y, Sano M, Mayeux R. Cumulative risks of developing extrapyramidal signs, psychosis, or myoclonus in the course of Alzheimer's disease. Arch Neurol 1991; 48: 1141–1143

53. Reisberg B, Borenstein J, Salob SP, Ferris SH, Franssen E, Georgotas A. Behavioral symptoms in Alzheimer's disease: Phenomenology and treatment. J Clin Psychiatry 1987; 48(5;suppl):9–15

54. Petry S, Cummings JL, Hill MA, Shapira S. Personality alterations in dementia of the Alzheimer type. Arch Neurol 1988; 45:1187–1190

55. Rubin EH, Morris JC, Berg L. The progression of personality changes in senile dementia of the Alzheimer's type. J Am Geriatr Soc 1987; 35:721–725

56. Wragg RE, Jeste DV. Overview of depression and psychosis in Alzheimer's disease. Am J Psychiatry 1989; 146:577–587

57. Brody E.M. The long haul: A family odyssey. In Jarvik LF, Winograd, CH, eds., Treatments for the Alzheimer Patient: The Long Haul. New York: Springer, 1988:107–122

58. Cohler BJ, Groves L, Borden W, Lazarus L. Caring for family members with Alzheimer's disease. In Light E, Lebowitz BD, eds., Alzheimer's Disease Treatment and Family Stress: Directions for Research. Washington, DC: U.S. Government Printing Office, 1989:50–105

59. Dura JR, Haywood-Niler E, Kiecolt-Glaser J.K. Spousal caregivers of persons with Alzheimer's and Parkinson's disease dementia: A preliminary comparison. Gerontologist 1990; 30:332–336

60. Williamson GM, Schulz R. Coping with specific stressors in Alzheimer's disease caregiving. Gerontologist 1993; 33:747–755

61. Cattanach L, Tebes JK. The nature of elder impairment and its impact on family caregivers' health and psychosocial functioning. Gerontologist 1991; 31:246–255

62. Gallagher D, Rose J, Rivera P, Lovett S, Thompson LW. Prevalence of depression in family caregivers. Gerontologist 1989; 29:449–456

63. George LK, Gwyther LP. Caregiver well-being: A multidimensional examination of family caregivers of demented adults. Gerontologist 1986; 26:253–259

64. Kiecolt-Glaser JK, Glaser R. Caregiving, mental health, and immune function. In Light E, Lebowitz BD, eds., Alzheimer's Disease Treatment and Family Stress: Directions for Research. Washington, DC: U.S. Government Printing Office, 1989:245–266

65. Kiecolt-Glaser JK, Glaser R, Shuttleworth EC, Dyer CS, Ogrocki P, Speicher CE. Chronic stress and immunity in family caregivers of Alzheimer's disease victims. Psychosomatic Med 1987; 49:523–535

66. Coyne AC, Reichman WE, Berbig LJ. The relationship between dementia and elder abuse. Am J Psychiatry 1993; 150:643–646

67. Mayeux R, Stern Y, Spanton S. Heterogeneity in dementia of the Alzheimer type: Evidence of subgroups. Neurology 1985; 35:453–461

68. Stern Y, Mayeux R, Sano M, Hauser WA, Rush T. Predictors of disease course in patients with probable Alzheimer's disease. Neurology 1987; 37:1649–1654

69. Huff FJ, Belle SH, Shim YK, Ganguli M, Boller F. Prevalence and prognostic value of neurologic abnormalities in Alzheimer's disease. Dementia 1990; 1:32–40

70. Drachman DA, O'Donnell BF, Lew RA, Swearer JM. The prognosis in Alzheimer's disease. Arch Neurol 1990; 47:851–856

71. Mirra S, Gearing M. The neuropathology of dementia. In: Morris JC, ed., Handbook of Dementing Illnesses. New York: Marcel Dekker, 1994:189–228

72. Koo EH, Price DL. The neurobiology of dementia. In: White-

house PJ, ed., Dementia. Philadelphia: FA Davis, 1993:55–56

73. Esiri MM, Wilcock GK. Cerebral amyloid angiopathy in dementia and old age. J Neurol Neurosurg Psychiatry 1986; 49: 1221–1226

74. Selkoe DJ. Altered structural proteins in plaques and tangles: What do they tell us about the biology of Alzheimer's disease? Neurobiol Aging 1986; 7:425–432

75. Iqbal K, Grundke-Iqbal I, Zaidi T, Merz PA, Wen GY, Shaikh SS, Wisniewski HM, Alafuzoff I, Winblad B. Defective brain microtubule assembly in Alzheimer's disease. Lancet 1986; 2(8504):421–426

76. Whitehouse PJ, Price DL, Clark AW, Coyle JT, DeLong MR. Alzheimer disease: Evidence for selective loss of cholinergic neurons in the nucleus basalis. Ann Neurol 1981; 10: 122–126

77. Whitehouse PJ, Price DL, Struble RG, Clark AW, Coyle JT, DeLong MR. Alzheimer's disease and senile dementia: Loss of neurons in the basal forebrain. Science 1982; 215:1237–1239

78. Whitehouse PJ. Neurotransmitter receptor alterations in Alzheimer disease: A review. Alzheimer Disease and Associated Disorders 1987; 1(1):9–18

79. Quirion R, Martel JC, Robitaille Y, Etienne P, Wood P, Nair NPV, Gauthier S. Neurotransmitter and receptor deficits in senile dementia of the Alzheimer type. Le Journal Canadien Des Sciences Neurologiques 1986; 13(4):503–510

80. Bowen DM, Allen SJ, Benton JS, Goodhardt MJ, Haan EA, Palmer AM, Sims NR, Smith CCT, Spillane JA, Esiri MM, Neary D, Snowdon JS, Wilcock GK, Davison AN. Biochemical assessment of serotonergic and cholinergic dysfunction and cerebral atrophy in Alzheimer's disease. J Neurochem 1983; 41(1):266–272

81. Mann DMA, Yates PO. Neurotransmitter deficits in Alzheimer's disease and in other dementing disorders. Human Neurobiol 1986; 5:147–158

82. Joachim CL, Selkoe DJ. The seminal role of β-amyloid in the pathogenesis of Alzheimer disease. Alzheimer Dis Assoc Disord 1992; 6(1):7–34

83. Nitsch RM, Slack BE, Wurtman RJ, Growdon JH. Release of

Alzheimer amyloid precursor derivatives stimulated by activation of muscarinic acetylcholine receptors. Science 1992; 258: 304–307

84. Shoji M, Golde TE, Ghiso J, Cheung TT, Estus S, Shaffer LM, Cai ZD, McKay DM, Tintner R, Frangione B, Younkint SG. Production of the Alzheimer amyloid β-protein by normal proteolytic processing. Science 1992; 258:126–129

85. Schellenberg GD, Bird TD, Wijsman EM, Orr HT, Anderson L, Nemens E, White JA, Bonnycastle L, Weber JL, Alonso ME, Potter H, Heston LL, Martin GM. Genetic linkage evidence for familial Alzheimer's disease locus on chromosome 14. Science 1992; 258:668–671

86. Goate AM, Haynes AR, Owen MJ, Farrall M, James LA, Lai LY, Mullan MJ, Roques P, Rossor MN, Williamson R, Hardy J. Predisposing locus for Alzheimer's disease on chromosome 21. Lancet 1989; 1:352–355

87. Clark RF, Goate AM. Molecular genetics of Alzheimer's disease. Arch Neuol 1993; 50:1164–1172

88. Tanzi RE, Gusella JF, Watkins PC, Bruns GA, St. George-Hyslop P, Van Keuren ML, Patterson D, Pagan S, Kurnit DM, Neve RL. Amyloid beta protein gene: cDNA, mRNA distribution, and genetic linkage near the Alzheimer locus. Science 1987; 235:880–884

89. Goldgaber D, Lerman MI, McBride OW, Saffiotti U, Gajdusek DC. Characterization and chromosomal localization of a cDNA encoding brain amyloid of Alzheimer's disease. Science 1987; 235:877–880

90. Goate A, Chartier-Harlin MC, Mullan M, Brown J, Crawford F, Fidani L, Giuffra L, Haynes A, Irving N, James L, Mant R, Newton P, Rooke K, Roques P, Talbot C, Pericak-Vance M, Roses A, Williamson R, Rossor M, Owen M, Hardy J. Segregation of a missense mutation in the amyloid precursor protein gene with familial Alzheimer's disease. Nature 1991; 349:704–706

91. Murrell J, Farlow M, Ghetti B, Benson MD. A mutation in the amyloid precursor protein associated with hereditary Alzheimer's disease. Science 1991; 254:97–99

92. Karlinsky H, Vaula G, Haines JL, Ridgley J, Bergeron C, Mortilla M, Tupler RG, Percy ME, Robitaille Y, Noldy NE, Yip TCK, Tanzi RE, Gusella JF, Becker R, Berg JM,

Crapper-McLachlan DR, St. George-Hyslop PH. Molecular and prospective phenotypic characterization of a pedigree with familial Alzheimer's disease and a missense mutation in codon 717 of the β-amyloid precursor protein gene. Neurology 1992; 42:1445–1453

93. Rosenberg RN. An introduction to the molecular genetics of neurological disease. Arch Neurol 1993; 50:1123–1128

94. Roses AD. Molecular genetics of neurodegenerative diseases (Review). Curr Opin Neurol Neurosurg 1993; 6(1):34–39

95. Corder EH, Saunders AM, Strittmatter WJ, Schmechel DE, Gaskell PC, Small GW, Roses AD, Haines JL, Pericak-Vance MA. Gene dose of apolipoprotein E type 4 allele and the risk of Alzheimer's disease in late onset families. Science 1993; 261:921–923

96. Tierney MC, Fisher RH, Lewis AJ, Zorzitto ML, Snow WG, Reid DW, Nieuwstraten P. The NINCDS-ADRDA Work Group criteria for the clinical diagnosis of probable Alzheimer's disease: A clinicopathologic study of 57 cases. Neurology 1988; 38:359–364

97. Folstein MF, Folstein SE, McHugh PR. "Mini-mental state": a practical method for grading the mental state of patients for the clinician. J Psychiatric Res 1975; 12:189–198

98. Blessed G, Tomlinson BE, Roth M. The association between quantitative measures of dementia and of senile changes in the cerebral grey matter of elderly subjects. Br J Psychiatry 1968; 114:797–811

99. Hughes CP, Berg L, Danziger WL, Coben LA, Martin RL. A new clinical scale for the staging of dementia. Br J Psychiatry 1982; 140:566–572

100. Prohovnik I, Mayeux R, Sackheim HA, Smith G, Stern Y, Alderson PO. Cerebral perfusion as a diagnostic marker of early Alzheimer's disease. Neurology 1988; 38:931–937

101. Schmitt FA, Shih WJ, Dekosky ST. Lateralized neuropsychological and SPECT findings in Alzheimer's disease. Neuropsychology 1992; 6:159–171

102. Celsis P, Agniel A, Puel M, Rascol A, Marc-Vergnes JP. Focal cerebral hypoperfusion and selective cognitive deficit in dementia of the Alzheimer type. J Neurol Neurosurg Psychiatry 1987; 50:1602–1612

103. Khachaturian ZS. Diagnosis of Alzheimer's Disease. Arch Neurol 1985; 42:1097–1105

104. Civil RH, Whitehouse PJ, Lanska DJ, and Mayeux R. Degenerative dementias. In Whitehouse PJ, ed., Dementia. Philadelphia: FA Davis, 993:167–176

105. Pomponi M, Giacobini E, Brufani M. Present state and future development of the therapy of Alzheimer disease. Aging 1990; 2:125–153

106. Volger BW. Alternatives in the treatment of memory loss in patients with Alkzheimer's disease. Clinical Pharmacy 1991; 10:447–456

107. Summers WK, Viesselman JO, March GM, Candelor K. Use of THA in treatment of Alzheimer-like dementia: Pilot study in twelve patients. Biological Psychiatry 1981; 16(2):145–153

108. Summers WK, Majovski LV, Marsh GM, Tachiki K, Kling A. Oral tetrahydroaminoacridine in long-term treatment of senile dementia, Alzheimer type. N Engl J Med 1986; 315: 1241–1245

109. Eagger SA, Levy R, Sahakian BJ. Tacrine in Alzheimer's disease. Lancet 1991; 337:989–992

110. Davis KL, Thal LJ, Gamzu ER, Davis CS, Woolson RF, Gracon SI, Drachman DA, Schneider LS, Whitehouse PJ, Hoover TM, Morris JC, Kawas CH, Knopman DS, Earl NL, Kumar V, Doody RS. Tacrine Collaborative Study Group. A double-blind, placebo-controlled multicenter study of tacrine for Alzheimer's disease. N Engl J Med 1992; 327(18): 1253–1259

111. Farlow M, Gracon SI, Hershey LA, Lewis KW, Sadowsky CH, Dolan-Ureno J. A controlled trial of tacrine in Alzheimer's disease. The Tacrine Study Group. JAMA 1992; 268(18):2523–2529

112. Gautheir S, Bouchard R, Lamontagne A, Bailey P, Bergman H, Ratner J, Tesfaye Y, St. Martin M, Bacher Y, Carrier L, Charbonneau R, Clarfield AM, Collier B, Dastoor D, Gautheir L, Germain, M, Kissel C, Krieger M, Kushnir S, Masson H, Morin J, Nair V, Neirinck L, Suissa S. Tetrahydroaminoacridine-lecithin combination treatment in patients with intermediate-stage Alzheimer's disease. N Engl J Med 1990; 322:1272–1276

113. Chatellier G, Lacomblez L. Tacrine (tetrahydroaminoacridine; THA) and lecithin in senile dementia of the Alzheimer type: A multicentre trial. Br Med J 1990; 300:495–499

114. Growdon, JH. Treatment for Alzheimer's disease. N Engl J Med 1992; 327(18):1306–1308

115. Mace NL, Rabins PV. The 36-Hour Day. Baltimore: The Johns Hopkins University Press, 1981

116. Salzman C. Treatment of the elderly agitated patient. J Clin Psychiatry 1987; 48(5 suppl):19–22

117. Risse SC, Barnes R. Pharmacologic treatment of agitation associated with dementia. J Am Geriatr Soc 1986; 34:368–376

118. Raskin MA, Risse SC, Lampe TH. Dementia and antipsychotic drugs. J Clin Psychiatry 1987; 48(5):16–18

119. Winograd CH, Jarvik LF. Physician management of the demented patient. J Am Geriatr Soc 1986; 34:295–308

120. Maletta GJ. Pharmacologic treatment and management of the aggressive demented patient. Psychiatric Annals 1990; 20(8): 446–455

121. Small GW. Psychopharmacological treatment of elderly demented patients. J Clin Psychiatry 1988; 49(5):8–13

122. Teri L, Logsdon R. Assessment and management of behavioral disturbances in Alzheimer's disease. Compreh Therapy 1990; 16(5):36–42

123. Yudofsky SC, Silver JM, Hales RE. Pharmacologic management of aggression in the elderly. J Clin Psychiatry 1990; 51(10):22–32

124. Devanand DP, Sackeim HA, Brown RP, Mayeux R. A pilot study of haloperidol treatment of psychosis and behavioral disturbance in Alzheimer's disease. Arch Neurol 1989; 46: 854–857

125. Stern RG, Duffelmeyer ME, Zemishlani Z, Davidson M. The use of benzodiazepines in the management of behavioral symptoms in demented patients. Psychiatr Clin North Am 1991; 14:375–384

126. Tiller JG. Short-term buspirone treatment in disinhibition with dementia. Lancet 1988; 1:1169

127. Colenda C. Buspirone in treatment of agitated demented patient. Lancet 1988; 1:1169

128. Leibovici A, Tariot PN. Carbamazepine treatment of agitation

associated with dementia. J Ger Psychiatry Neurol 1988; 1: 110–112

129. Gleason RP, Schneider LS. Carbamazepine treatment of agitation in Alzheimer's outpatients refractory to neuroleptics. J Clin Psychiatry 1990; 51:115–118

130. Mellow AM, Solano-Lopez C, Davis S. Sodium valproate in the treatment of behavioral disturbance in dementia. J Ger Psychiatry Neurol 1993; 6:205–209

131. Simpson DM, Foster D. Improvement in organically disturbed behavior with trazodone treatment. J Clin Psychiatry 1986; 47:191–193

132. Pinner E, Rich CL. Effects of trazodone on aggressive behavior in seven patients with organic mental disorders. Am J Psychiatry 1988; 145(10):1295–1296

133. Weiler PG, Mungas D, Bernick C. Propranolol for the control of disruptive behavior in senile dementia. J Geriatr Psychiatry Neurol 1988; 1:226–230

134. Greendyke RM, Schuster DB, Wootton JW. Propranolol in the treatment of assaultive patients with organic brain disease. J Clin Psychopharmacol 1984; 4:282–285

135. Coyne AC. Information and referral service usage among caregivers for dementia patients. Gerontologist 1991; 31: 384–388

136. Kahan J, Kemp B, Staples FR, Brummel-Smith K. Decreasing the burden in families caring for a relative with a dementing illness: A controlled study. J Am Geriatr Soc 1985; 33:664–670

137. Shope JT, Holmes SB, Sharpe PA, Goodman C, Izenson S, Gilman S, Foster NL. Services for persons with dementia and their families: A survey of information and referral agencies in Michigan. Gerontologist 1993; 33:529–533

138. Silverstein NM, Kennedy K, McCormick D. A telephone helpline for Alzheimer's disease: Information, referral, and support. Amer J Alz Care Related Disord Res 1993; 8:28–36

139. Toseland RW, Labrecque MS, Goebel ST, Whitney MH. An evaluation of a group program for spouses of frail elderly veterans. Gerontologist 1992; 32:382–390

140. Tune LE, Lucas-Blaustein MJ, Rovner BW. Psychosocial interventions. In Jarvik LF, Winograd CH, eds., Treatments for

the Alzheimer Patient: The Long Haul. New York: Springer, 1988:123–136

141. Knight BG, Lutzky SM, Macofsky-Urban F. A meta-analytic review of interventions for caregiver distress: Recommendations for future research. Gerontologist 1993; 33:240–248

142. Brown LJ, Potter JF, Foster BG. Caregiver burden should be evaluated during geriatric assessment. J Am Geriatr Soc 1990; 38:455–460

143. Zarit SH. Issues and directions in family intervention research. In Light E, Lebowitz BD, eds. Alzheimer's Disease Treatment and Family Stress: Directions for Research. Washington, DC: U.S. Government Printing Office, 1989:458–486

144. Zarit SH, Reever KE, Bach-Peterson J. Relatives of the impaired elderly: Correlates of feelings of burden. Gerontologist 1980; 20:649–655

145. Zarit SH, Todd PA, Zarit JM. Subjective burden of husbands and wives as caregivers: A longitudinal study. Gerontologist 1986; 26:260–266

146. Zarit SH, Anthony CR, Boutselis M. Interventions with care givers of dementia patients: Comparison of two approaches. Psychol Aging 1987; 2:225–232

147. Kinney JM, Stephens MAP. Caregiving Hassles Scale: Assessing the daily hassles of caring for a family member with dementia. Gerontologist 1989; 29:328–332

148. Poulshock SW, Deimling GT. Families caring for elders in residence: Issues in the measurement of burden. J Gerontol 1984; 39:230–239

149. Robinson B. Validation of a caregiver strain index. J Gerontol 1983; 38:344–348

150. Pearlin LI, Mullan JT, Semple SJ, Skaff MM. Caregiving and the stress process: An overview of concepts and their measures. Gerontologist 1990; 30:583–594

151. Zung WWK. A self-rating depression scale. Arch Gen Psychiatry 1965; 12:63–70

152. Derogatis LR, Spencer PM. The Brief Symptom Inventory (BSI): Administration and Procedures Manual I. Baltimore, MD: Johns Hopkins, 1982

153. Zarit SH, Zarit JM. Families under stress: Interventions for caregivers of senile dementia patients. Psychother: Theory, Res and Practice 1982; 19:461–471

154. Thompson EH, Futterman AM, Gallagher-Thompson D, Rose
      JM, Lovett SB. Social support and caregiving burden in fam-
      ily caregivers of frail elders. J Gerontol: Social Sciences
      1993; 48:S245–S254
155. Gwyther L. Introduction: What is respite care? Pride Institute
      J Long Term Home Health Care 1986; 5:4–6
156. Buckwalter K.C. Applied services research: Clinical issues
      and directions. In Light E, Lebowitz BD, eds. Alzheimer's
      Disease Treatment and Family Stress: Directions for Re-
      search. Washington, DC: U.S. Government Printing Office,
      1989:434–457

2

Non-Alzheimer Dementing Disorders

Brian R. Ott
Brown University School of Medicine and
Roger Williams Medical Center
Providence, Rhode Island

I. DEMENTIA

A. Introduction

Dementia is a clinical state in which acquired cognitive impairments produce dysfunction in a person's occupational and social life. The *Diagnostic and Statistical Manual of Mental Disorders, Third Edition* (DSM-III-R), criteria for the diagnosis of dementia (see Table 1) emphasize that memory impairment is a central aspect of the disorder, and that other impairments such as problems with abstract thinking, judgment, altered personality, and other disturbances of higher cortical function also exist (1). It should be noted, however, that certain dementias such as frontal lobe dementia may present initially with altered personality and behavior despite relative preservation of memory function. Dementia is usually of gradual onset and progressive; however, it may be acute in onset, static, or resolving in its clinical course.

There are over 70 different causes of dementia (2). A review of clinical series including 2889 subjects reported prevalence figures for the most common dementias as follows: Alzheimer's disease (56.8%), multi-infarct (13.3%), depression (4.5%), alcoholic (4.2%), and drug toxicity (1.5%) (3).

Table 1 Diagnostic Criteria for Dementia

Impaired short and long-term memory
Other cognitive disturbances must be present
    Impaired abstract thinking
    Impaired judgment
    Personality change
    Other cognitive deficits (aphasia, apraxia, agnosia, constructional
       impairment)
Impairments significantly interfere with occupational or social function
Delirium excluded as the sole etiology
An organic disorder is etiologically related or no functional disturbance such as major depression is etiologically related

Source: Adapted from Ref. 1.

Autopsy series have reported figures of 40–75% for Alzheimer's disease, 8–15% for multi-infarct dementia, and 8–30% for mixed Alzheimer's disease and vascular dementia (4). Differences in diagnostic criteria, genetic, and other cultural factors have resulted in considerable variation in reported prevalence figures in other countries (5–7). For example, a recent epidemiologic study from Sweden of 494 elderly subjects found that 43.5% had Alzheimer's disease and 46.9% had vascular dementia (8).

The frequency of specifically treatable or reversible dementia ranges from 13.2% (3) to 30% (9), with most reports describing a frequency of about 20% (10). The most common etiologies include medication toxicity, depression, and metabolic disorders. Such classifications as treatable or reversible dementia, however, are vague. Furthermore, they may lead to an inappropriate bias toward abandoning the important management issues that affect all persons with dementia (11).

Differential diagnosis of dementia requires a thorough medical, neurologic, and psychiatric evaluation that begins with the history and physical examination. Attention to characteristic historical features, risk factors, and classification based on specific neurobehavioral characteristics provides a firm basis on which to focus the diagnostic work-up.

B.   Mode of Onset and Clinical Course

Mode of onset and subsequent temporal course are variable features of dementia. Because patients with dementia commonly have impaired awareness for their illness as well as amnesia, determination of dementia onset may be particularly difficult. Historical information from spouses, other family members, friends, or work associates is essential, as well as review of medical records. Quantitative tests of cognitive function as well as scales assessing daily living activities and behavior are useful in following disease course once a baseline level has been established. A number of clinical scales have been developed for this purpose (12).

Although there are significant variations in onset and temporal course, typical patterns seen with some disorders may suggest a specific disease or group of diseases that need to be ruled out. Acute onset of dementia is seen most commonly related to trauma, stroke, or a more generalized vascular insult such as hypoxic-ischemic encephalopathy. Hypoglycemia, Wernicke's encephalopathy, drug toxicity, and encephalitis are in the differential diagnosis. Prompt attention to correction of these disorders is of paramount importance to avoid chronic sequelae of dementia with fixed deficits. An example is the chronic amnestic state of Korsakoff's psychosis seen in alcoholics in whom thiamine deficiency was overlooked or inadequately treated.

Subacute onset developing over periods of days rather than hours is sometimes seen in stroke. A subacute onset over days to weeks without evidence of delirium is seen in depression, Creutzfeldt-Jakob disease, progressive multifocal leukoencephalopathy, and obstructive hydrocephalus, as well as occasionally in cases of neoplasm and certain chronic infections such as cryptococcal meningitis or AIDS encephalopathy. Rapid progression of dementia over a course of weeks is typical of such cases.

Dementias with a fluctuating course are often related to toxic and metabolic cases and are among those most likely to be correctable with specific treatment of the underlying disorder. Examples include encephalopathies related to end-organ failure such as hepatic and uremic encephalopathy, respiratory failure, drug toxicity, and electrolyte imbalance. A stepwise course is seen in cases of vascular dementia, where there may be partial or no remission of dementia symptoms with each acute event.

An insidious presentation, where one cannot accurately date disease onset, is typically seen in the cerebral degenerations such as Alzheimer's disease, Binswanger's encephalopathy, normal-pressure hydrocephalus, vitamin B_{12} deficiency, and hypothyroidism. Usually such disorders follow a slow progressive course, with changes being observable over a span of many months or from year to year.

C. Risk Factors for Dementia

A thorough history may reveal medical or psychiatric illnesses that can be identified as risk factors for dementia. Hypertension, hyperlipidemia, diabetes, atherosclerosis, cardiac disease, stroke, and transient ischemic attacks are seen in patients with vascular dementia. Homosexuality and intravenous drug use remain major risk factors for AIDS-associated infections of the CNS and AIDS dementia complex. Alcohol abuse is associated with Korsakoff psychosis, hepatic encephalopathy, subdural hematoma, Marchiafava-Bignami disease, and alcoholic dementia. Malignancies are associated with limbic encephalitis, progressive multifocal leukoencephalopathy, neoplastic meningitis, and cerebral metastases. Prior history of major depression may be an important clue to recurrent depression as the cause of memory complaints.

Certain dementias may be associated with a family history of the same disorder. Age of onset and pattern of inheritance are useful clues from the history in refining the differential diagnosis of such patients.

D. Neurobehavioral Profiles

Because of diverse etiologies for the dementia syndrome, certain patterns of cognitive and behavioral abnormalities can be identified as distinctive when comparing different diseases. These patterns of brain behavior can be used to formulate hypotheses regarding the regional anatomic pathology affecting the patient with dementia (13).

One popular attempt to establish a working link between cognitive-behavioral patterns and pathology is the cortical-subcortical classification of dementia. The impetus for this approach came from the descriptions of subcortical dementia in progressive supranuclear palsy by Albert and colleagues in 1974 (14) and Huntington's disease by McHugh and Folstein in 1975 (15). Besides basal ganglia and thalamic degenerative diseases, the subcortical dementia syndrome has been related to vascular dementia from subcortical ischemic infarctions, demyelinating illnesses such as multiple sclerosis and AIDS encephalopathy, and hydrocephalus. The clinical features of dementia in such patients are distinguished from diseases in which the major pathology is in cerebral cortex such as Alzheimer's disease, Pick's disease, Creutzfeldt-Jakob disease, and vascular dementia from multiple cortical infarctions (16). A comparison of the two syndromes is presented in Table 2.

Although this descriptive classification is recognizable in clinical practice and serves as a useful starting point in differential diagnosis, the division of dementias into cortical or subcortical types is controversial and neuropathologically imprecise. "Cortical" diseases like Alzheimer's disease also have disease of subcortical structures in the basal forebrain and rostral brainstem, and some clinical features of "subcortical" dementia are also seen with diseases involving frontal cortex, probably reflecting the important interconnections of this area with subcortical structures such as the basal ganglia.

This simple dichotomy can be further subdivided into cognitive-behavioral syndromes related to regional disease involving association cortex and limbic structures (13). For

Table 2 Neurobehavioral Profiles: Cortical vs. Subcortical Dementia

Characteristic	Subcortical dementia	Cortical dementia
Language	No aphasia (anomia and comprehension deficit when dementia syndrome is severe)	Aphasia early
Memory	Recall impaired; recognition normal or better than recall	Recall and recognition impaired
Visuospatial skills	Impaired	Impaired
Calculation	Preserved until late	Involved early
Frontal system abilities	Disproportionately affected compared with other neuropsychological abilities	Impaired to a degree consistent with involvement of other abilities
Speed of cognitive processing	Slowed early	Normal until late in disease course
Personality	Apathetic, inert	Unconcerned
Mood	Depressed	Euthymic
Speech	Dysarthric	Normal articulation until late
Posture	Bowed or extended	Upright
Coordination	Impaired	Normal until late
Adventitious movements	Present: chorea, tremor, tics, dystonia	Absent (myoclonus occurs in some cases of Alzheimer's disease)
Motor speed	Slowed	Normal

Source: Ref. 16.

example, although in their final stages patients with Alzheimer's disease and Pick's disease are clinically indistinguishable, early behavioral manifestations differ sufficiently to draw conclusions regarding differential diagnosis. In Alzheimer's disease, amnesia, aphasia, dyscalculia, and visuospatial impairments are early manifestations due to involvement of hippocampi, temporal and parietal cortex. In Pick's disease, the "frontal lobe syndrome" is seen early as the result of prefrontal cortex degeneration. This syndrome consists of perseveration, apathy, irritability, disinhibition, euphoria or jocularity, loss of insight, and impaired judgment. Behavior may be inappropriate and antisocial. Cognitive function is most impaired for executive abilities, such as planning and sequencing, as well as attention. Abulia, or slowness of thought and responsiveness, may occur. Bilateral disease in the orbito-basal regions tends to produce an irritable disinhibited euphoric state, while dorsolateral bifrontal disease tends to produce an apathetic state with abulia or features resembling depression (17,18). Features of Klüver-Bucy syndrome (hyperorality, hypersexuality, placidity, and sensory agnosia) also occur in the early stage of Pick's disease due to involvement of bilateral temporal lobes (19).

Further correlations between neurobehavioral syndromes and neuroimaging abnormalities have led to recognition of asymmetric or focal cortical degeneration syndromes such as primary progressive aphasia.

E. Diagnostic Work-up

The primary focus of the initial evaluation of dementia is to exclude the more common and treatable diagnostic possibilities. When present, specific findings on the neurologic examination such as pyramidal and extrapyramidal signs, focal signs, gait disorder, and other abnormalities of movement are important clues to the diagnosis of non-Alzheimer-type diseases.

Screening laboratory tests are routinely employed to assess the presence of systemic disorders that could account for dementia. In 1987 a consensus panel of the National Institutes of Health offered recommendations for the work-up of dementia (20). Computed tomography (CT) was regarded as ancillary and particularly indicated in cases of suspected mass lesion, in the presence of focal neurologic signs, and in dementia of brief duration.

Controversy still exists regarding the clinical utility of routinely ordering CT or magnetic resonance imaging (MRI) scans, particularly for patients with advanced dementia in which there is no reasonable hope of finding a reversible cause. In most cases, brain images should be performed, however, to exclude treatable diseases such as neoplasm, chronic subdural hematoma, and hydrocephalus, as well as to exclude preventable diseases such as stroke. Such information also offers more definitive information regarding prognosis by refining the diagnostic accuracy of dementia diagnosis. MRI is more sensitive than CT for demonstration of small infarcts, white-matter disease, and focal atrophy; however, it is more expensive and less well tolerated by the confused individual. Therefore, it is probably less desirable as a routine screening test. A list of commonly used standard and ancillary diagnostic studies is presented in Table 3.

While regions of lobar and focal atrophy may be seen on CT and MRI, functional neuroimaging studies of brain metabolism—positron emission tomography (PET)—and blood flow—single photon emission computed tomography (SPECT)—are more sensitive for demonstration of such abnormalities. Diminished metabolism and blood flow in bilateral frontal regions are typically seen in Pick's disease and frontal lobe dementia, in bilateral temporoparietal regions in Alzheimer's disease, and in the left temporal region in primary progressive aphasia. Normal PET and SPECT studies, however, do not exclude these diagnoses. When focal or regional abnormalities are seen, comparison with CT or MRI is required to rule out other structural brain disease such as stroke.

Table 3 Diagnostic Evaluation of Dementia

History	Tests
Medical/psychiatric/social	Laboratory: chemistry profile, B_{12}, RPR,
Drug and alcohol use	T4, TSH, blood count, ESR
HIV and stroke risk factors	Radiologic: chest radiograph, brain CT
Family history of dementia	Ancillary: neuropsychometric tests, electro-
Medications	encephalogram, magnetic resonance,
Physical examination	functional imaging (SPECT/PET),
General	lumbar puncture, HIV
Neurologic	
Extrapyramidal features	
Gait	
Focal signs	
Mental status	

Source: Ref. 21.

Electroencephalography (EEG) often shows nonspecific slowing of background activity in dementia and is normal in primary major depression. Approximately 80% of patients with Creutzfeldt-Jakob disease will show an EEG pattern of periodic activity consisting of triphasic waves or slow-wave burst suppression (22).

Lumbar puncture is not done routinely, but is reserved for cases in which there is a clinical suspicion of immunologic disease (e.g., vasculitis, sarcoidosis, Lyme disease) or CNS infection (e.g., tertiary syphilis, cryptococcal meningitis).

Detailed neuropsychometric testing can provide useful information regarding the presence of typical patterns of performance in dementia (e.g., prominent executive deficits in the frontal lobe syndrome) as well as quantitative information that can be used to follow the clinical course of dementia over time.

II. DISEASES CAUSING DEMENTIA

A. Non-Alzheimer Cerebral Degenerations

1. *Lobar degenerations*

Pick's disease was described by Arnold Pick in 1892. Grossly, the brain in Pick's disease shows circumscribed atrophy of frontal and temporal lobes. The hippocampi are typically involved. Involvement of subcortical structures is variable. The nucleus basalis of Meynert is relatively unaffected by the degeneration process, and markers of cortical cholinergic function are usually normal, unlike in Alzheimer's disease. Histologic findings include argentophilic intraneuronal inclusions called Pick bodies, swollen (ballooned), pale-staining (achromatic) neurons, and often white-matter gliosis.

Clinical features have been described above. Usual onset is in the presenile period from age 40 to 60 years, ranging from the 20s to late 80s. Family history of an affected relative may be seen in half of cases, with an autosomal-dominant inheritance pattern occurring in 10–20% of cases.

The course is slowly progressive over 5–10 years. Typically the dementia begins predominantly as a breakdown of social propriety and personality—unlike in Alzheimer's disease, in which these are later features of disease. Some patients are withdrawn and apathetic whereas others are more disinhibited and inappropriate. Stereotyped behaviors and obsessions may occur. Features suggestive of the Klüver-Bucy syndrome such as hypersexuality, hyperorality, and visual agnosia are seen as manifestations of bilateral temporal lobe involvement (23). Disorganization of thought, loss of insight and judgment, and perseveration are seen. Memory, calculations, and visuospatial functions are relatively preserved early in the disease; however, deficits in these areas develop as disease progresses. Stereotyped speech, diminished speech output, and eventual muteness in the terminal state are seen in distinction to the fluent aphasia and the palilalia in terminal state seen in Alzheimer's disease. Seizures are uncommon (19).

A recent series of 21 pathologically proven cases of Pick's disease and 42 cases of Alzheimer's disease reported that 44% of CT scans showed atrophy in the frontal lobes, temporal lobes, or both in Pick's cases, compared to no such findings in the Alzheimer's disease cases. Distinguishing clinical characteristics favoring a diagnosis of Pick's disease in those with normal CTs included onset prior to age 65, personality change at onset, hyperorality, disinhibition, and roaming behavior (24).

There are no strictly defined diagnostic criteria for Pick's disease. Cases may be suspected based on the neurobehavioral syndrome described, and supported by findings of frontotemporal atrophy on CT or MRI (see Figure 1A), or similar regional abnormalities on functional brain images such as PET and SPECT.

Infrequently one encounters atypical patients with a relatively circumscribed neurobehavioral syndrome, who may go on to develop dementia over time. Unlike Alzheimer's disease, memory dysfunction is not the predominant cognitive

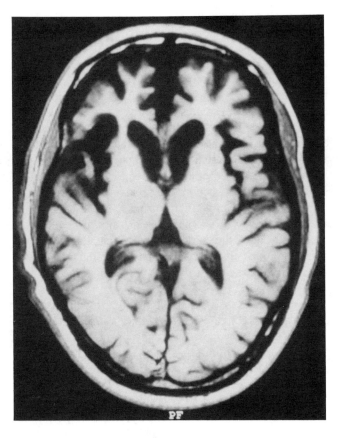

Figure 1A   MRI: Bilateral frontal and temporal lobe atrophy in a patient with Pick's disease.

impairment. Neuroimaging studies often reveal evidence of focal or asymmetric atrophy. A classification scheme for these cases has been referred to as asymmetric cortical degeneration syndrome and defined by Caselli and Jack (25) as "a slowly progressive (i.e., a period of years), localizable neurologic deficit or cortical syndrome that was not caused by a focal structural lesion, such as tumor, vascular impairment or

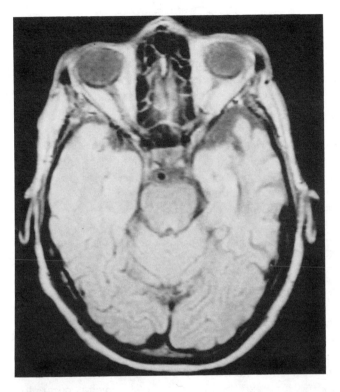

Figure 1B MRI: Left temporal atrophy in a patient with primary progressive aphasia syndrome.

anomaly, demyelination, trauma or infection." Although these neurobehavioral syndromes are heterogeneous in their underlying pathology, recognition of their characteristic neurobehavioral patterns serves a clinically useful purpose in distinguishing them from the more common and typical presentation of probable Alzheimer's disease (26).

The most commonly recognized focal or asymmetric lobar degeneration syndrome is *primary progressive aphasia*. In contrast to Alzheimer's disease patients, in whom aphasia occurs following or concurrent with memory impairment, these cases are characterized by slowly progressive aphasia, often of a nonfluent type. In the early years of the illness there is no dementia. Neuroimaging studies may show evidence of lobar atrophy of the left temporal perisylvian region (see Figure 1B). Postmortem studies in a small number of patients have shown asymmetric atrophy, predominantly in the left frontotemporal region with nonspecific gliosis and spongiform degeneration in at least half of cases. The remainder have shown evidence of Alzheimer- or Pick-type pathologic changes (27). Distinction of patients with primary progressive aphasia from Alzheimer's or Pick's disease is of prognostic importance, since those with focal degeneration appear to follow a more benign course (28).

Patients with progressive *posterior cortical atrophy* affecting the parieto-occipital regions have been described in whom deficits such as agnosia, alexia, agraphia, and anomia are prominent along with relative preservation of memory function (25,29). Progressive asymmetric atrophy of the frontal and parietal lobes and basal ganglia is associated with the syndrome of *corticobasal ganglionic degeneration*. The underlying pathology resembles Pick's disease without the presence of Pick bodies. Clinical features include akinesia, rigidity, postural-action tremor, dystonia, reflex myoclonus, cortical sensory loss, apraxia, and hyperreflexia. Dementia occurs in 43% of cases, but is not a prominent feature compared with typical Pick's disease (30,31).

Another group of patients have been described in whom frontal lobe degeneration is the dominant feature—*frontal lobe dementia* is characterized prominently by the frontal lobe syndrome. Pick bodies, neuritic plaques, or neurofibrillary tangles are absent on postmortem examination. Investigators have labeled such cases "progressive neuropsychiatric syndrome" (25), "dementia of frontal-lobe type" (32) or "frontal lobe degeneration of non-Alzheimer type" (33). Like Pick's disease, unusual cases of frontal lobe dementia have been associated with motor neuron disease (34). Whether such cases represent a variant of Pick's disease without Pick bodies (35) or a separate nosologic entity remains to be clarified.

2. *Extrapyramidal system disorders*

The prevalence of dementia in patients with *Parkinson's disease* is at least 10–15% (36), although some studies report a much higher frequency of 30–50% (37). Distinction must be made between the potentially reversible delirium caused by anticholinergic medications, psychosis due to levodopa, and depression related to the disease, and irreversible progressive dementia. Risk factors for development of dementia in Parkinson's disease include age greater than 70 years, depression, and levodopa-induced psychosis or confusion (38).

Several possible etiologies for dementia with Parkinson's disease are to be considered. A postmortem series of 100 cases of Parkinson's disease found a prevalence of dementia of 44%: 29% had Alzheimer's disease, 10% had diffuse Lewy body disease, 6% possible vascular dementia, and 55% no definite pathologic cause for dementia (39). Parkinson patients often exhibit relatively mild or circumscribed cognitive impairments such as bradyphrenia and amnesia as well as mood disturbance. A more pervasive subcortical dementia secondary to dysfunction of basal ganglia, amygdala, and thalamus has been ascribed to Parkinson's disease (40).

The co-occurrence of Parkinson's disease and Alzheimer's disease is well recognized (37,41). Furthermore, there is a higher than expected frequency of Alzheimer's disease in Parkinson's disease. Both diseases share degeneration of the nucleus basalis of Meynert along with deficiencies in markers of cortical cholinergic function, and degeneration of ascending noradrenergic projections from the locus ceruleus. These observations suggest that there may be a common pathogenetic mechanism between the two disorders (37).

In some patients with clinical features of Parkinson's disease and dementia, postmortem examination reveals cellular loss and eosinophilic inclusion bodies called Lewy bodies in the substantia nigra as seen in typical Parkinson's disease as well as Lewy bodies in significant numbers in the cerebral cortex. Neuritic plaques and small numbers of neurofibrillary tangles are also present as in Alzheimer's disease. This entity has been referred to as *diffuse Lewy body disease* (42), idiopathic diffuse cortical Lewy body disease or Lewy body dementia (43), Lewy body variant of Alzheimer's disease (44), and senile dementia of Lewy body type (45). As in other degenerative diseases, definite diagnosis rests on postmortem evidence. There are no generally accepted clinical diagnostic criteria. The initial symptoms of diffuse Lewy body disease may consist of parkinsonism or dementia. Fluctuating cognitive deficits including memory and in particular, visuospatial function may suggest recurrent delirium or vascular dementia in the differential diagnosis. Exaggerated adverse response to neuroleptics is often seen (46,47). Other antemortem clues to the diagnosis include rapid progression, gait disturbance, psychosis with hallucinations or delusions, and background slowing with a frontally predominant burst pattern on EEG early in the course of dementia (48).

As previously mentioned, the concept of subcortical dementia was originally described in patients with *progressive supranuclear palsy* (PSP) (14). This disorder accounts for approximately 4% of cases of parkinsonism. Unlike dementia associated with idiopathic Parkinson's disease and diffuse Lewy body disease, in which pathology is found in both cortex and subcortical structures, degeneration in PSP is generally confined to the basal ganglia, brainstem, and cerebellar nuclei. Neuropathologic changes include neuronal loss, granulovacuolar degeneration, gliosis, and neurofibrillary tangles. Forgetfulness, unsteady gait, backward falls, and slurred speech are early clinical features. Dementia, bradykinesia, axial rigidity, and supranuclear gaze palsy of downgaze are also characteristic. Tremor is uncommon. The temporal course is marked by slow progressive decline with a median duration from onset to death of 5.9 years (49,50). Response to L-dopa and dopamine agonists is usually poor, although some benefit may be seen in patients early in their disease.

Huntington's disease is an autosomal-dominant hereditary disease characterized by the triad of progressive chorea, behavioral disturbances, and dementia. It was first described in a classic report on a kindred from Long Island by George Huntington in 1872 (51). The most common presenting feature is personality change with inappropriate or antisocial behavior. Psychiatric disturbances are common, particularly depression; suicide accounts for about 7% of deaths. Delusions and hallucinations are common as well. Dementia of the subcortical type with prominent features of the frontal lobe syndrome may occur early and precede the movement disorder. Dystonia is sometimes seen along with choreic movements. Dysphagia is a complication that may lead to aspiration. Terminally the patient is rigid and mute. Age of onset is 35–45, with a range of 10–70 years. The usual course of the disease is 10–15 years (19).

Inheritance is autosomal dominant with complete penetrance. Prediction of relatives at risk has been possible through genetic linkage testing; recently, the Huntington's disease gene was identified (52), which should allow for simpler and more accurate genetic testing. On gross pathology atrophy involves frontal and parietal lobes, thalamus, caudate nucleus, globus pallidus, and putamen. Neuronal loss and gliosis are seen microscopically to involve the caudate and striatum most severely, which are important centers for inhibition of movement. Evidence of caudate atrophy may be seen on CT and MRI images; however, the diagnosis is generally made on the basis of the typical clinical features and family history.

Neuroleptic drugs such as haloperidol are used frequently to control chorea; however, treatment with such agents is complicated by the development of tardive dyskinesia and rigidity, which often lead to tapering and discontinuing the drug. Antidepressants, lithium, and electroconvulsive therapy are used for management of depression. Anxiety may be treated with benzodiazepine medications.

Wilson's disease is an autosomal-recessive degenerative disease in which dementia is associated with hepatic dysfunction. Clinical onset is usually in childhood or early adulthood, with rare cases being reported as late as the sixth decade (53). Failure to excrete copper normally leads to deposition in the liver and brain associated with cirrhosis and degeneration of the putamen and globus pallidus. Along with hepatic abnormalities, neurologic features include tremor, bradykinesia, dysarthria, dysphagia, hoarseness, chorea, and dystonic postures of the limbs. Muteness, rigidity, and subcortical dementia are late features. Nearly all cases show a brownish discoloration of the peripheral cornea called Kayser-Fleischer rings, which may require slit-lamp examination to visualize. Confirmatory laboratory studies include low serum ceruloplasmin, low serum copper, and increased urinary copper excretion. Chelation treatment with D-penicillamine, particularly if instituted early, is effective in reversing neurologic signs.

3. *Cerebellar degenerations*

In heterogeneous group of diseases referred to as *olivopontocerebellar atrophy,* progressive cerebellar ataxia and parkinsonism are prominent features. Pathologic findings include loss of neurons in cerebellar cortex, ventral pons, and inferior olives. Depigmentation and cell loss are seen in the substantia nigra, accounting for the parkinsonian features. Atrophy of the brainstem and cerebellum may be seen on neuroimaging studies. These disorders are frequently associated with dementia, which in some cases has been related to cortical neuronal loss. Among cases with dementia, ophthalmoplegia is another typical finding. Onset ranges from childhood to age 50, usually in the third to fifth decade.

The majority of cases of olivopontocerebellar atrophy are inherited in an autosomal-dominant pattern, including the cases reported in association with dementia (54). Some families have followed an autosomal-recessive pattern and other cases appear to be sporadic. The ataxia is untreatable. Parkinsonian features may respond partially to dopaminergic drugs.

Dementia of a subcortical type probably occurs as a late sign in many cases of *Friedreich's ataxia*, a hereditary disorder characterized by progressive signs of cerebellar, corticospinal, posterior column, and peripheral nerve dysfunction. Pathological changes are most severe in the spinal cord. Onset is from age 10 to 20, with unusual cases presenting in adulthood. Inheritance is autosomal recessive.

Other forms of primary *cerebellar degeneration* occur, which are clinically heterogeneous and may be associated with ophthalmoplegia, optic atrophy, retinitis pigmentosa, extrapyramidal signs, dysarthria, and polyneuropathy. Onset is in the fourth to sixth decades. If dementia occurs, it is usually a late sign of the disease. Cases are commonly sporadic or inherited in an autosomal-dominant pattern (55).

4. *Dementia with motor neuron disease*

Classic *amyotrophic lateral sclerosis* is a progressive disease of motor neurons, corticobulbar and corticospinal tracts, which produces severe and eventually fatal muscular weakness, wasting, and spasticity. Rarely, such cases are associated with dementia, parkinsonism, or both. The co-occurrence of these three disorders is found with a particularly high frequency in certain islands of the western Pacific, including Guam, New Guinea, and the Kii Peninsula of Japan. Neurofibrillary degeneration, but not neuritic plaques, are seen throughout the brain and spinal cord. In non-Guamanian cases, pathology consists of cerebral cortex atrophy, with loss of neurons, spongiform changes, and mild gliosis, but no plaques, tangles, or inclusion bodies.

Clinically the dementia may resemble Alzheimer's disease (56), but more often it is of the frontal lobe type (34). Hudson's review suggests that ALS-parkinsonism-dementia complex is a universal condition representing variant cases of the same illness in which the degenerative process extends to cortex and subcortical basal ganglia structures (57). Motor neuron disease has also been described as a concurrent disease in patients with Pick's disease, Creutzfeldt-Jakob disease, and Parkinson's disease (58).

B. Vascular Dementia

Although vascular dementia is generally recognized as the second leading cause of dementia, considerable controversy exists regarding how to diagnose the disorder (59–61). Problems arise from the co-occurrence of stroke in patients with Alzheimer's disease, the frequent findings of incidental radiologic signs suggesting cerebral ischemia in patients with slowly progressive decline in function, pathologic heterogeneity of the underlying disease, and the difficulties encountered in correlating stroke with cognitive deficits in the individual patient. Recognition of stroke as a contributing cause of dementia is of great importance since appropriate medical interventions to prevent recurrence may impede progression of disease.

Information from the history and physical examination of the patient with dementia yields important information that identifies patients at significant risk for stroke as a cause of their dementia. In 1975 Hachinski and colleagues (62) described an ischemic score to identify such patients. A modified version of the score, presented in Table 4, has been shown to be useful in discriminating Alzheimer's disease from cases of vascular dementia or mixed Alzheimer's disease with

Table 4   Modified Hachinski Ischemic Score

	Absent	Present
Abrupt onset	0	2
Stepwise deterioration	0	1
Somatic complaints	0	1
Emotional incontinence	0	1
History or presence of hypertension	0	1
History of strokes	0	2
Focal neurologic signs	0	2
Focal neurologic symptoms	0	2

A total score >3 suggests vascular dementia.
Source: Adapted from Ref. 63.

vascular dementia, but not for discriminating mixed cases from "pure" vascular dementia (63). Fischer and colleagues (64) reported that the use of this score provided an accuracy of 81.3% in discriminating primary degenerative dementia from multi-infarct/mixed cases.

An attempt to define diagnostic criteria for ischemic vascular dementia, including information from radiologic studies, was proposed by the State of California Alzheimer's Disease Diagnostic and Treatment Centers based on a probability classification strategy used previously by the NIH for Alzheimer's disease (65). The central diagnostic features for "probable ischemic vascular dementia" under this classification system are shown in Table 5. Evidence of infarcts in brain regions known to cause cognitive deficits, history of transient ischemic attacks, vascular risk factors, and elevated ischemic score are features supportive of the diagnosis.

Although the occurrence of multiple discrete cortical or subcortical ischemic infarctions, i.e., *multi-infarct dementia*, is the most widely recognized cause of vascular dementia, multiple mechanisms are recognized (66). A more encompassing set of criteria for diagnosis of vascular dementia was proposed by the NINDS-AIREN International Workshop, which accounts for heterogeneity of pathologic mechanisms and includes cases of dementia related to global hypoperfusion and intracranial hemorrhages (67).

Table 5 Proposed Diagnostic Criteria for Vascular Dementia

1. Dementia
2. Evidence of two or more ischemic strokes by history, neurologic signs, and/or neuroimaging studies (CT or T1-weighted MRI)   or   Occurrence of a single stroke with a clearly documented temporal relationship to the onset of dementia
3. Evidence of at least one infarct outside the cerebellum by CT or T1-weighted MRI

Source: Adapted from Ref. 65.

Vascular dementia may result from multiple infarctions in cortical, subcortical, or both locations. Although the multi-infarct state is usually divided into (1) multiple cortical infarcts as seen in thromboembolism or (2) multiple subcortical lacunar infarcts related to small vessel disease such as lipo-hyalinosis, the two types of infarction often coexist. The term *ischemic vascular dementia* encompasses both.

Probably the most crucial factor in producing dementia is location of stroke. Since amnesia is an important component of the dementia syndrome, strategic locations for production of dementia include the hippocampus and thalamus. Most commonly, amnesia from unilateral stroke involves ischemia of the left infero-medial temporal lobe or thalamus. These are supplied by anterior choroidal and posterior cerebral arteries, and thalamic penetrating arteries, respectively (68). An example is seen in Figure 2. In a study of 251 stroke patients, dementia was present in 66 (26.3%) cases. Infarcts were cortical and subcortical, predominantly left hemispheric, and in the vascular territories of the left posterior cerebral and anterior cerebral arteries (69).

Volume and number of infarctions are also felt by many to be significant although difficult to define, factors in the production of dementia, either by causing total injury that exceeds the brain's cognitive reserve or by more specific additive effects on cognitive function. In a quantitative MRI study of normals and stroke patients, Liu and coworkers (70) found a strong relationship between dementia and total area of cortical and subcortical infarction. Cortical infarction was more likely to produce dementia than subcortical infarction, and left-hemisphere infarction was more likely to be associated with dementia than right-hemisphere infarction.

Co-occurrence of Alzheimer's disease as well as other degenerative disorders results in mixed cases wherein the specific contribution of either alone cannot be readily determined. Mixed dementia is particularly suspected when a patient follows a steadily progressive deterioration following or concurrent with an isolated stroke, that itself does not fully explain the cognitive impairment.

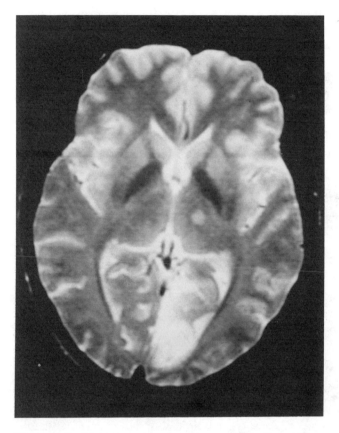

Figure 2A MRI: Posterior circulation stroke causing infarction of left thalamus, occipital, and medial temporal lobes in a patient with amnesia and anomic aphasia.

A host of different cerebrovascular disorders may produce multiple ischemic infarctions including atherosclerotic thromboembolism, cardiac embolism (endocarditis, atrial fibrillation, myocardial infarction, cardiomyopathy), fat embolism, lipohyalinosis, amyloid angiopathy, coagulopathy, dysproteinemia, and arteritis. Multiple cerebral hemorrhages may occur

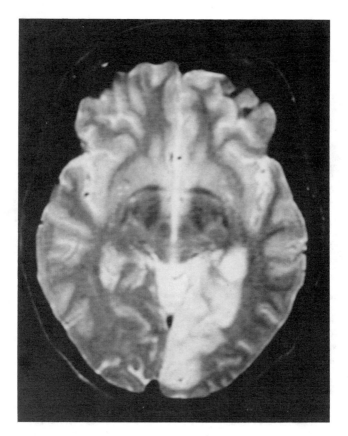

Figure 2A Continued

in septic embolism or mycotic aneurysms from endocarditis, vasculitis, thrombocytopenia, and amyloid angiopathy. A thorough evaluation for the cause of vascular dementia should include a search for risk factors, historical evidence, and physical signs of these disorders. A complete blood count, platelet count, prothrombin and partial thromboplastin times, sedimentation rate, electrocardiogram, and CT or MRI are essential to the diagnostic work-up. Noninvasive studies to

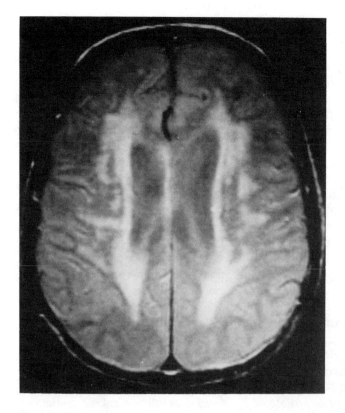

Figure 2B MRI: Leuko-araiosis in a patient with Binswanger's disease.

search for cardiac embolism source include transthoracic and transesophageal echocardiography as well as Holter monitor. Noninvasive studies of the cerebral arteries include carotid ultrasonography and magnetic resonance angiography. In cases of suspected arteritis and surgically amenable carotid stenosis, angiography is usually performed.

Determination of the etiology of stroke is a prerequisite to planning an effective preventive strategy for patients with vascular dementia as well as nondemented stroke patients.

Usually antiplatelet agents such as aspirin and ticlopidine are used. Pentoxifylline, a drug that lowers blood viscosity, has been suggested to benefit cognition in patients with vascular dementia (71); however, studies of this drug as well as other experimental trials using metabolic enhancement, vasodilator, and nootropic agents have not produced conclusive evidence of efficacy.

Binswanger's disease is a form of ischemic vascular dementia in which decline is often slowly progressive rather than marked by the more typical abrupt onset with stepwise course of the multi-infarct state. Binswanger's cases were first described in 1894; however, it was not until the advent of CT and MRI that the disease became increasingly recognized pre-mortem. MRI has been found to be more sensitive than CT in demonstrating the pathologic changes radiographically. Pathologic studies have consistently reported patchy but relatively symmetric confluent areas of white-matter discoloration most commonly in the occipital and periventricular regions. Discrete lacunar infarctions occur in 93% of cases. Microscopic evidence of demyelination is associated with astrocytic gliosis; extremely affected areas consist of white-matter rarefaction or cavitation with microcystic areas of infarction. Microscopic vascular changes are most prominent in the white-matter arterioles (72).

The radiologic appearance of subcortical white-matter decreased density, called leuko-araiosis (73), is typically seen extensively in the subcortical and periventricular regions of persons with Binswanger's disease (see Figure 2A). As discussed in Section III, this radiographic appearance is relatively nonspecific. Consequently, diagnosis must rely on recognizing risk factors and clinical features of the disease in patients with this radiographic pattern.

Although the neuropathologic and radiologic features of this relatively uncommon disease are well defined, there is no consensus on the essential clinical features. Babikian and Ropper (72) noted that a slow rather than abrupt onset occurred in 66% of cases. The temporal course was gradually progressive without acute deficits in 43%, gradually progressive with acute exacerbations in 43%, and acute without progression in 14%. Most patients have a history of longstanding or poorly controlled hypertension. Besides dementia, focal motor signs, pseudobulbar palsy, gait disturbance, and incontinence are common. The diagnosis is most appropriately based on the combination of vascular risk factors, evidence of systemic and focal cerebral vascular disease, clinical features of subcortical dementia, and support from radiologic studies showing leuko-araiosis (74).

Another mechanism for vascular dementia is diffuse bihemispheric ischemia due to hypotension. In the case of cardiopulmonary arrest a mixed cerebral insult occurs called *hypoxic-ischemic encephalopathy*. Particularly if severe carotid artery stenosis is present, less severe hypotensive insults may produce *watershed infarctions* in the border zones between major vessel territories of the anterior, middle, and posterior cerebral arteries as well as subcortical regions in the territories of deep penetrating vessels. Another mechanism of generalized or focal insult occurs from *hyperviscosity* related to hematologic disorders (66).

Among vasculitic disorders affecting the elderly, *temporal arteritis* is the most common and has been reported as a treatable cause of dementia (75). Headaches and ophthalmologic deficits, including permanent visual loss, are common; however, neuropsychiatric disorders were reported in only 3% and stroke in 7% in one series of 166 cases (76).

Vascular dementia may result from multiple intracerebral hemorrhages. A common cause of multiple cerebral hemorrhages in the elderly is *amyloid angiopathy*. Typically the hemorrhages are cortically located in different lobes of the brain and occur at different times. Although amyloid angiopathy occurs frequently in patients with Alzheimer's disease, this is not a uniform finding. A rapidly progressing dementia has been associated with amyloid angiopathy, and in such cases there are often prominent subcortical white-matter changes (77).

C. Infectious Disease

Among the bacterial infections that may produce dementia, one must consider chronic meningoencephalitis from syphilis, Lyme disease, and tuberculosis. General paresis, the form of tertiary *syphilis* presenting as dementia, is one of the classic treatable diseases causing dementia. Cases of syphilis affecting the nervous system are still rarely encountered and in fact may be increasing in recent years (78). The incidence of syphilis in this country has risen threefold since its low point in 1956 to about 4 cases per 100,000 (79). Signs and symptoms of tertiary syphilis occur 15–20 years after the initial infection. Chronic basilar meningitis may occur and is manifested by cranial nerve palsies and obstructive hydrocephalus. A similar picture is seen in association with other granulomatous diseases such as tuberculosis as well as fungal meningitis. Involvement of the spinal cord produces tabes dorsalis, in which there is thickening of the spinal meninges and degeneration of the spinal cord, particularly affecting dorsal nerve roots and posterior columns. Clinical symptoms that result include lightening pains in the extremities, ataxia, sensory loss affecting vibration and position sense, and bladder dysfunction.

Subacute encephalitis and arteritis due to direct treponemal infection of the brain is seen in about one-third of cases of tertiary syphilis. Tremor, dysarthria, and seizures are common. The Argyll Robertson pupil (accommodates, but does not react directly to light) is present in over 90% of cases. Early in the course, prominent changes in personality are seen followed by progressive decline in cognitive abilities. A positive blood serologic test from a patient with dementia should be further evaluated by lumbar puncture. A positive serology test and cell count showing a lymphocytic pleocytosis should prompt treatment with intravenous penicillin. A positive FTA-ABS, increased cell count, and negative serology test should also be considered indications for treatment (80).

Another disease produced by a spirochete, *Borrelia burgdorferi*, is *Lyme disease*. Neurologic manifestations of the

disease are extremely variable and include cranial neuropathies, radiculopathy, mononeuritis multiplex, polyneuropathy, and aseptic meningitis (81). Cases of severe encephalitis have been reported in which MRI reveals multiple
sclerosis–like lesions in the white matter (82,83). In some
cases antibodies to *B. burgdorferi* are found. Spinal fluid
shows a lymphocytic pleocytosis. Chronic neuropsychiatric
symptoms including dementia appear to be relatively resistant
to treatment with antibiotics.

Tuberculosis and *cryptococcus* infections of the CNS may
produce a chronic meningitis with similar clinical features.
Mental-status changes are common and may result from meningitis or the secondary effects of obstructive hydrocephalus.
Other common symptoms include headache, nuchal rigidity,
cranial nerve palsies, and ataxia. Spinal fluid studies typically
show a low-glucose, high-protein, and lymphocytic pleocytosis.

In one comparative study, 25% of patients did not seek
medical attention until symptoms were present for 4 weeks.
Abnormalities such as miliary pattern on chest films and inappropriate antidiuretic hormone were helpful clues to the
presence of tuberculosis. Cryptococcal antigen was a sensitive
and specific indicator of cryptococcus. Tuberculosis was seen
more often in patients with alcoholism and heart disease, while
cryptococcus was seen in patients with immunosuppressive
conditions such as lymphoma and renal transplantation (84).
Delay in diagnosis may be particularly common in cryptococcal meningitis in which 50% of patients lack fever (84,85).
In recent times cryptococcal infection is commonly seen in
patients with AIDS.

The approach to diagnosis of the etiology of chronic
meningitis requires a thoughtful evaluation for multiple possible etiologies. Organisms implicated in chronic neutrophilic
meningitis include the bacteria nocardia, actinomyces,
arachnia, brucella, and the fungi blastomyces, coccidioides,
candida, aspergillus, zygomycetes, cladosporium, and
pseudallescheria. A similar picture may be seen with chemi-

cal meningitis from epidermoid tumors, and craniopharyn-giomas, exogenous chemical meningitis from contrast agents, and lupus meningitis. Chronic lymphocytic meningitis may be secondary to syphilis, actinomyces, nocardia, brucella, Lyme disease, leptospirosis, tuberculosis, various fungi, carcinoma, sarcoidosis, and granulomatous arteritis (86).

Protozoans and parasites may produce the dementia syndrome by producing multifocal areas of abscess or cerebritis. An example is *toxoplasmosis*, a disease often seen in patients with AIDS. The causative organism is *Toxoplasma gondii*, an obligate intracellular protozoan. Clinical manifestations include focal and diffuse meningoencephalitis as well as necrotizing granulomas containing encysted organisms, seen as enhancing mass lesions on CT or MRI. Symptoms of altered mental status occur in 70% of cases, often accompanied by headache and focal signs and symptoms. Symptoms may be present for several weeks before coming to recognition. Serologic tests are usually positive, particularly in immunocompetent individuals. Spinal fluid shows a mild lymphocytic pleocytosis. Mass lesions may require biopsy for definite diagnosis (87).

Neurocysticercosis results from CNS infection by the encysted larvae of *Taenia solium*, the pork tapeworm. The disease is endemic to Mexico, Hispanic America, and Southeast Asia. The most common signs are seizures, hydrocephalus, and focal deficits. Dementia is a presenting feature in 3% of cases (88). Hydrocephalus can occur due to chronic meningitis or ventriculitis. CT and MRI typically show multiple cystic lesions that are frequently calcified, thin walled, and located at the gray–white-matter junction. Serologic studies of blood and spinal fluid should be performed to support the diagnosis (89).

Viruses that produce an acute encephalitis may leave a state of chronic fixed mental impairment. Survivors of *Herpes simplex* encephalitis may have a persistent dementia characterized by amnesia and prominent behavioral disturbances due to necrosis of bilateral frontal and temporal lobes.

Viruses producing a more insidious subacute or rapidly progressing dementing illness include the *AIDS dementia complex* and *progressive multifocal leukoencephalopathy* (PML). The human immunodeficiency virus (HIV-1) affects the nervous system in 60–90% of cases of AIDS. A subacute viral encephalitis may occur, which usually develops during the full-blown stage of the disease when opportunistic infections occur, although occasionally the dementia may precede the diagnosis of systemic AIDS. Clinical manifestations include tremor, rigidity, and cotton wool spots in the retina. Apathy or depression lead to progressive dementia characterized by social withdrawal, amnesia, and finally terminal mutism and rigidity over the course of weeks to months. Brain imaging studies are normal or show evidence of diffuse disease in the white matter. Spinal fluid shows no cells or a small number of lymphocytes with elevated protein. Secondary infections of the CNS must be ruled out, such as cryptococcal meningitis and toxoplasmosis (90,91). Reports from a few small studies suggest that dementia may be responsive to zidovudine therapy (92).

PML is an unusual rapidly progressive demyelinating disease frequently attributed to opportunistic infection by the JC virus. Clinical features include multifocal neurologic signs often accompanied by memory disturbance or aphasia. Spinal fluid examination is generally normal. CT and MRI show large patches of demyelination in white matter. The diagnosis is confirmed by biopsy or postmortem examination, but may be suspected in patients with AIDS or other immunosuppressive conditions such as lymphoma and chronic lymphocytic leukemia. The disease is fatal and untreatable (93).

D. Prion Diseases

The four diseases in humans caused by prions are kuru, fatal familial insomnia, Gerstmann-Sträussler-Scheinker disease, and Creutzfeldt-Jakob disease. All are associated with dementia. Kuru was found to be transmitted by cannibalism among natives of New Guinea and is now virtually non-existent due to abandonment of the practice. Creutzfeldt-Jakob disease is typically a sporadic disorder. Fatal familial insomnia, Gerstmann-Sträussler-Scheinker disease, and familial Creutzfeldt-Jakob disease are inherited in autosomal-dominant form (94,95).

The infectious agent is a protein coded for by the prion protein gene. The role of this protein in normal cellular function is unknown. It appears that the pathogenic form of the protein is the result of altered conformation (96).

The most common of the prion diseases is *Creutzfeldt-Jakob disease*. The annual incidence of the disease is one per million. Rapid onset occurs in 20% and rapid progression with death by one year in 90% of cases. Dementia occurs at onset in 64% and at some point in 100% of cases. Other frequent neurologic signs include cerebellar ataxia, visual disturbances, pyramidal signs, and extrapyramidal rigidity. Myoclonus is seen usually late in the course in 88% of cases. Periodic EEG abnormalities are seen in 80% of cases. The full triad of dementia, myoclonus, and 1–2 cycle/second periodic EEG activity occurs in 51% (22). Spinal fluid and CT are generally normal. MRI may show hyperintensity in the basal ganglia and thalamus.

E. Noninfectious Inflammatory and Demyelinating Diseases

Patients with *multiple sclerosis*, who usually have severe or longstanding chronic progressive disease, occasionally exhibit features of subcortical dementia. Affective disorders including euphoria and depression also occur. There has been no proof that immunosuppressive treatment reverses the dementia associated with multiple sclerosis.

Another group of subcortical diseases affecting white matter that may cause dementia are the leukodystrophies. These typically begin in childhood and early adult years. The adult form of *metachromatic leukodystrophy* may present with dementia or psychiatric disorder (97).

Marchiafava-Bignami disease is a rare idiopathic demyelinating disorder affecting the corpus callosum and adjacent midline structures, which is seen predominantly in alcoholics. Dementia may be abrupt in onset and is often progressive.

Behçet's disease is an idiopathic inflammatory disorder that is most common in Eastern and Middle Eastern countries. Young adults with recurrent aphthous stomatitis are affected by genital ulcers, uveitis, vasculitis, synovitis, and meningoencephalitis. The chronic relapsing and remitting course with multiple neurologic signs simulates multiple sclerosis. Subcortical gray- and white-matter structures are most affected. Early diagnosis and treatment with immunosuppressive drugs may prevent chronic sequelae such as dementia (98).

Sarcoidosis is a systemic idiopathic granulomatous inflammatory disease that often affects the CNS early in the course of disease. Characteristics of sarcoidosis include hilar adenopathy, hypercalcemia, uveitis, and arthralgias. Chronic basilar meningitis and intraventricular granulomas may result in obstructive hydrocephalus. Cerebral granulomatous mass lesions and stroke are less common. Dementia may arise from these mechanisms or metabolic disorder such as hypercalcemia. Spinal fluid reveals a lymphocytic pleocytosis with elevated protein and low glucose. Biopsy of skeletal muscle or other affected tissues provides definitive diagnosis. Response of neurologic deficits to steroid therapy is unpredictable and may be dramatic (99,100).

F. Toxic and Metabolic Disorders

A wide variety of toxic and metabolic disorders may produce a confusional state. Often the confusional state is relatively acute or fluctuating and marked by disturbances of consciousness, and hence is more appropriately considered under the category of *delirium* rather than dementia. Etiologies include electrolyte disturbances, dehydration, sepsis, drug toxicity, and alcoholism. Endocrine disturbances include thyroid disorder, hypercalcemia (e.g., hyperparathyroidism and malignancy), hypocalcemia, Addison's disease, and Cushing's syndrome.

Major *organ failure* may produce acute, intermittent, or chronic mental impairments. Examples are transient severe hypoxia, chronic hypercapnia-hypoxia, congestive heart failure, severe anemia, and hyperviscosity syndromes. Hepatic and uremic encephalopathy are major and common causes of metabolic encephalopathy. *Dialysis dementia* is usually attributed to aluminum toxicity from dialysate and aluminum-containing antacids. Stuttering dysarthria is associated with myoclonus, seizures, and rapidly progressive dementia usually terminating in death within 2 years (101).

Hypoglycemic encephalopathy is usually transient; however, dementia may result when the insult is severe or prolonged. *Wernicke's encephalopathy* from thiamine deficiency is a preventable and treatable disease seen most commonly in alcoholics, but also in other malnourished patients. Pathologic changes consist of softening and petechial hemorrhages in the periventricular gray matter of the third and fourth ventricles, dorsal medial thalamus, and mamillary bodies. The classic triad of signs and symptoms consisting of global confusion, ataxia, and ophthalmoplegia may not be seen completely in all patients. Onset is usually acute, although 20% of cases develop gradually. Signs of neurologic dysfunction can remit dramatically with parenteral thiamine; however, a chronic amnestic state with confabulation called *Korsakoff's psychosis* may be a permanent sequela (102).

Niacin deficiency may contribute to dementia in alcoholics as well as other malnourished states and is associated with signs of diarrhea and dermatitis. *Cobalamin deficiency* is a common disorder, particularly in the elderly; however, controversy exists regarding how often dementia is the result of this deficiency when the typical features of pernicious anemia and combined systems degeneration are absent.

G. Other Dementias

1. *Neoplasms*

With the routine use of CT and MRI, identification of patients with dementia related to *primary and metastatic tumors* is usually easily made. Involvement of single tumors in the left temporal lobe or thalamus may mimic a rapidly progressive degenerative disease. Diffuse spread of primary glial cell malignancy throughout one or both hemispheres is referred to as *gliomatosis cerebri*, and may present as a global rapidly progressive dementia without well-defined focal lesions on brain imaging. *Neoplastic meningitis* should be considered in any patient with a subacute or rapidly progressive confusional state in whom there is a known primary or metastatic carcinoma, leukemia, or lymphoma. Clinical features of this illness include confusion, low grade fever, meningismus, cranial nerve palsies, spinal pain, limb weakness, and radiculopathy, usually at multiple levels of the neuraxis (103). Meningeal enhancement may be seen on MRI (104). Definite diagnosis is based on demonstration of malignant cells on spinal fluid examination. Although radiation and intrathecal chemotherapy may be used, death usually ensues within 1 to 3 months after diagnosis.

In 1968 Corsellis et al. (105) coined the term *limbic encephalitis* to describe a paraneoplastic disorder related to bronchial carcinoma manifested as a severe amnestic state and rapidly progressive dementia. Inflammation and degeneration were found predominantly in the temporal lobe limbic gray matter. Subsequent cases have been related to bronchogenic carcinoma 70% of the time, with oat cell being the most common histology (106).

2. *Hydrocephalus*

A number of disorders causing dementia via the mechanism of obstructive hydrocephalus have already been mentioned including sarcoidosis, tuberculosis, cryptococcus, and cysticercosis. To this list of primary causes of hydrocephalus should be added subarachnoid hemorrhage and head trauma. When hydrocephalus is recent and an underlying cause can be identified, response of neurologic symptoms, including to ventricular shunt procedures, is often good.

In 1965 Adams and coworkers (107) described a syndrome of hydrocephalus with normal spinal fluid pressure associated with gait disturbance, urinary incontinence, and dementia. Often of idiopathic origin and seen particularly in elderly persons, the term *normal pressure hydrocephalus* was applied to such cases, and in some a satisfactory response to shunting was reported. Although it is still recognized as a diagnostic entity, controversy exists regarding how to diagnose the disorder and how to select persons likely to respond to shunting. The issue of diagnostic uncertainty is particularly important since complications from ventricular shunt procedures occur in about one-third of cases, including shunt infection, subdural hematoma, seizures, and shunt malfunction (108). Radionuclide cisternography has fallen out of favor, since it is a poor predictor of shunt response (109). CT and MRI show dilation of all ventricles out of proportion to cortical atrophy. Clinical response to removal of 40–50 milliliters of spinal fluid has been recommended as a predictor of shunt response (110). Patients with gait disorder preceding dementia and in whom cognitive impairment is relatively mild may be regarded as surgical candidates, particularly if a primary cause has been identified for the hydrocephalus. Elderly patients with symptoms of hydrocephalus for less than 2 years are more likely to benefit from shunting (111); patients with longstanding and severe dementia are unlikely to benefit and should not be subjected to the risks of the procedure.

Normal-pressure hydrocephalus must be distinguished from the irreversible disorder of Binswanger's disease. Both may show ventricular dilation on CT or MRI and be associated with a subcortical type of dementia along with gait disturbance. In one comparative series, patients with NPH had a later age of onset, more frequent gait disturbance at onset, shorter duration of illness, rare signs of vascular disease, and more severe dementia. Focal neurologic signs and symptoms suggest Binswanger's disease rather than NPH (112).

3. *Trauma*

Among the traumatic causes of dementia are those arising from direct cerebral trauma producing multiple contusions or shearing lesions of white matter, multiple secondary strokes, normal-pressure hydrocephalus, chronic subdural hematoma, and dementia pugilistica. *Chronic subdural hematoma* may present with relatively minor or no localizing neurologic signs along with mental-status abnormalities, which may be mistaken for degenerative dementia. History of head trauma may be minor or absent. Elderly persons are particularly prone to subdural hemorrhage because of the fragility of bridging veins stretched across the subdural space due to brain atrophy. Mildly or nonsymptomatic subdurals, particularly if thin, may be managed conservatively and monitored for spontaneous resorption (19). Symptomatic large subdurals are generally surgically drained. Unfortunately, recurrence of fluid in the subdural sac is not uncommon.

Dementia pugilistica is seen in a large percentage of boxers. Repeated traumatic brain injuries lead to pathologic changes, including widespread neuronal degeneration with large numbers of neurofibrillary tangles in the cerebral cortex. Clinically patients develop bradykinesia, clumsiness, dysarthria, ataxic gait, tremor, rigidity, spasticity, memory impairment, slowed mentation, and personality change. Dementia may progress even after cessation of the boxing career. Dementia pugilistica represents a potentially preventable form of dementia (113,114).

III. ISSUES RELATED TO AGING

A. Hereditary Dementia and Aging

Dementia secondary to inherited metabolic disorders is seen most commonly in children, but occasionally may be seen in adults (115). Among the inherited dementias, very few have their onset after age 65, as can be seen in Table 6. Diseases that may be considered in the elderly population with a strong family history of dementia include Alzheimer's disease, Pick's disease, Creutzfeldt-Jakob disease, Gerstmann-Sträussler-Sheinker disease, and fatal familial insomnia.

Table 6 Hereditary Dementias in Adults

Disease	Inheritance pattern[a]	Age of onset[b]
Acute intermittent porphyria	AD	A, B
Adrenoleukodystrophy	XLR	A
Alzheimer's disease	S, AD	B, C
Ataxia telangiectasia	AR	A
Cerebellar and spinocerebellar ataxias	AR, AD, S	A, B
Cerebrotendinous xanthomatosis	AR	A
Creutzfeldt-Jakob disease	S, AD	B, C
Dentatorubral-pallidoluysian atrophy	AD	A, B
Fabry's disease	XLR	A
Familial cerebral calcification	AR, AD	A, B
Fatal familial insomnia	AD	B
Gangliosidoses GM1, GM2	AR	A
Gaucher's disease	AR	A
Gerstmann-Sträussler-Scheinker disease	AD	B

Hallervorden-Spatz disease	AR, S	A, B
Huntington's disease	AD	A, B
Kuf's disease (neuronal ceroid lipofuscinosis)	AR, AD	A
Lafora's disease	AR	A
Leigh's disease	AR, S	A
Mast syndrome	AR	A
Membranous lipodystrophy	AR	A, B
Metachromatic leukodystrophy	AR	A, B
Mucopolysaccharidosis type III B	AR	A
Myotonic dystrophy	AD	A, B
Neuroacanthocytosis	AR, S	A, B
Neuronal intranuclear inclusion disease	AD	A
Niemann-Pick disease	AR	A
Pick's disease	S, AD	B, C
Progressive myoclonus epilepsy	AR	A
Wilson's disease	AR	A

[a]AD, autosomal dominant; XLR, X-linked recessive; S, sporadic; AR, autosomal recessive.
[b]A, usually <35 years; B, 35–65 years; C, >65 years.
Source: Adapted from Ref. 115.

The hereditary basis of some cases of familial Alzheimer's disease is covered in the preceding chapter. Among families with Pick's disease and the prion diseases, autosomal dominance has been the reported inheritance pattern. Familial cases in these disorders seldom have their onset beyond the sixth decade.

B.   Co-morbid Disorders of Aging

In the evaluation of demented patients, one often encounters disorders of the elderly that may cause dementia themselves or accompany degenerative diseases of aging such as Alzheimer's disease. When slowly progressive dementia resembling Alzheimer's disease occurs in an elderly person with such a disorder, the terms *mixed dementia* or *possible Alzheimer's disease* are often applied. Because these disorders are specifically treatable and may be at least contributory to functional and cognitive impairment, their recognition is important.

Vascular disease, hypothyroidism, cobalamin deficiency, and depression deserve particular attention as common contributing or comorbid disorders of aging, which will be covered as separate topics.

1.   *The contribution of aging to vascular dementia*

Dementia and cerebrovascular disease both occur with increasing frequency with aging. Stroke and degenerative disease, therefore, may both contribute to dementia in the same patient. The pathologic changes of Alzheimer's disease are seen in small degree in normal elderly without dementia. In parallel to the presence of Alzheimer-type pathology seen in normal elderly persons, incomplete ischemic lesions are also seen in normal elderly without dementia. Ferrer and associates (117) have called such lesions "arteriosclerotic leucoencephalopathy in the elderly" to emphasize the common association with atherosclerosis and hypertension as well as similarities to pathologic findings in Binswanger's disease and multi-infarct dementia. White-matter disease may be seen in up to 100% of postmortem cases who reach the age of 80.

There has been a great deal of recent interest in the frequent finding of decreased density of white matter on CT, and particularly MRI, images of the brains of elderly persons both with and without dementia. As noted above, this radiographic finding has been called leuko-araiosis (73) and is demonstrated in Figure 2B. The finding on MRI is often referred to as white-matter hyperintensities (WMH), being seen particularly well on T2-weighted images. This is a nonspecific finding that includes a differential diagnosis of over 50 disorders, the most common of which are multiple or diffuse vascular ischemic lesions, demyelinating diseases, Alzheimer's disease, and normal aging (118).

Leuko-araiosis is seen to some extent in 10–89% of healthy elderly persons (119,120). One risk factor study of stroke patients and normals related WMH to age and diabetes but not to clinical ischemic events (121). WMH on MRI is more prevalent in vascular than in Alzheimer's disease, and more severe cognitive impairment has been related to changes in the posterior periventricular regions (122). Mirsen and associates (123) found WMH to be twice as prevalent in Alzheimer's disease as in normal elderly controls, whereas others have found no difference (124). Kozachuk and associates (125) found correlations between age and WMH for both healthy subjects and Alzheimer's disease subjects without vascular risk factors, although systolic blood pressure correlated with WMH in the elderly controls. A relationship has also been shown between WMH and late-life depression (126,127). In a study of a mixed population of psychiatric and healthy elderly, Sullivan and associates (128) found age and history or evidence of stroke to be independent risk factors for the presence and severity of WMH.

Conflicting results have been found between numerous studies correlating white-matter abnormalities on CT or MRI and neuropsychological measures. Positive studies have linked white-matter changes on MRI to speed of mental processing (119,129), and global (130,131) as well as specific tests of cognition (131) in normal elders. Boone and associates (132) found a relationship between tests of frontal lobe dysfunction and WMH in normal elders. Similarly, Wolfe and associates (133) found impaired performance on executive tests of frontal system function to be related to multiple subcortical lacunes. Negative results, however, have also been found in several studies of normal elders (122,123,134,135).

Clinicopathologic correlation studies have recently shed further light on the significance of the radiologic findings of WMH. Brun and Englund (136) found white-matter disease, which they characterized as "incomplete infarction," in 60% of patients with Alzheimer's disease, which was moderate to severe in one-third of cases. They hypothesized a vascular mechanism of underlying vascular disease plus systemic hypotension in the pathogenesis. Areas of increased T2 signal in the centrum semiovale (deep hemispheric subcortical white-matter regions) showed nonspecific white-matter pallor on histologic stains without infarction in a study of seven elderly persons without history of stroke (137).

In another postmortem study of seven elderly subjects without neurologic disease, four patterns of white-matter lesions were defined: periventricular rims and caps, punctate lesions, and patches. The MRI appearance was attributed to myelin pallor, and evidence of arteriosclerosis was present in some but not all lesions (138). Leifer and associates (139) found that periventricular "caps" of increased T2 signal on MRI corresponded to normal subependymal glial accumulations. These were often associated with fibrotic small vessels. The study of Fazekas and associates (140) confirmed that periventricular halos and caps were most likely normal. They observed further that patchy and diffuse confluent WMH was likely related to ischemic tissue damage. The postmortem study of Munoz and associates (141) confirmed previous reports that punctate WMH lesions often represent normal dilated perivascular spaces in the elderly. Extensive confluent areas were associated with white-matter pallor, which they speculated was the result of leakage of serum proteins from cerebral vessels, rather than incomplete infarction.

In summary, leuko-araiosis or WMH abnormalities on brain imaging studies in the elderly have been associated with stroke, vascular risk factors, hypertension, hypotension, vascular dementia, late-life depression and Alzheimer's disease. The finding is pathogenetically nonspecific and may be primarily related to normal aging effects, particularly when mild in severity and affecting the regions immediately adjacent to the ventricles. Attention to the particular patterns of radiologic abnormality may be of some clinical significance in sorting out common age-related effects from infarction with secondary cognitive impairment. Correlation of radiologic findings with the history, physical, and mental-status examination, however, is essential if a diagnosis of vascular dementia is to be made with any degree of confidence in elderly patients.

2. *Thyroid disorders*

Thyroid dysfunction is common but often unrecognized in the elderly due to atypical presentations. Hyperthyroidism in the elderly is more likely to produce an apathetic state characterized by lethargy or depression than the euphoric or hyperactive state seen in younger patients. Other features include heart failure, anorexia, unexplained weight loss, and muscle weakness (142).

Hypothyroidism probably ranks as the second most common metabolic cause of dementia after drug toxicity. It has been estimated that 2% of patients over age 65 in hospitals have unsuspected hypothyroidism (143). The usual physical features of hypothyroidism include hoarseness, cold dry skin, alopecia, scarcity of lateral eyebrows, periorbital edema, pasty complexion, and depressed deep tendon reflexes. Mental changes include diminished attention, paranoia, hallucinations, and irritability. Myxedema coma is rare. In elderly patients, the associated dementia may closely mimic Alzheimer's disease (144).

In the elderly, T3 serum levels decline. Effects of non-thyroid disease, starvation, and drugs may alter other thyroid measurements by affecting thyroid hormone binding and conversion of T4 to T3. Diagnosis of hypothyroidism is usually based on the presence of a low T4 level and elevated TSH level, except in the rare instance of pituitary or hypothalamic failure, when TSH is not elevated. Elevation of TSH is the earliest sign of a failing thyroid (143).

Early treatment of hypothyroidism in the elderly is important. Infections are poorly tolerated in elderly hypothyroid patients. Furthermore, the hypometabolic state leads to decreased drug metabolism, making them particularly sensitive to side effects of sedating drugs, which may result in life-threatening coma (143). Treatment should be instituted at half the usual dosage (e.g., equivalent to ½ grain desiccated thyroid) in the elderly because of cardiac intolerance (143,145).

3. *Cobalamin deficiency*

Cobalamin (vitamin B_{12}) deficiency is a common condition in the elderly, estimated to occur in 3–10% of patients over the age of 65 (146). There are two major clinical syndromes associated with the deficiency: megaloblastic anemia and a neurologic disorder referred to as subacute combined degeneration. Neurologic symptoms often begin as paresthesias in the hands and feet due to effects on the peripheral nervous system. Degeneration of posterior columns produces a sensory ataxia and loss of position and proprioception sense, while degeneration of lateral columns, including the corticospinal tracts, produces spastic weakness with hyperreflexia and Babinski signs. Cerebral involvement produces a spectrum of neuropsychiatric manifestations including delirium, paranoia, psychosis, irritability, depression, personality change, and dementia. Clinical features may present in the elderly in atypical fashion with symptoms such as fatigue, apathy, anorexia, lightheadedness, and breathlessness (146,147).

Most cases are the result of malabsorption, including the classic disease pernicious anemia, a disease predominantly seen in the elderly. Pernicious anemia results from intrinsic factor deficiency arising from autoantibodies to the gastric parietal cells. Other common etiologies include diseases of the stomach, gastrectomy, small intestinal disease, and ileal resection.

Neurologic signs may precede hematologic abnormalities. The definitive test for diagnosis of pernicious anemia is the Schilling test; however, collection of a reliable 24-hour urine specimen may be impractical or impossible in a demented elderly patient. Measurement of anti-intrinsic factor antibody may also be done. The radioimmunoassay for cobalamin is very reliable and, along with complete blood count analysis, this test has become routine in the evaluation of treatable causes of dementia in the elderly. There is some evidence that cobalamin measurements may decrease with normal aging (148). This may be related to decreased binding of transcobalamin II. Additional testing is particularly useful in elderly patients with borderline levels of 150–200 pg/ml. Another group of diagnostically challenging patients are those with dementia or other neuropsychiatric symptoms but no evidence of anemia.

Commercially available assays have become available that measure serum levels of methylmalonic acid and homocysteine. These are felt to be reliable measures of functional cobalamin deficiency, since they depend on cobalamin as an essential coenzyme for catabolism. Lindenbaum and coworkers (147) found that elevated levels of methylmalonic acid and homocysteine were highly associated with the presence of neuropsychiatric disorders. Furthermore, the levels decreased along with symptoms after treatment with cobalamin. Normal hematocrit was seen in 85% and normal cell volume in 63% of cases with cobalamin deficiency.

A standard replacement regimen consists of 1000 micrograms by intramuscular injection weekly for 4 weeks followed by monthly maintenance injections of the same dose. The biologic half-life of cobalamin in the liver is 12 months; hence, monthly injections are probably not necessary. A regimen of maintenance injections every 3–4 months may be adequate to prevent symptoms of deficiency once hepatic stores have been replenished (146).

Often dementia does not improve with replacement therapy. This may be due to a number of factors such as incorrect diagnosis of cobalamin deficiency through laboratory error; falsely low cobalamin levels due to folate deficiency, antibiotics, radionuclides, or presence of myeloma; irreversible pathologic damage to the nervous system or to the presence of another disease causing dementia. Low serum cobalamin and elevated methylmalonic levels are encountered in patients with clinically diagnosed Alzheimer's disease (149). In such cases cobalamin deficiency may be a treatable contributing factor to dementia or an unrelated factor in patients with primary degenerative dementia.

4. *Depression*

Depression is a common disorder among the elderly, with an estimated incidence of 2–20% in the community setting (150–152). The prevalence of depression among persons over age 60 appears to be greater than in younger age groups (153). Whereas signs and symptoms of depression often accompany dementia, lack of mental effort and forgetfulness in the patient with a primary depressive disorder may be misdiagnosed as dementia. In the past, this latter clinical presentation has been referred to as *pseudodementia*, a term that may be misleading. Some patients with depression may go on to develop progressive decline in cognition consistent with true dementia, and some may have functional impairments akin to those with dementia. More recently the term *depressive dementia* has been used (154). In these cases, cognitive deficits are expected to respond to antidepressant treatment.

Prolonged reactive depression in the form of grief over loss of loved ones is more common in the elderly than the young. Prior history of depression may be an important clue to depression as a cause of cognitive complaints in an elderly person. Due to increased sensitivity to side effects on cognition and mood, a careful medication history is important to exclude a predisposing or causative factor for depression.

As with dementia, medication side effects may aggravate or precipitate symptoms of depression in the elderly. Such medications include antihypertensive agents (e.g., alphamethyldopa, propranolol), appetite suppressants, indomethacin, corticosteroids, antipsychotics, barbiturates, and other sedatives. Depression in the elderly may present in atypical fashion with predominantly somatic complaints. Depressed mood is not always evident (153).

In patients in whom cognitive impairments progressively worsen over time in a steady and consistent fashion, depression is usually secondary to an organic illness or is a co-existing illness. Depression as a concurrent illness may be present in cases of Parkinson's disease, stroke, Alzheimer's disease, thyroid disease, cobalamin deficiency, Cushing's and Addison's disease, hyperparathyroidism, and other medical illnesses. Focal brain lesions producing depression are seen more commonly in the left frontal region. The presence of aphasia, apraxia, or visuospatial deficits as well as relatively rapid progression are helpful features in the history and mental-status examination that point to the presence of an underlying organic illness.

A number of scales and interview techniques have been developed to assess for depression and dementia in late life (155). The Geriatric Depression Scale is a popular self-rated instrument that has been validated in nondemented elderly outpatients (156). Because loss of insight and aphasia commonly seen in patients with dementia may result in discrepancy between the patient's self-assessment and observations by others of depressive signs and symptoms, diagnosis of depression in this population is problematic. The use of a clinician-rated scale that incorporates observations of others may be more appropriate (157). An example is the Cornell Scale of Depression (158), which was developed and validated in an institutional setting for use with elderly and demented patients.

Five major areas of depressive signs and symptoms are covered, including mood-related signs, behavioral disturbances, physical signs, cyclic functions, and ideational disturbances.

Because depression in demented patients is often transitory and recurrent due to psychological stressors in the environment, nonpharmacologic treatment may be particularly beneficial. Such approaches include environmental changes, exercise and social activities, and provision of companionship. The addition of antidepressant medication may also be of benefit in some patients.

C. Compliance, Drug Toxicity, and Medical Management Issues

The first approach to treatment of dementia is a thorough diagnostic work-up with treatment of the etiology. The second arm of therapy is treatment of concurrent medical and psychiatric illness. In a postmortem case control study of patients with degenerative dementia by Chandra and coworkers (159), preventable or treatable conditions were found to be quite common. These included infections, trauma, nutritional deficiency, chronic skin ulcers, aspiration of foreign body, cataracts, glaucoma, blindness, deafness, Parkinson's disease, and epilepsy.

Because specific treatment to alleviate the underlying etiology of dementia is often not possible, symptomatic treatment constitutes the third and often the predominant arm of therapy, particularly in the primary cerebral degenerations. Target symptoms commonly treated include depression, anxiety, sleep disturbance, agitation, psychosis, and seizures.

Pharmacologic treatment is made difficult by noncompliance due to forgetfulness or refusal to take medication on the part of the patient. Indeed, noncompliance may produce situations of delirium from overdosage or withdrawal effects that can magnify the confusional state of the patient. Caregiver supervision is essential to safe medication. Aids to monitoring compliance include daily-dose medicine boxes and serum drug levels.

The dosage of psychotropic drugs must take into account the special pharmacokinetic effects of aging on absorption, distribution, metabolism, and elimination of drugs. In aging hepatic metabolism of drugs is decreased, renal clearance is decreased, and protein binding may be decreased. As a rule of thumb, decreasing the dosage of psychotropic drugs in the elderly by 50% is often prudent. Dividing dosages into two or three daily doses may lessen side effects by minimizing large rises in blood levels (160).

Due to limited cognitive reserve and concurrent metabolic disturbances or other brain disorders, sensitivity to mental side effects is greater in the elderly as well. Table 7 lists some of the more well tolerated and widely used drugs for symptomatic treatment of dementia symptoms in the elderly. No drug has been approved specifically by the FDA for treatment of aggression and violence; however, limited clinical experience and reports of success have been seen with several drugs listed (161).

Among the antidepressants, tricyclic agents are often poorly tolerated due to anticholinergic side effects such as constipation, bladder retention, blurred vision, and dry mouth. The elderly are particularly susceptible to the central anticholinergic side effects, which may aggravate or precipitate amnesia as well as global confusion (162).

The newer antidepressant drugs including trazodone, and the selective serotonin reuptake inhibitors fluoxetine, sertraline, and paroxetine, appear to be better tolerated and have minimal anticholinergic side effects. Perhaps due to its sedative side effects, trazodone has been reported to be of benefit in control of aggression and agitation as well in patients with dementia (163). Another potential advantage of trazodone is that its pharmacokinetic profile is not significantly affected by aging. Among the selective serotonin reuptake inhibitors, sertraline may be preferable because it has relatively few age-related effects on metabolism and a lowe likelihood for drug–drug interactions (164).

Among the anxiolytics, short-acting benzodiazepines such as lorazepam and oxazepam are probably better tolerated than

Table 7 Symptomatic Medications Used in the Treatment of Dementia in the Elderly

Drug	Target symptom	Side effects	Geriatric daily dosage (mg)
Antidepressants			
Tricyclics		Anticholinergic, confusion, hypotension, arrhythmia	
Nortriptyline	Depression		20–100
Doxepin	Depression		25–150
Fluoxetine	Depression	Anxiety, insomnia, anorexia headaches, dizziness	10–40
Sertraline	Depression	Nausea, diarrhea, tremor, dizziness, insomnia, sedation	25–100
Trazodone	Depression, anxiety, agitation, insomnia	Sedation, hypotension, sexual dysfunction, arrhythmia	50–300
Anxiolytics			
Benzodiazepines	Anxiety, agitation, insomnia	Sedation, habituation, amnesia, confusion, agitation	
Lorazepam			0.5–2
Buspirone	Anxiety, agitation	Dizziness, headaches, insomnia, anxiety	15–60

Hypnotics			
Chloral hydrate	Insomnia	Sedation, habituation, confusion, dizziness, ataxia, nightmares	500–1000
Diphenhydramine	Insomnia	Sedation, confusion, anticholinergic	25–50
Neuroleptics			
Haloperidol	Psychosis, agitation, aggression	Extrapyramidal, anticholinergic, confusion	0.5–3
Loxapine	Psychosis, agitation, aggression	Extrapyramidal, anticholinergic, confusion	5–50
Thioridazine	Psychosis, anxiety, agitation, aggression	Sedation, anticholinergic, hypotension, extrapyramidal, confusion	10–100
Anticonvulsants			
Phenytoin	Seizures	Ataxia, nausea, dizziness, confusion	200–300
Carbamazepine	Seizures, aggression	Ataxia, nausea, dizziness,	400–800
Valproic acid	Seizures	Nausea, hepatic dysfunction, sedation, tremor, hair loss, altered bleeding time	500–2,500
Other			
Propranolol	Aggression	Bradycardia, hypotension, depression	40–320

those with longer half-lives such as diazepam and chlordiazep-oxide. Paradoxical anxiety or rage reactions may occur in elderly demented patients. This class of drugs may be useful, however, particularly in patients intolerant of neuroleptic drugs, in the treatment of mild agitation and anxiety (161,165). Chloral hydrate or diphenhydramine may be used instead of benzodiazepines when the primary target symptom is insomnia.

The use of neuroleptics is ubiquitous in the management of agitation, psychosis, and hallucinosis. These drugs are modestly effective, and no single agent appears to be significantly better than another (166). The choice of drug should take into account the side-effect profile. Extrapyramidal signs, including parkinsonism, akathisia, dystonia, and tardive dyskinesia, are more frequent and severe with high-potency neuroleptics like haloperidol, fluphenazine, and trifluoperazine. Low-potency drugs such as thioridazine or atypical neuroleptics such as clozapine may be more appropriate for patients with parkinsonian features, whereas high-potency drugs should be chosen when sedation, anticholinergic effects, and hypotension need to be minimized.

Psychoactive medications of all types tend to be poorly tolerated by elderly demented patients. If such medications are used, the lowest starting dose should be used, upward titration done very gradually, and the minimal maintenance dose used for as long as symptoms need to be controlled. Once controlled, the drug may be gradually tapered to intermittent use as needed.

It is important to emphasize that successful management of behavioral symptoms in dementia requires attention to behavioral interventions even when pharmacologic intervention is chosen. Behavioral approaches include minimization of inciting or aggravating factors in the environment, adjusting staff behaviors in reaction to the patient, and maximizing positive aspects of behavior (161). Caregivers can help to alleviate stress by providing routine activity in a structured environment, frequent reassurance, and redirection in situations of distress. Physical exercise, music, and social activities such as meals are important.

The comprehensive approach to management of the dementia patient must include integration of a wide range of community support systems and social, mental health, nursing, legal, and other professional services (167). The physician must have a working relationship with others in these areas in order to offer optimal treatment.

State departments of elderly affairs and the local chapter of the Alzheimer's Association offer helpful advice and guidance as well as educational materials regarding access to community services. Family support groups offer educational, discussion, and counseling opportunities for caregivers. Social stimulation may be available for patients in the form of senior centers and adult day-care facilities. Visiting nurses may assist in monitoring and delivering home health care. Homemaker and home health aide services as well as visiting family members and neighbors can assist with activities of daily living and monitor safety in a nonthreatening manner. Nutrition services such as Meals-On-Wheels offer valuable assistance in maintaining a healthy diet. Hospice services are available for the terminally ill.

Assisted-living housing offers some degree of supervision and homemaking support that may be appropriate for some patients with mild dementia. Respite programs in nursing homes and other long-term-care facilities may help to alleviate the burden of daily caregiving and allow a trial experience in the institutional environment. Nursing homes vary according to the levels of care they will deliver. Some offer specialized units for dementia patients. Selection of a nursing home requires a thoughtful evaluation of the options available in the community, which should be undertaken with the assistance of a licensed social worker. Professional advice regarding legal and financial issues, such as providing for payment for long-term-care services and guardianship issues, should be sought from a trusted attorney. Elder-care law is growing as a legal subspecialty to deal with these common, important, and increasingly complex issues.

REFERENCES

1. American Psychiatric Association. Diagnostic and Statistical Manual of Mental Disorders, Third Edition, Revised. Washington, DC: American Psychiatric Association, 1987:103–106.
2. Katzman R. Diagnosis and management of dementia. In: Katzman R, Rowe JW, eds., Principles of Geriatric Neurology, vol. 38. Contemporary Neurology Series. Philadelphia: FA Davis, 1992:170.
3. Clarfield AM. The reversible dementias: Do they reverse? Ann Intern Med 1988;109:476–486.
4. Barclay L. Postmortem examination in dementia. In: Barclay L, ed., Clinical Geriatric Neurology. Philadelphia: Lea & Febiger, 1993:108–109.
5. Boller F, Saxton J. Comparison of criteria for diagnosing Alzheimer's disease in the United States and Europe. In: Wurtman RJ, Corkin S, Growdon JH, Ritter-Walker E, eds., Alzheimer's Disease, vol. 51. Advances in Neurology. New York: Raven Press, 1990:1–5.
6. Henderson AS. Epidemiology of dementia disorders. In: Wurtman RJ, Corkin S, Growdon JH, Ritter-Walker E, eds., Alzheimer's Disease, Vol. 51. Advances in Neurology. New York: Raven Press, 1990:15–25.
7. Mortimer JA. Epidemiology of dementia: Cross-cultural comparisons. In: Wurtman RJ, Corkin S, Growdon JH, Ritter-Walker E, eds., Alzheimer's Disease. Vol. 51. Advances in Neurology. New York: Raven Press, 1990:27–33.
8. Skoog I, Nilsson L, Palmartz B, Andreasson L, Svanborg A. A population-based study of dementia in 85-year-olds. N Engl J Med 1993; 328:153–158.
9. Freemon FR. Evaluation of patients with progressive intellectual deterioration. Arch Neurol 1976; 33:658–659.
10. Beck JC, Benson DF, Scheibel AB, Spar JE, Rubinstein LZ. Dementia in the elderly: The silent epidemic. Ann Intern Med 1982; 97:231–241.
11. Maletta GJ. The concept of "reversible" dementia: How nonreliable terminology may impair effective treatment. J Am Geriatr Soc 1990; 38:136–140.
12. Applegate WB, Blass JP, Williams TF. Instruments for the functional assessment of older patients. N Engl J Med 1990; 322:1207–1214.

13. Chui HC. Dementia: A review emphasizing clinicopathologic correlation and brain behavior relationships. Arch Neurol 1989; 46:806–814.

14. Albert ML, Feldman RG, Willis AL. The "subcortical dementia" of progressive supranuclear palsy. J Neurol Neurosurg Psychiatry 1974; 37:121–130.

15. McHugh PR, Folstein ME. Psychiatric syndromes in Huntington's disease. In: Benson DF, Blumer D, eds., Psychiatric Aspects of Neurologic Disease. New York: Grune and Stratton, 1975:267–285.

16. Cummings JL. Introduction. In: Cummings JL, ed., Subcortical Dementia. New York: Oxford University Press, 1990:3–16.

17. Strub RL, Black FW. The Mental Status Examination in Neurology. Philadelphia: FA Davis, 1993:16–18.

18. Mesulam MM. Patterns in behavioral neuroanatomy: Association areas, the limbic system, and hemispheric specialization. In: Mesulam MM, ed., Principles of Behavioral Neurology, vol. 26. Contemporary Neurology Series. Philadelphia: FA Davis,1985:27–30.

19. Cummings JL, Benson DF. Dementia: A Clinical Approach. Boston: Butterworths,1983.

20. Consensus Conference. Differential diagnosis of dementing diseases. JAMA 1987; 258:3411–3416.

21. Ott BR. Alzheimer's disease. In: Feldmann E, ed., Current Diagnosis in Neurology. Philadelphia: Mosby-Year Book, 1994.

22. Brown P, Cathala F, Castaigne P, Gajdusek C. Creutzfeldt-Jakob Disease: Clinical analysis of a consecutive series of 230 neuropathologically verified cases. Ann Neurol 1986; 20:597–602.

23. Lilly R, Cummings JL, Benson DF, Frankel M. The human Kluver-Bucy syndrome. Neurology 1983; 33:1141–1145.

24. Mendez MF, Selwood A, Mastri AR, Frey WH. Pick's disease versus Alzheimer's disease: A comparison of clinical characteristics. Neurology 1993; 43:289–292.

25. Caselli R, Jack CR. Asymmetric degeneration syndromes: A proposed clinical classification. Arch Neurol 1992; 49:770–780.

26. McKhann G, Drachman D, Folstein M, Price D, Stadlan E. Clinical diagnosis of Alzheimer's disease: Report of the

NINCDS-ADRDA Work Group under the auspices of the Department of Health and Human Services Task Force on Alzheimer's disease. Neurology 1984; 34:939–944.

27. Mesulam MM, Weintraub S. Spectrum of primary progressive aphasia. In: Rossor MN, ed., Unusual Dementias, vol. 1, number 3. Balliere's Clinical Neurology. Philadelphia: Balliere Tindall, 1992:583–609.

28. Mesulam MM. Primary progressive aphasia—Differentiation from Alzheimer's disease. Ann Neurol 1987; 22:533–534.

29. Benson DF, Davis RJ, Snyder BD. Posterior cortical atrophy. Arch Neurol 1988; 45:789–793.

30. Riley DE, Lang AE, Lewis A, Resch L, Ashby P, Hornykiewicz, Black S. Cortical-basal ganglionic degeneration. Neurology 1990; 40:1203–1212.

31. Thompson PD, Marsden CD. Corticobasal degeneration. In: Rossor MN, ed., Unusual Dementias, vol. 1, number 3. Balliere's Clinical Neurology. Philadelphia: Balliere Tindall, 1992:677–686.

32. Neary D. Non-Alzheimer's disease forms of cerebral atrophy. J Neurol Neurosurg Psychiatry 1990; 53:929–931.

33. Gustafson L, Brun A, Passant U. Frontal lobe degeneration of non-Alzheimer type. In:Rossor MN, ed., Unusual Dementias, vol. 1, number 3. Balliere's Clinical Neurology. Philadelphia: Balliere Tindall, 1992:559–582.

34. Neary D, Snowden JS, Mann DMA, Northern B, Goulding PJ, Macdermott N. Frontal lobe dementia and motor neuron disease. J Neurol Neurosurg Psychiatry 1990; 53:23–32.

35. Case records of the Massachusetts General Hospital (Case 16-1986). N Engl J Med 1986; 314:1101–1111.

36. Mayeux R, Chen J, Mirabello E, Marder K, Bell K, Dooneief G, Cote L, Stern Y. An estimate of the incidence of dementia in idiopathic Parkinson's disease. Neurology 1990; 1513–1517.

37. Boller F. Alzheimer's disease and Parkinson's disease: Clinical and pathological associations. In: Reisberg B, ed., Alzheimer's Disease: The Standard Reference. New York: Free Press,1983:295–302.

38. Stern Y, Marder K, Tang MX, Mayeux R. Antecedent clinical features associated with dementia in Parkinson's disease. Neurology 1993; 43:1690–1692.

39. Hughes AJ, Daniel SE, Blankson S, Lees AJ. A clinicopatho-
     logic study of 100 cases of Parkinson's disease. Arch Neurol
     1993; 50:140–148.
40. De la Monte SM, Wells SE, Hedley-Whyte ET, Growdon
     JH. Neuropathological distinction between Parkinson's
     dementia and Parkinson's plus Alzheimer's disease. Ann
     Neurol 1989; 26:309–320.
41. Rajput AH, Rozdilsky B, Rajput A. Alzheimer's disease and
     idiopathic Parkinson's disease coexistence. J Geriatr Psychia-
     try Neurol 1993; 6:170–176.
42. Byrne EJ, Lennox G, Lowe J, Godwin-Austen RB. Diffuse
     Lewy body disease: Clinical features in 15 Cases. J Neurol
     Neurosurg Psychiatry 1989; 52:709–717.
43. Gibb WRG, Esiri MM, Lees AJ. Clinical and pathological
     features of diffuse cortical Lewy body disease (Lewy body
     dementia). Brain 1985; 110:1131–1153.
44. Hansen L, Salmon D, Galasko D, Masliah E, Katzman R,
     DeTeresa R, Thal L, Pay MM, Hofstetter R, Klauber M,
     Rice V, Butters N, Alford MA. The Lewy body variant of
     Alzheimer's disease: A clinical and pathologic entity. Neurol-
     ogy 1990; 40:1–8.
45. Perry RH, Irving D, Blessed G, Perry EK, Smith CJ,
     Fairbairn AF. Senile dementia of Lewy body type: A clini-
     cally and neuropathologically distinct form of Lewy body
     dementia in the elderly. J Neurol Sci 1990; 95(2):119–139.
46. McKeith IG, Perry RH, Fairbairn AF, Jabeen S, Perry EK.
     Operational criteria for senile dementia of Lewy body type.
     Psychol Med 1992; 22:911–922.
47. Byrne EJ, Lennox GG, Godwin-Austen RB, Jefferson D,
     Lowe J, Mayer RJ, Landon M, Doherty FJ. Dementia asso-
     ciated with cortical Lewy bodies: Proposed clinical diagnos-
     tic criteria. Dementia 1991; 2:283–284.
48. Crystal HA, Dickson DW, Lizardi JE, Davies P, Wolfson LI.
     Antemortem diagnosis of diffuse Lewy body disease. Neurol-
     ogy 1990; 40:1523–1528.
49. Steele JC, Richardson JC, Olszewski J. Progressive supra-
     nuclear palsy. Arch Neurol 1964; 10:333–358.
50. Maher ER, Lees AJ. The clinical features and natural history
     of Steele-Richardson- Olszewski syndrome (progressive
     supranuclear palsy). Neurology 1986; 36:1005–1008.

51. Huntington G. On chorea. Medical and Surgical Reporter 1872; 26:317–321.

52. The Huntington's Disease Collaborative Research Group. A novel gene containing a trinucleotide repeat that is expanded and unstable on Huntington's disease chromosomes. Cell 1993; 72:971–983.

53. Ross ME, Jacobson, Dienstag JL, Martin JB. Late-onset Wilson's disease with neurological involvement in the absence of Kayser-Fleischer rings. Ann Neurol 1985; 17:411–413.

54. Konigsmark BW, Weiner LP. The olivopontocerebellar atrophies: A review. Medicine 1970; 19:227–241.

55. Civil RH, Whitehouse PJ, Lanska DJ, Mayeux R. Degenerative dementias. In: Whitehouse PJ, ed., Dementia, vol. 40. Contemporary Neurology Series. Philadelphia: FA Davis, 1993:167–214.

56. Wilkstrom J, Paetau A, Palo J, Sulkava R, Haltia M. Classic amyotrophic lateral sclerosis with dementia. Arch Neurol 1982; 39:681–683.

57. Hudson AJ. Amyotrophic lateral sclerosis and its association with dementia and other neurological disorders: A review. Brain 1981; 104:217–247.

58. Bonduelle M. Amyotrophic lateral sclerosis. In: Vinken PJ, Bruyn GW, eds. Handbook of Clinical Neurology. System Disorders and Atrophies, part 2, vol 22. New York: North-Holland Publishing Company,1975:313–318.

59. Brust JC. Vascular dementia is overdiagnosed. Arch Neurol 1988; 45:799–801.

60. Drachman DA. New criteria for the diagnosis of vascular dementia: Do we know enough yet? Neurology 1993; 43:243–245.

61. O'Brien MD. Vascular dementia is underdiagnosed. Arch Neurol 1988; 45:797–798.

62. Hachinski VC, Iliff LD, Zilhka E, et al. Cerebral blood flow in dementia. Arch Neurol 1975; 32:632–637.

63. Rosen WG, Terry RD, Fuld PF, Katzman R, Peck A. Pathological verification of ischemic score in differentiation of dementias. Ann Neurol 1980; 7:486–488.

64. Fischer P, Jellinger K, Gatterer G, Danielczyk. Prospective neuropathological validation of Hachinski's Ischemic Score in dementias. J Neurol Neurosurg Psychiatry 1991; 54:580–583.

65. Chui HC, Victoroff JI, Margolin D, Jagust W, Shankle R, Katzman R. Criteria for the diagnosis of ischemic vascular dementia proposed by the state of California Alzheimer's Disease Diagnostic and Treatment Centers. Neurology 1992; 42:473–480.

66. Wallin A, Blennow K. Heterogeneity of vascular dementia: Mechanisms and subgroups. J Geriatr Psychiatry Neurol 1993; 6:177–188.

67. Roman GC, Tatemichi TK, Erkinjutti T, et al. Vascular dementia: Diagnostic criteria for research studies. Report of the NINDS-AIREN International Workshop. Neurology 1993; 43:250–260.

68. Ott BR, Saver JL. Unilateral amnesic stroke: Six new cases and a review of the literature. Stroke 1993; 24:1033–1042.

69. Tatemichi TK, Desmond DW, Paik M, Figueroa M, Gropen TI, Stern Y, Sano M, Remien R, Williams JBW, Mohr JP, Mayeux R. Clinical determinants of dementia related to stroke. Ann Neurol 1993; 33:568–575.

70. Liu CK, Miller BL, Cummings JL, Mehringer CM, Goldberg MA, Howng SL, Benson DF. A quantitative MRI study of vascular dementia. Neurology 1992; 42:138–143.

71. Black RS, Barclay LL, Nolan KA, Thaler HT, Hardiman ST, Blass JP. Pentoxifylline in cerebrovascular dementia. J Am Geriatr Soc 1992; 40:237–244.

72. Babikian V, Ropper AH. Binswanger's disease: A review. Stroke 1987; 18:2–12.

73. Hachinski VC, Potter P, Lee D, Merskey H. Leuko-araiosis. Arch Neurol 1987; 44:21–23.

74. Bennett DA, Wilson RS, Gilley DW, Fox JH. Clinical diagnosis of Binswanger's disease. J Neurol Neurosurg Psychiatry 1990; 53:961–965.

75. Pascuzzi RM, Roos KL, Davis TE. Mental status abnormalities in temporal arteritis: A treatable cause of dementia in the elderly. Arth Rheum 1989; 32:1308–1311.

76. Caselli RJ, Hunder GG, Whisnant JP. Neurologic disease in biopsy-proven giant cell (temporal) arteritis. Neurology 1988; 38:352–359.

77. Greenberg SM, Vonsattel JPG, Stakes JW, Gruber M, Finklestein SP. The clinical spectrum of cerebral amyloid angiopathy: Presentations without lobar hemorrhage. Neurology 1993; 43:2073–2079.

78. Case records of the Massachusetts General Hospital (Case 32-1991). N Engl J Med 1991; 325:414–422.

79. Tramont EC. Syphilis in the AIDS era. N Engl J Med 1987; 316:1600–1601.

80. Hart G. Syphilis tests in diagnostic and therapeutic decision making. Ann Intern Med 1986; 104:368–376.

81. Steere A. Lyme disease. N Engl J Med 1989; 321:586–596.

82. Kohler J, Kern U, Kasper J, Rhese-Kupper B, Thoden U. Chronic central nervous system involvement in Lyme borreliosis. Neurology 1988; 38:863–867.

83. Reik L, Burgdorfer W, Donaldson JO. Neurologic abnormalities in Lyme disease without erythema chronicum migrans. Am J Med 1986; 81:73–77.

84. Stockstill MT, Kauffman CA. Comparison of cryptococcal and tuberculous meningitis. Arch Neurol 1983; 40:81–85.

85. Lewis JL, Rabinovich S. The wide spectrum of cryptococcal infections. Am J Med 1972; 53:315–322.

86. Swartz MN. "Chronic meningitis"—Many causes to consider. N Engl J Med 1987; 317:957–959.

87. Townsend JT, Wolinsky JS, Baringer JR, Johnson PC. Acquired toxoplasmosis: A neglected cause of treatable nervous system disease. Arch Neurol 1975; 32:335–343.

88. Scharf D. Neurocysticercosis—238 cases from a California hospital. Arch Neurol 1988; 45:777–780.

89. McCormick GF, Chi-Shing Z, Heiden J. Cysticercosis: Review of 127 cases. Arch Neurol 1982; 39:534–539.

90. Ho DD, Bredesen DE, Vinters HV, Daar ES. The acquired immunodeficiency syndrome (AIDS) dementia complex. Ann Intern Med 1989; 111:400–410.

91. Navia BA, Jordan BD, Price RW. The AIDS dementia complex: I. Clinical features. Ann Neurol 1986; 19:517–524.

92. Sidtis JJ, Gatsonis C, Price RW, et al. Zidovudine treatment of the AIDS dementia complex: Results of a placebo-controlled trial. Ann Neurol 1993; 33:343–349.

93. Krupp LB, Lipton RB, Swerdlow ML, Leeds NE, LLena J. Progressive multifocal leukoencephalopathy: Clinical and radiologic features. Ann Neurol 1985; 17:34–349.

94. Prusiner SB. Genetic and infectious prion diseases. Arch Neurol 1993; 50:1129–1153.

95. Manetto V, Medori R, Cortelli P, et al. Fatal familial insom-

nia: Clinical and pathological study of five new cases. Neurology 1992; 42:312-319.

96. Clinton J, Roberts GW. Prion disease: The essential facts. Int J Geriatr Psychiatry 1992; 7:853-864.

97. Finelli PF. Metachromatic leukodystrophy manifesting as a schizophrenic disorder: Computed tomographic correlation. Ann Neurol 1985; 18:94-95.

98. Herskovitz S, Lipton RB, Lantos G. Neuro-Behçet's disease: CT and clinical correlates. Neurology 1988; 38:1714-1720.

99. Delaney P. Neurologic manifestations in sarcoidosis: Review of the literature, with a report of 23 cases. Ann Intern Med 1977; 87:336-345.

100. Scott TF. Neurosarcoidosis: Progress and clinical aspects. Neurology 1993; 43:8-12.

101. O'Hare JA, Callahan NM, Murnaghan DJ. Dialysis encephalopathy: Clinical electroencephalographic and interventional aspects. Medecine 1983; 62:129-141.

102. Victor M, Adams RD, Collins GH. The Wernicke-Korsakoff Syndrome. Philadelphia: FA Davis,1989.

103. Olsen ME, Chernik NL, Posner JB. Infiltration of the leptomeninges by systemic cancer: A clinical and pathologic study. Arch Neurol 1974; 30:122-137.

104. Chamberlain MC, Sandy AD, Press GA. Leptomeningeal metastasis: A comparison of gadolinium-enhanced MR and contrast-enhanced CT of the brain. Neurology 1990; 40:435-438.

105. Corsellis JAN, Goldberg GJ, Norton AR. "Limbic encephalitis" and its association with carcinoma. Brain 1968; 91:481-496.

106. Case records of the Massachusetts General Hospital (Case 30-1985). N Engl J Med 1985; 313:249-257.

107. Adams RD Fisher CM, Hakim S, Ojemann RG, Sweet WH. Symptomatic occult hydrocephalus with "normal" cerebrospinal fluid pressure. A treatable syndrome. N Engl J Med 1965; 273:117-126.

108. Anderson M. Normal pressure hydrocephalus. Br Med J 1986; 293:837-838.

109. Vanneste J, Augustijn P, Davies GAG, Dirven C, Tan WF. Normal-pressure hydrocephalus: Is cisternography still useful in selecting patients for a shunt? Arch Neurol 1992; 49:366-370.

110. Wikkelso C, Andersson H, Blomstrand C, Lindqvist G. The clinical effect of lumbar puncture in normal pressure hydrocephalus. J Neurol Neurosurg Psychiatry 1982; 45:64–69.

111. Petersen RC, Bahram M, Laws ER. Surgical treatment of idiopathic hydrocephalus in elderly patients. Neurology 1985; 35:307–311.

112. Gallassi R, Morreale A, Montagna P, Sacquegna T, DiSarro R, Lugaresi E. Binswanger's disease and normal-pressure hydrocephalus: Clinical and neuropsychological comparison. Arch Neurol 1991; 48:1156–1159.

113. Richards NG. Ban boxing. Neurology 1984; 34:1485–1486.

114. Ross R, Cole M, Thompson JS, Kim KH. Boxers—computed tomography, EEG, and neurological examination. JAMA 1983; 249:211–213.

115. Coker SB. The diagnosis of childhood neurodegenerative disorders presenting as dementia in adults. Neurology 1991; 41:794–798.

116. Friedland RP. Alzheimer's disease: Clinical features and differential diagnosis. Neurology 1993; 43(suppl 4):S45–S51.

117. Ferrer I, Bella R, Serrano M, et al. Arteriosclerotic leucoencephalopathy in the elderly and its relation to white matter lesions in Binswanger's disease, multi-infarct encephalopathy and Alzheimer's disease. J Neurol Sci. 1990; 98:37–50.

118. Knobler RL. Demyelinating disorders of the aged brain. In: Duckett S, ed. The Pathology of the Aging Human Nervous System. Philadelphia: Lea & Febiger, 1991:317–335.

119. Ylikoski R, Ylikoski A, Erkinjuntti, Sulkava R, Raininko R, Tilvis R. White matter changes in healthy elderly persons correlate with attention and speed of mental processing. Arch Neurol 1993; 50:818–824.

120. van Sweiten JC, van Den Hout JHW, van Ketel BA, et al. Periventricular lesions in the white matter on magnetic resonance imaging in the elderly. A morphometric correlation with arteriosclerosis and dilated perivascular spaces. Brain 1991; 114:761–774.

121. Schmidt R, Fazekas F, Kleinert G, Offenbacher H, Gindl K, Payer F, Freidl W, Niederkon K, Lechner H. Magnetic resonance imaging signal hyperintensities in the deep and subcortical white matter: A comparative study between stroke patients and normal volunteers. Arch Neurol 1992; 49:825–827.

122. Almkvist O, Lars-Olof W, Andersson-Lundman G, Basun H, Backman L. White-matter hyperintensity and neuropsychological functions in dementia and healthy aging. Arch Neurol 1992; 49:626–632.

123. Mirsen TR, Lee DH, Wong CJ, Diaz JF, Fox AJ, Hachinski VC, Merskey H. Clinical correlates of white matter changes on magnetic resonance imaging scans of the brain. Arch Neurol 1991; 48:1015–1021.

124. Leys D, Soetaert G, Petit H, Fauquette A, Pruvo JP, Steinling M. Periventricular and white matter magnetic resonance imaging hyperintensities do not differ between Alzheimer's disease and normal aging. Arch Neurol 1990; 47:524–527.

125. Kozachuk WE, DeCarli C, Schapiro MB, Wagner EE, Rapoport SI, Horwitz B. White matter hyperintensities in dementia of Alzheimer's type and in healthy subjects without cerebrovascular risk factors: A magnetic resonance imaging study. Arch Neurol 1990; 47:1306–1310.

126. Zubenko GS, Sullivan P, Nelson JP, Belle SH, Huff FJ, Wolf GL. Brain imaging abnormalities in mental disorders of late life. Arch Neurol 1990; 47:1107–1111.

127. Coffey C, Figiel GS, Djang WT, Weiner RD. Subcortical hyperintensity on magnetic resonance imaging: A comparison of normal and depressed elderly subjects. Am J Psychiatry 1990; 147:187–189.

128. Sullivan P, Pary R, Telang F, et al. Risk factors for white matter changes detected by magnetic resonance imaging in the elderly. Stroke 1990; 21:1424–1428.

129. Junque C, Pujol J, Vendrell P, Bruna O, Jodar M, Ribas JC, Vinas J, Capdevila A, Marti-vilalta JL. Leuko-araiosis on magnetic resonance imaging and speed of mental processing. Arch Neurol 1990; 47:151–156.

130. Matsubayashi K, Shimada K, Kawamoto A, Ozawa T. Incidental brain lesions on magnetic resonance imaging and neurobehavioral functions in the apparently healthy elderly. Stroke 1992; 23:175–180.

131. van Sweiten JC, Geyskes GG, Derix MMA, Peeck MA, Ramos LMP, van Latum JC, van Gijn J. Hypertension in the elderly is associated with white matter lesions and cognitive decline. Ann Neurol 1991; 30:825–830.

132. Boone KB, Miller BL, Lesser IM, Mehringer CM, Hill-Gutierrez E, Goldberg MA, Berman NG. Neuropsychological correlates of white-matter lesions in healthy elderly subjects: A threshold effect. Arch Neurol 1992; 49:549–554.

133. Wolfe N, Linn R, Babikian VL, Knoefel JE, Albert M. Frontal systems impairments following multiple lacunar infarcts. Arch Neurol 1990; 47:129–132.

134. Tupler LA, Coffey E, Logue P, Djang WT, Fagan SM. Neuropsychological importance of subcortical white matter hyperintensity. Arch Neurol 1992; 49:1248–1252.

135. Hunt AL, Orrison WW, Yeo RA, Haaland KY, Rhyne RL, Garry PJ, Rosenberg GA. Clinical significance of MRI white matter lesions in the elderly. Neurology 1989; 39:1470–1474.

136. Brun A, Englund E. A white matter disorder in dementia of the Alzheimer type: A pathoanatomical study. Ann Neurol 1988; 19:253–262.

137. Grafton ST, Sumi SM, Stimac G, Ellsworth CA, Cheng-Mei S, Nochlin D. Comparison of postmortem magnetic resonance imaging and neuropathologic findings in the cerebral white matter. Arch Neurol 1991; 48:293–298.

138. Chimowitz MI, Estes ML, Furlan AJ, Awad IA. Further observations on the pathology of subcortical lesions identified on magnetic resonance imaging. Arch Neurol 1992; 49:747–752.

139. Leifer D, Buonanno FS, Richardson EP. Clinicopathologic correlations of cranial magnetic resonance imaging of periventricular white matter. Neurology 1990; 40:911–918.

140. Fazekas F, Kleinert R, Offenbacher H, Schmidt R, Kleinert G, Payer F, Radner H, Lechner H. Pathologic correlates of incidental MRI white matter signal hyperintensities. Neurology 1993; 43:1683–1689.

141. Munoz DG, Hastak SH, Harper B, Lee D, Hachinski VC. Pathologic correlates of increased signals of the centrum ovale on magnetic resonance imaging. Arch Neurol 1993; 50:492–497.

142. McGee RR, Whittaker RL, Tullis IF. Apathetic hyperthyroidism: Review of the literature and report of four cases. Ann Intern Med 1959; 50:1418–1432.

143. Blum M. Thyroid function and disease in the elderly. Hosp Practice 1981; Oct:105–116.

144. Swanson JW, Kelly JJ, McConahey WM. Neurologic aspects of thyroid dysfunction. Mayo Clin Proc 1981; 56:504–512.

145. Refetoff S. Thyroid hormone therapy. Symposium on Current Concepts of Thyroid Disease. Med Clin N America 1975; 59(5):1147–1161.
146. Carethers M. Diagnosing vitamin B_{12} deficiency, a common geriatric disorder. Geriatrics 1988; 43:89–112.
147. Lindenbaum J, Healton EB, Savage DG, Brust JCM, Garrett TJ, Podell ER, Marcell PD, Stabler SP, Allen RH. Neuropsychiatric disorders caused by cobalamin deficiency in the absence of anemia or macrocytosis. N Engl J Med 1988; 318:1720–1728.
148. Fairbanks VF, Elveback LR. Tests for pernicious anemia: Serum vitamin B_{12} assay. Mayo Clin Proc 1983; 58:135–137.
149. Kristensen MO, Gulmann NC, Christensen JEJ, Ostergaard K, Rasmussen K. Serum cobalamin and methylmalonic acid in Alzheimer's dementia. Acta Neurol Scand 1993; 87:475–481.
150. Gurland BJ. The comparative frequency of depression in various age groups. J Gerontol 1976; 31:283–292.
151. Weissman MM, Myers JK. Affective disorders in a US urban community: The research diagnostic criteria in an epidemiological survey. Arch Gen Psychiatry 1978; 35:1304–1311.
152. Blazer D. Depression in the elderly. N Engl J Med 1989; 320:164–166.
153. Haggerty JJ, Golden RN, Evans DL, Janowsky DS. Differential diagnosis of pseudodementia in the elderly. Geriatrics 1988; 43:61–74.
154. Emery VO, Oxman TE. Update on the dementia spectrum of depression. Am J Psychiatry 1992; 149:305–317.
155. Thompson LW, Gong V, Haskins E, Gallagher D. Assessment of depression and dementia during the late years. Ann Rev Gerontol Geriatrics 1987; 7:295–324.
156. Yesavage JA, Brink TL. Development and validation of a geriatric depression screening scale: A preliminary report. J Psychiatr Res 1983; 22:165–170.
157. Ott BR, Fogel BS. Measurement of depression in dementia: Self vs clinician rating. Int J Geriatr Psychiatry 1992; 7:899–904.
158. Alexopoulos GS, Abrams RC, Young RC, Shamoian CA. Cornell scale for depression in dementia. Biol Psychiatry 1988; 23:271–284.
159. Chandra V, Bharucha NE, Schoenberg BS. Conditions associated with Alzheimer's disease at death: Case control study. Neurology 1986; 36:209–211.

160. Peabody CA, Whiteford HA, Hollister LE. Antidepressants and the elderly. J Am Geriatr Soc 1986; 34:869–874.

161. Maletta GJ. Treatment of behavioral symptomatology of Alzheimer's disease, with emphasis on aggression: Current clinical approaches. Int Psychogeriatr 1992; 4(suppl 1): 117–130.

162. Davies RK, Tucker GJ, Harrow M, et al. Confusional episodes and antidepressant medication. Am J Psychiatry 1971; 128:127–132.

163. Pinner E, Rich CL. Effects of trazodone on aggressive behavior in seven patients with organic mental disorders. Am J Psychiatry 1988; 145:1295–1296.

164. Preskorn SH. Recent pharmacologic advances in antidepressant therapy for the elderly. Am J Med 1993; 94(suppl 5A): 2–11.

165. Small GW. Psychopharmacological treatment of elderly demented patients. J Clin Psychiatry 1988; 49(suppl 5):8–13.

166. Schneider LS, Pollock VE, Lyness SA. A metaanalysis of controlled trials of neuroleptic treatment in dementia. J Am Geriatr Soc 1990; 38:553–563.

167. Cairl RE, Middleton L. Longterm care in geriatrics: Ancillary services for patients and caregivers. In: Barclay L, ed., Clinical Geriatric Neurology. Philadelphia: Lea & Febiger, 1993:467–474.

3

Acute Confusion and Delirium

David S. Geldmacher
Case Western Reserve University School of Medicine and
University Hospitals of Cleveland
Cleveland, Ohio

I. DEFINITIONS AND TERMINOLOGY

Acute confusional states are transient disturbances of consciousness and behavior that have many causes. These states are of particular importance in the elderly because older individuals are prone to develop confusion rapidly, in response to a wide variety of illness states. The term *confused* is nonspecific and may be applied to any state of clouded consciousness or muddled thought, regardless of cause or duration. The term *acute confusional state* has been popularized to denote a syndrome of impaired attention or arousal with disturbed cognition, and is often used interchangeably with other terms such as *delirium* or *metabolic encephalopathy* (1). Clinically, the syndrome is often described as a "change in mental status."

The American Psychiatric Association has selected *delirium* as the term to refer to this broad grouping of clinical states (DSM-III-R) (2). Delirium, as used to describe the condition accompanying acute confusion, dates to Celsus in the first century A.D., and is derived from the Latin for "out of the furrow" (i.e., off the intended path). Confusion can thus be viewed as a symptom of delirium. Some authors reserve *delirium* for states that include hallucinations or hyperactivity (3) and use *acute confusion* to describe patients with normal or depressed levels of cognition and psychomotor activity. A similar division of delirium syndromes into *activated* and *somnolent* types has been proposed as having clinical utility (4). These distinctions address some of the variability that is the hallmark of confusional states, but these two presentations have overlapping features and may even alternate in the same patient. Furthermore, the clinical symptom patterns in delirium are not specific to any particular causation. Therefore, as a general descriptor, delirium is historically appropriate, concise, and clearly defined. For these reasons, delirium is used in place of its many synonyms throughout this chapter.

II. CLINICAL FEATURES

The DSM-III-R diagnostic criteria for delirium are listed in Table 1 and the ICD-10 (5) criteria are presented in Table 2. These diagnostic schemes provide an overview of the basic elements of the clinical state and underscore the variability of the syndrome. The variable nature and course of the symptoms are perhaps the greatest challenge in diagnosing the source of the confusional symptoms. They reflect not only the many causes of delirium, which are explored later in this chapter, but also interindividual differences that become magnified with the aging process.

A. Behavioral Manifestations

1. *Attentional impairments*
A cardinal feature of delirium is impaired attention (6). Attention is a mental process of specific alertness to internal or external stimuli that involves multiple interrelated component functions. The derangement of attention in delirium may become manifest as impairment in any of its functional components, including vigilance, selectivity, sustainability, capacity, and shifting (7). Although attention as a whole is dysfunctional, vigilance may be heightened, with an accompanying sensitivity to environmental cues. Alternatively, vigilance may

Table 1 DSM-III-R Diagnostic Criteria for Delirium

A. Reduced ability to maintain attention to external stimuli (e.g., questions must be repeated because attention wanders) and to appropriately shift attention to new external stimuli (e.g., perseverates answer to a previous question).

B. Disorganized thinking, as indicated by rambling, irrelevant, or incoherent speech.

C. At least two of the following:
   (1) reduced level of consciousness, e.g., difficulty keeping awake during examination
   (2) perceptual disturbances: misinterpretations, illusions, or hallucinations
   (3) disturbance of sleep/wake cycle with insomnia or daytime sleepiness
   (4) increased or decreased psychomotor activity
   (5) disorientation to time, place, or person
   (6) memory impairment, e.g., inability to learn new material, such as the names of several unrelated objects after 5 minutes, or to remember past events, such as history of current episode of illness

D. Clinical features develop over a short period of time (usually hours to days) and tend to fluctuate over the course of a day.

E. Either (1) or (2):
   (1) evidence from the history, physical examination, or laboratory tests of a specific organic factor (or factors) judged to be etiologically related to the disturbance.
   (2) in the absence of such evidence, an etiologic organic factor can be presumed if the disturbance cannot be accounted for by any nonorganic mental disorder, e.g., manic episode, accounting for agitation and sleep disturbance.

Source: Ref. 3. Reprinted with permission.

be reduced, with a lack of responsiveness to pertinent stimuli (i.e., a familiar face). Selectivity, capacity, and sustainability of attention are invariably impaired (8). Deficits in these components lead to an inability to maintain a focus of mental processes on a task and result in easy distractibility. The in-

Table 2 ICD 10 Diagnostic Criteria for Delirium

For a definite diagnosis, symptoms, mild or severe, should be present in each one of the following areas:

(A) impairment of consciousness and attention (on a continuum from clouding to coma; reduced ability to direct, focus, sustain, and shift attention)

(B) global disturbance of cognition (perceptual distortions, illusions, and hallucinations—most often visual; impairment of abstract thinking and comprehension, with or without transient delusions, but typically with some degree of incoherence; impairment of immediate recall and of recent memory but with relatively intact remote memory; disorientation for time as well as in more severe cases, for place and person)

(C) psychomotor disturbances (hypo-or hyperactivity and unpredictable shifts from one to the other; increased reaction time; increased or decreased flow of speech; enhanced startle reaction)

(D) disturbance of the sleep/wake cycle (insomnia or, in more severe cases, total sleep loss or reversal of the sleep/wake cycle; daytime drowsiness; nocturnal worsening of symptoms; disturbing dreams or nightmares, which may continue as hallucinations after awakening)

(E) emotional disturbances, for example, depression, anxiety or fear, irritability, euphoria, apathy, or wondering perplexity

The onset is usually rapid, the course diurnally fluctuating, and the total duration of the condition less than 6 months. The above clinical picture is so characteristic that a fairly confident diagnosis of delirium can be made even if the underlying cause if not firmly established. In addition to a history of an underlying physical or brain disease, evidence of cerebral dysfunction (such as an abnormal electroencephalogram, usually but not invariably showing a slowing of the background activity) may be required if the diagnosis is in doubt.

Source: Ref. 5. Reprinted with permission.

ability to stop attending to a stimulus or shift attention away from a task contributes to perseverations and intrusionary responses. Because attention is required for the organization of thought and mental activity, disordered attentional processes largely account for the disorganized thinking so characteristic of delirium.

2. *Alterations of arousal*

Arousal is a physiologic condition of alertness or receptiveness to stimulation. Unlike attention, it is not stimulus-specific, but rather represents an underlying physiologic state integral to attentional processing. In delirium, arousal may be suppressed or heightened. Depressed arousal is manifest by reduced consciousness and responsiveness to the environment. Lethargy, stupor, and coma are other clinical descriptors for the low arousal states characteristic of somnolent types of delirium. Agitation, restlessness, and hypervigilance are psychomotor manifestations of increased arousal. Physical signs of increased arousal may also be present in activated forms of delirium, and include tachycardia, hypertension, and diaphoresis. Disordered diurnal patterns of arousal present as aberrant sleep/wake cycles or nighttime confusion with agitation, often referred to as "sun-downing."

3. *Perceptual disturbances*

Alterations of visual perception are common and typically manifest as illusions or misperceptions. Fluctuating awareness may produce incomplete sensory registration of the environment. Also, lapses in attention can lead to the substitution of an inappropriate context for intact perceptions or distortion of perceptual information. As a result, visual inputs may be perceived as large (macropsia), small (micropsia), repeated (palinopsia), or otherwise distorted (dysmorphopsia) (9).

Hallucinations may also occur. The sources of hallucination in delirium are unclear, but confabulation in the presence of impaired perception and disordered thought processes probably contributes. Visual hallucinations are most common. They are influenced by low arousal states and impairments of attention that distort the continuity of time. Such hallucinations can be quite vivid and laden with emotion, and are often frightening. They are usually brief in duration. Tactile hallucinations, especially formication (the sense of crawling skin), are common in agitated delirious states, particularly those induced by alcohol or cocaine withdrawal.

The threatening and directive auditory hallucinations common to acute psychotic breaks are rare in delirium. Delusions are frequently present but are usually incomplete or transitory. Since they are often provoked by environmental cues, inaccurate processing of sensory information probably contributes to their expression.

4. *Disorders of cognition*

Many aspects of cognitive function may be impaired in delirium. Deficits in attention are an important contributor to the cognitive disturbances (10). Language abnormalities include anomia, disordered fluency, alexia, and agraphia. Chedru and Geshwind (11) have suggested agraphia as the most sensitive cognitive indicator of delirium. Breakdowns in the complex sequencing and integrative processes necessary to produce written language suggest that attentional impairments and arousal disturbances contribute to the inability to write. Other integrative tasks such as construction and mental calculation are similarly impaired.

Memory is disturbed, often in a hierarchical pattern. Disorientation to time, and subsequently place, is typical early in the course. Primary or immediate memory also becomes disrupted with worsening delirium, which then reduces learning of new information. The lack of learning constitutes an anterograde amnesia, such that many patients will not recall their delirium. Although poor attention contributes to the memory problems, basic memory processes are also disrupted (10).

B. Presentation and Course

Since delirium can arise from many sources, there is no uniform presentation. Very often there is a prodrome of irritability, restlessness, sleep disturbance, or dysphoria for a day or two prior to the development of overt behavioral disturbances. Fluctuations in functional ability, often with lucid intervals, are common early in the course, and variability in the degree of cognitive dysfunction may continue throughout the illness. When no causes of the delirium are identified and treated, there is progression toward less fluctuation and more severe symptoms. Fluctuating hypoarousal states frequently evolve to coma, but persistent activated (hyperkinetic) delirium may result in sudden cardiovascular collapse. When causative factors are identified and treated appropriately, the prognosis for recovery is generally good (12). Nonetheless, the mortality rate for delirium is 25–33% within one month, roughly twice the rate of similar nondelirious patients (13–15).

Key features in the diagnosis of delirium are the course at onset and the duration. Dementia also presents with confusion as a prominent symptom, but the course is typically long and of gradual onset. Dementia is not associated with alterations in basic arousal. About 5% of Bedford's (13) series of 4000 patients who exhibited delirium on admission remained confused after 6 months (i.e., progressed into dementia). Delirium is a common complicating factor in dementia and should be approached similarly to delirium in the nondemented patient.

III. EPIDEMIOLOGY

Although the point prevalence of delirium in community-dwelling adults aged 18–64 has been calculated to be 0.4%, this figure increases to 1.1% over age 55 (16). Among hospitalized populations the figures are remarkably higher. Delirium has been reported as occurring in up to 17% of all patients on a medical ward at some point during their hospitalization, with over 13% meeting diagnostic criteria on admission (17). A number of risk factors have been identified for the development of delirium (Table 3).

Table 3 Risk Factors for the Development of Delirium

Increased age
Impaired sensory function
Multiple therapeutic drugs (polypharmacy)
Preexisting brain disease
Psychosocial stressors

Among adults, there is a distinct relationship between advancing age and prevalence of delirium (8). Age may be the basis of most other risk factors as well, since sensory dysfunction, multiple medical conditions, and brain disease are all more prevalent in the elderly. In addition, because of diminished cognitive flexibility in older individuals, psychosocial stressors play a greater role among the causes of delirium in the aged population.

IV. PATHOGENESIS

No single anatomical or biochemical disruption accounts for the cognitive and behavioral changes in delirium. Romano and Engel characterized delirium as a disorder of "functional metabolism" of the cerebral cortex (18). They determined that the severity of the delirium correlated with the degree of abnormality of a patient's electroencephalograph (EEG), and that the EEG changes were reversible when the delirium and its underlying factors could be improved. The changes were not, however, diagnostic of the etiologic process in any given patient (18). Given the disturbances of attention observed clinically, and the dynamic, yet nonspecific, EEG changes, dysfunction in cerebral structures responsible for maintaining and directing cortical arousal is likely. These include the mesencephalic reticular formation and nonspecific thalamic nuclei, such as the intralaminar and reticular nuclei. In conjunction with polymodal association cortex, these structures regulate the activation of regions of the cerebral cortex for selective information processing. Functional disruption of this system leads to the characteristic disorganization of sensory processing, thought, and memory in delirium. The pathophysiologic mechanism that leads to the dysfunction in these brain areas is not clear. The activating and polymodal systems may be the most vulnerable to metabolic stressors because they have the most polysynaptic pathways (19). If all synaptic function were compromised to a fixed extent, then those processes requiring the most synapses would be the most vulnerable to cumulative deleterious effects.

Neurotransmitter imbalances, particularly involving acetylcholine (ACh), have been hypothesized as contributing to delirium (1). ACh plays an important regulatory role in cortical arousal, including modulating neuronal response to other transmitters. The ability to induce delirious symptoms with anticholinergic agents (20) supports the hypothesis of an important role for ACh in delirium, as does the reversibility of symptoms with physostigmine, a cholinomimetic cholinesterase inhibitor (21). It is also interesting to note that anticholinergic agents reduce frontal lobe metabolism (22), since frontal polymodal association cortex is vital in maintaining and shifting the focus of attention. The absolute levels of ACh may be less important than the relative balance of cholinergic and other neurotransmitter functions. For instance, in activated delirious states, such as delirium tremens, there is increased central noradrenergic activity relative to ACh (23). Dynamic perturbations and compensations in metabolic and synaptic function may well account for the fluctuating symptoms common in delirium.

V. ETIOLOGY

The list of possible causes of delirium is expansive and grows as new understanding is gained and new therapeutic agents are introduced. Table 4 provides a summary of the major etiologic categories. Some areas will be discussed in more detail, focusing on the common systemic and primary neurologic states.

Table 4 Diagnostic
Groups in Delirium

Systemic
  Toxic
    Drug intoxication
    Drug withdrawal
    Poisons
    Physical agents
  Metabolic
  Nutritional
  Hypoxic/ischemic
  Infectious
  Neoplastic
Primary neurologic
  Vascular
  Trauma
  Seizures
  Degenerative
  Infectious/inflammatory
  Neoplastic

A role for psychosocial stressors in the pathogenesis of delirium has been debated (8). Although psychological distress
clearly acts as a predisposing factor, perhaps through modulation of cortical neurotransmitter systems by limbic system,
delirium must be considered an acute medical illness state.

A. Systemic Causes

1. *Toxic events*

Drug intoxication frequently causes delirium in the general
population and is even more common in the elderly. Nonprescription and illicit agents should not be overlooked, regardless of a patient's age. These include ethanol, cocaine, cough
and cold remedies, and stimulant appetite suppressants. In
addition, many prescription drugs interact with each other and
nonprescription agents. These combinations can trigger de-

lirium at both toxic and therapeutic dosages. The mechanism of drug-induced delirium can be via direct central nervous system effects, as with psychotropic agents, or indirect through the drug's primary systemic action (e.g., antihypertensive-induced hypotension) and side effects (e.g., diuretic-induced hypokalemia). Treatment with multiple drugs increases also the risk for delirium (24). A partial listing of agents associated with drug-induced delirium is shown in Table 5. The most common offenders are drugs with anticho-

Table 5 Some Drug Types Associated with Delirium

Anticholinergic	Antipsychotics
Benztropine	Antihypertensives
Diphenhydramine	Alphamethyldopa
Promethazine	Propranolol
Scopolamine	Antiepileptics
Trihexphenidyl	Phenobarbital
Anti-inflammatory	Phenytoin
ACTH	Valproic acid
Nonsteroidals	Sedatives
Steroids	Alcohol
Antimicrobials	Barbiturates
Amphotericin B	Benzodiazepines
Chloroquine	Sympathomimetics
Isoniazid	Aminophylline
Metronidazole	Appetite suppressants
Quinacrine	Caffeine
Rifamipicin	Decongestants
Antiparkinsonian	Theophylline
Amantadine	Analgesics
Levodopa	Anesthetic gases
Antidepressants (especially amitriptyline)	Opiates
Antarrhythmics	Salicylates
Digoxin	Miscellaneous
Lidocaine	Chlorpropamide
Procainamide	Cimetidine
Quinidine	

Table 6   Metabolic and Nutritional Disorders Associated with
Delirium

Blood sugar	Endocrine
Hyperglycemia	Hyperinsulinism
Hypoglycemia	Hyper/Hypothyroidism
	Hyper/Hypocortisolism
Fluid and electrolytes	Hyper/Hypoparathyroidism
Dehydration	Hypopituitarism
Water intoxication	Paraneoplastic (SIADH)
pH disturbances	Carcinoid
Hyper/Hyponatremia	Porphyria
Hyper/Hypokalemia	Nutritional
Hyper/Hypocalcemia	Vitamin deficiency
Hyper/Hypomagnesemia	Nicotinic acid
System failure	Thiamine
Hepatic	B_{12}
Renal	Folate
Pancreatic	Hypervitaminosis
Pulmonary	Vitamin A
	Vitamin D

linergic effects, narcotic analgesics, and psychotropic agents.
Nonetheless, any drug that affects neurotransmitters, cell
membranes, cellular metabolism, or homeostatic regulation
must be considered as contributory in delirious patients.

Withdrawal and drug rebound effects are also common.
Withdrawal from ethanol is a common cause of delirium in
hospitalized patients, and need not be expressed as frank *delirium tremens*. Confusion and agitation may also occur as
rebound effects after discontinuation of sedative agents, including the commonly prescribed benzodiazepine hypnotics
(e.g., flurazepam).

Subtle occupational intoxications with agents such as
heavy metals, organic solvents, and organophosphates can
cause delirium. Inadvertent dietary poisonings also occur, with
plant products such as alkaloid-rich roots (25) and mush-

rooms. These contributors can be very hard to identify without corroborating history.

2. *Metabolic disorders*

The spectrum of metabolic disorders that can lead to delirium is broad. Some examples are listed in Table 6. Correction of the basic process and its effects, such as hyperinsulinemia with secondary hypoglycemia, is vital to reversing the delirium. There is often a lag between correction of the inciting metabolic derangements and the return of normal cognition. It is also important to recognize that a laboratory's normal reference range may not represent the "normal" or compensated baseline for any given patient, and that delirium can persist if metabolic corrections are inappropriate for the patient. Paraneoplastic effects, such as inappropriate secretion of antidiuretic hormone (SIADH) and carcinoid syndromes, should not be overlooked. Intermittent delirium without identification of typical causes can suggest porphyria.

Wernicke's encephalitis is a primary neurologic expression of a systemic nutritional deficiency (thiamine). It is a delirium accompanied by oculomotor pareses, nystagmus, and ataxia. Even when appropriately treated, residual amnesia may be prominent (Korsakoff's syndrome).

3. *Hypoxic and ischemic states*

Any clinical situation that reduces effective oxygen delivery to the brain may account for delirium. Besides overt hypoxia and hypotension, more subtle factors such as mildly decompensated congestive heart failure may be sufficient to cause a change in the patient's clinical state. Anemia can also be a significant factor. Although not directly hypoxic in nature, ventilatory inadequacy following surgery may lead to CO_2 narcosis in the postoperative phase with concomitant delirium. Slow clearance of inhalant anesthetics can complicate this picture, which would not be evident on isolated measures of oxygenation, such as those provided by noninvasive pulse oximetry.

4. *Infections*

Infections are a common source of delirium in hospitalized
and long-term-care patients. Individuals with preexisting brain
damage are particularly prone to the effects of systemic infections. Urinary tract infections and pneumonia are among the
most frequently recognized causes. The mechanisms of infection as the cause of delirium are not completely understood.
There are frequently secondary effects such as hypoxia in
pneumonia and hepatic encephalopathy in hepatitis, but primary effects such as the so-called septic encephalopathy also
occur (26).

B. Primary Neurologic Causes

1. *Vascular disease*

Delirium can occur acutely with cerebral infarctions or hemorrhages. Most often the confusional symptoms are transient
and represent secondary events such as increased intracranial
pressure. Sometimes, however, delirium can continue beyond
the acute phase. Although strokes in the anterior, middle, or
posterior cerebral artery distributions have been reported as
causing delirium, lesions involving the right middle cerebral
artery (MCA) are particularly likely to cause a persistent state
of confusion that would eventually be characterized as
dementia (27). Such lesions can be difficult to identify early
in the clinical course, because they may be small and not
associated with hemiparesis. The inferior parietal lobule is
frequently involved. This area is one of the polymodal association cortices responsible for attentional processing (27). The
other lesion site commonly associated with persistent delirium
involves the fusiform gyrus at the occipitotemporal junction
and associated deep temporal lobe structures supplied by the
posterior cerebral artery (PCA) (28,29). The delirium is associated with the sudden development of partial to complete
visual loss, and is typically activated in nature. The causative
lesions may be unilateral or bilateral. Unlike the MCA lesions, PCA distribution strokes causing delirium more often

involve the left hemisphere (30). Infarctions in the antero-medial thalamus produce delirium as well (31,32).

Paroxysmal confusion has been attributed to migraine, especially in children (33). The acute period of transient global amnesia may be associated with agitation, anxiety, and confusion suggestive of delirium.

Transient confusional symptoms are often attributed to vertebrobasilar insufficiency. Careful analysis clearly indicates, however, that transient cerebral ischemia should not be considered the cause of confusion or delirium unless supported by appropriate time course and focal neurological signs (34). Fluent aphasias are disorders of cerebrovascular origin that are frequently misdiagnosed as delirium. They may be differentiated on the basis of frequent paraphasic errors, as well as basically preserved attention and arousal mechanisms.

2. *Trauma*

Head trauma can cause severe but transient delirium as well as permanent dementia. Traumatic brain injury (TBI) induces delirium by primary mechanisms, such as functional disruption of the reticular-activating system, or secondary means, including cerebral edema and intracranial hemorrhage. In cases of diffuse axonal injury, one focus of parenchymal disruption is in the dorsolateral midbrain contiguous with the mesencephalic reticular formation (35). This lesion site would account for alterations, which may be transient, in consciousness and arousal following TBI. The excitotoxic mechanisms proposed to be active in TBI would furthermore predispose to the widespread, but transient, cerebral dysfunction characteristic of post-concussive delirium.

3. *Seizures*

Delirium has been associated with seizures. The delirium can arise before, during, and immediately after ictal events. A state of increasing agitation and dysphoria prior to the expression of seizures has been called epileptic delirium (36). Status epilepticus, of the partial complex, absence, and tonic types, causes delirium that may persist for days, or possibly weeks, if unrecognized and therefore not appropriately treated (37,38). Periodic lateralized epileptiform discharges (PLEDs) are EEG phenomena that are also associated with confusional symptoms (39). They commonly accompany other neurologic or systemic causes of delirium. Postictal confusion is a well-recognized clinical state that occasionally meets criteria for delirium. It can be particularly difficult to identify in patients with subtle seizures and persistent postictal cognitive deficits. Finally, antiepileptic drugs can themselves cause confusional symptoms, which may complicate treatment of seizure-related delirium.

4. *Degenerative disorders*

Any of the neurodegenerative disorders that lead to decline in cognitive capabilities may present with delirium. A common scenario is that of individuals who compensate for their deficits in predictable environments and with overlearned behaviors, but who become delirious in unfamiliar surroundings brought on by travel or hospital admission. On careful evaluation, subtle hints of ongoing impairment, such as voluntary constriction of home and community activities or disordered finances, are frequently apparent. Since the underlying degenerative diseases progress slowly, the patient who acutely develops delirium in the presence of dementia still warrants a full evaluation for reversible environmental, metabolic, and neurologic causes for the acute decline in mental state.

5. *Infection and inflammation*

Infections of the brain or meninges frequently lead to confusional symptoms and delirium. *Herpes simplex* encephalitis must be considered in cases of delirium with an acute onset associated with fever, agitation, and prominent memory impairments. Bacterial meningitis also frequently causes delirium and need not be associated with meningeal signs, especially in children and the elderly. Acute postinfectious or idiopathic diffuse demyelinating processes commonly cause significant alterations of arousal and attention that may meet full criteria for the diagnosis of delirium. Exacerbations of multiple sclerosis, even without widespread acute lesions, have been associated with delirium, perhaps because of a susceptibility to cognitive dysfunction entailed by preexisting brain lesions. Other infectious/inflammatory processes such as the vasculitides and intracerebral abscesses may cause confusional symptoms.

6. *Neoplasm*

Rapidly expanding or multifocal tumors frequently cause alterations in basic mental functioning consistent with delirium. They can directly involve neuroanatomical sites vital for attention and arousal, or operate by secondary mechanisms such as cytotoxic edema and obstructive hydrocephalus. Treatment of the neoplasm or its effects can reverse the delirium. A more unusual source of confusional symptoms is the paraneoplastic process known as limbic encephalitis. It is commonly associated with small-cell lung cancer, although other tumors have also been linked to the process (40). The confusional symptoms may predate the diagnosis of carcinoma by years, and evolution to dementia is inevitable if the course is sufficiently long.

VI. SPECIAL CONSIDERATIONS IN THE ELDERLY

The recognition of delirium as an illness state, distinguishable from dementia, with a predilection for the elderly dates back over 100 years. Although estimates of the prevalence of delirium in all hospitalized patients is 15–20%, the rate among the elderly has been reported from that range up to 80% (15). The question of incidence has been evaluated in many ways, but it appears that from one-third to one-half of all acutely ill elderly patients in the hospital will demonstrate delirium during their stay (8). Although those with dementia and previous brain lesions are at risk for developing delirium, up to 25% of cases occur in elderly patients judged to be cognitively intact on admission (15). Delirium is most likely to develop in the first few days of hospitalization for medical patients (41) and in the days immediately following surgery for surgical patients. These temporal patterns represent the combined effects of acute illness, iatrogenic factors, and psychological stressors associated with hospitalization and surgery (41).

A. Clinical Features

Blass and Plum (1) identified three ways in which the course of delirium is different in the elderly. They noted that (1) the onset can be more subtle, as the delirium may gradually blend with previously acquired, fixed limitations in ability; (2) the symptoms are more prominent, even at the same degree of physiologic disturbance; and (3) the course of recovery can be much prolonged. Since delirium occurs in up to 50% of hospital admissions among dementia patients (42), the diagnosis and evaluation of the delirium's course may be further complicated by baseline abnormalities in behavior, cognition, and personality.

Organic causes are identified in 80–95% of all cases of delirium in the elderly (8), but many cases have multiple contributing factors. The rates for specific causes vary widely by study and population. In a neurologic consultation population, the most frequent causes were drug effects, fluid and electrolyte disturbances, and hypoxia/hypotension, with only 8% due to a primary neurologic event such as stroke (43).

B. Systemic Physiologic Changes

The rate of delirium in elderly patients is influenced by a number of physiologic changes that occur in association with healthy aging. There is an increase in the proportion of body fat with advancing age, accompanied by a decrease in lean body mass; there may also be changes in the proportion of intracellular and extracellular fluids (44). A smaller volume of distribution for hydrophilic substances, such as electrolytes, is therefore available. This causes greater fluctuations in response to any given perturbation in the system. The increased proportion of body fat is of importance in that lipid-soluble drugs have a proportionally increased volume of distribution. Such agents are better able to cross into the brain, allowing the body's relatively increased fat content to act as a larger functional reservoir for drugs that alter neuronal function. Both renal excretion and hepatic catabolism diminish with aging, which further contributes to increased susceptibility to inadvertent intoxications and adverse effects from poly-pharmacy among the elderly.

Age-related changes in dynamic homeostatic processes probably also contribute to the higher rate of delirium in the elderly. Lye (44) has proposed three ways in which the time course of the homeostatic response to a metabolic perturbation is altered by the aging process: (1) the amplitude of the response is inappropriate (either exaggerated or insufficient); (2) the initiation of the response is delayed; and (3) the response is prolonged. These alterations may account for the prominence of delirium as a result of physiologic stressors in the elderly (Figure 1).

C. Neurologic Changes

There are changes in basic neuroanatomy, neurochemistry, and brain metabolism associated with the aging process that are also important in the susceptibility of elderly individuals to delirium.

1. *Anatomy*

Brain weight decreases throughout adulthood, by up to 18% of the youthful size through the ninth decade; this can represent over 250 g of lost brain mass in males (1). In comparison, acute surgical resection of 120–150 g of brain tissue produced frank dementia in young adults (45). There are also losses in the richness of dendritic arborization and dendritic spine density with aging (46). Not surprisingly then, synaptic density is reduced within the cortex with advancing age (47). Commensurate with these changes, clinical imaging studies, such as computed tomography (CT), show both cortical atrophy and ventricular enlargement with aging. These

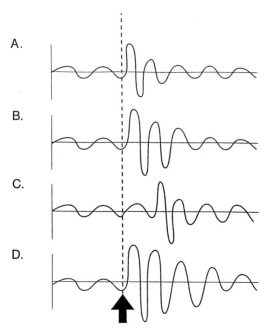

Figure 1 Depiction of typical temporal patterns of normal and impaired homeostasis in the elderly. The horizontal line represents the mean physiologic norma. The arrow and dashed line represent the onset of a metabolic perturbation. (A). Normal or youthful pattern. (B). Exaggerated response. (C). Delayed response. (D). Prolonged response. (Adapted with permission from Ref. 44.)

changes are not obligately associated with underlying dementia, nor can they be used as a sole explanation of delirium.

2. Neurotransmitter changes

The literature on age-related changes in neurotransmitter levels and activity in aging is complex. Because of differences in populations and methods, it is full of contradiction and controversy. Although consensus is limited, there are clearly identified trends toward decline in some aspects of activity for several transmitters. A modest decline in markers of acetyl-choline activity, such as choline acetyltransferase, occurs with aging. This reduction is predominantly located in frontal regions (48). The major intrinsic inhibitory transmitter of the cortex, gamma-aminobutyric acid (GABA) also appears to decline with age (49). There are accompanying losses in the major GABA synthetic enzyme, glutamic acid decarboxylase (48). There are no consistently reported changes in human cerebral cortex and variable results in subcortical structures for the monoaminergic transmitters dopamine, norepinephrine, and serotonin (48). Given the important modulatory roles of acetylcholine in cortical arousal and GABA in inhibition, it is plausible that age-related changes in those systems play a role in the prevalence of delirium among the elderly.

3. *Cerebral blood flow and metabolism*

Cerebral blood flow (CBF) has been reported to decline with age (50), though there has been disagreement. While CBF to the white matter is preserved with age, gray matter CBF and metabolism show clear declines in older age groups (51). In addition, cerebral autoregulation becomes impaired over the age of 60 (52). Neurotransmitter activity, particularly ACh synthesis, is dramatically affected by otherwise metabolically insignificant degrees of hypoxia (1). Age-related changes in CBF, metabolism, and autoregulation would therefore cumulatively leave elderly patients with less functional cerebral metabolic reserve to maintain normal neuronal communication during systemic insults. This increases the likelihood of developing delirium in response to small physiologic derangements.

D. Diagnostic Approach in the Elderly

Because of its high mortality and the seriousness of the disorders that lead to it, the diagnosis and initial management of delirium require an aggressive approach. A careful history from collateral informants with emphasis on possible intoxicants and exposures, as well as any recent changes in medication, is the first step. A thorough general physical examination looking for indications of infection, pain, and metabolic dysfunction (e.g., fever, pallor, dehydration) is required. The neurologic examination should be focused toward the detection of focal or lateralized central nervous system (CNS) signs and deficits of discrete cognitive functions, such as language. The absence of localizing CNS signs usually suggests a systemic cause. The presence of focal neurologic signs, however, does not necessarily indicate an acute structural brain lesion. Through a phenomenon known as *unmasking*, previously compensated CNS dysfunction can become apparent in the face of metabolic stressors. Also, nonketotic hyperglycemia is a condition common in the elderly that often presents with completely reversible, novel, and often mixed bilateral focal signs on neurologic exam.

Initial laboratory screening studies should include complete blood counts, looking for markers of systemic illness such as leukocytosis and anemia. Major and minor electrolytes (Na, K, Cl, CO_2, Ca, Mg, PO_4), blood urea nitrogen (BUN), and creatinine will provide some sense of homeostatic balance and renal function. Blood glucose concentration should always be screened, preferably first with a rapid ("finger-stick") determination. Liver function tests are also necessary. Toxicologic screens are necessary (in both blood and urine) when the history is either incomplete or suggestive of drug intoxication. Blood levels of any therapeutic agents the patient has had prescribed are useful when available. Urinalysis should be routinely performed. Arterial blood gas assessment is usually indicated as well, and should be considered requisite in postanesthesia cases of delirium. If arterial sampling is unavailable, digital pulse oximetry is the minimum required. Other laboratory measures may also be useful if screening reveals no obvious cause for the delirium. These include thyroid studies, vitamin B_{12} levels, sedimentation rate, acute phase reactants, and autoimmune screens such as antinuclear antibodies.

Chest x-ray to screen for subclinical heart failure, pneumonia, or neoplasm may be useful in diagnosis. Electrocardiography should also be performed to identify possible sources for cerebral or systemic hypoperfusion.

Therapeutic trials of oxygen, glucose (only after thiamine administration and screening for hyperglycemia), and the opiate-reversing agent naloxone (Narcan) may be of value in some cases based on history and physical findings. Flumazenil (Mazicon) is a benzodiazepine antagonist, but is *not* indicated as a diagnostic agent in delirium of unknown cause, because of the risk for inducing acute withdrawal complications such as seizures or increased intracranial pressure.

CT or magnetic resonance imaging (MRI) of the head should be performed emergently in any patient with focal neurologic signs, a history of trauma, or no available history, in order to screen for immediately life-threatening events such as subarachnoid or epidural hemorrhage. In cases without focal signs, CT or MRI remains indicated, but not necessarily on an emergent basis. Lumbar puncture should be accomplished after cranial imaging if there are signs of infection without obvious source. Electroencephalography can be a useful adjunct to diagnosis, in that it is the only bedside diagnostic procedure that demonstrates cerebral function, rather than structure.

E. Management of the Delirious Elderly Patient

Management of the patient with delirium requires multiple simultaneous approaches. Obviously, the identification and treatment of any causative factor must be undertaken. It is important to recognize, however, that there are frequently several concurrent processes contributing to the delirium and that the identification of one factor should not obviate the need to look for others. Possible contributory drugs, especially those with anticholinergic or psychotropic properties, should be discontinued or tapered. Supportive care is required while the search for, and treatment of, the primary causes is under way. This usually involves maintenance of respiration, hydration, and nutrition, with optimization of the patient's cardiopulmonary status. Management of abnormal and disruptive behaviors is also required, especially in activated forms of delirium. In all cases, use of physical restraints and psychotropic drugs (i.e., chemical restraints) should be minimized. This approach requires a very active role for nursing care and may exceed the available nursing resources.

If behavioral and other nonpharmacologic interventions prove inadequate, medications are required. Neuroleptics are the first choice for most new cases of delirium with hyperkinetic features, unless antipsychotic drugs are implicated as a cause. Haloperidol (Haldol) 0.5–2 mg IM or PO is often sufficient to reduce delusions and agitation to manageable levels. The acutely ill elderly often respond quite well to such small doses, without excessive sedation. The low dosages minimize acute side effects and the doses may be repeated as needed. A further reason for advocating the use of neuroleptics is that they produce no significant respiratory suppression at usual doses. This drug class, however, is not without its drawbacks. Neuroleptic agents lower the seizure threshold in experimental models, but the clinical significance of this finding in patients without preexisting seizure disorders is low. Extrapyramidal side effects also occur. Nonetheless, they are usually not a detriment to the patient during an acute delirium. Nor are the long-term neuroleptic-related tardive side effects of major concern in the typical time-limited low-dose treatment of delirium. The risk of neuroleptic malignant syndrome, which in itself causes delirium and can be life-threatening, is a more serious disadvantage to their use.

The benzodiazepine class of anxiolytic sedatives is frequently used in the treatment of delirium, but significant caution is warranted. Benzodiazepines, especially short-acting agents with a minimum of active metabolites such as lorazepam (Ativan), are the agents of choice in treating drug and alcohol withdrawal states. They can also be of value in other dangerous hyperautonomic delirious states such as thyroid storm and hypertensive crisis with encephalopathy. It is important to recognize, however, that they are primarily anxiolytics with sedative side effects (rather than primary sedatives), and that their use should be minimized unless anxiety is prominent. Members of this class of medication produce respiratory suppression and may reduce cardiac output at clinically sedating doses. Because of long half-lives and active metabolites, repeated doses frequently lead to late cumulative effects that can be difficult to identify and manage. Their use is further complicated by a high incidence of paradoxical hyperkinetic responses and rebound/withdrawal agitation. Benzodiazepines also place the patient at risk for seizures as treatment is withdrawn

Regulation of sleep/wake cycles can be achieved with behavioral measures such as bright/dark lighting schedules. Should pharmacologic intervention become necessary, pure soporifics, such as choral hydrate 250–1000 mg PO can be useful in short courses.

VII. CONCLUSION

Delirium is among the most common and most serious acute neurologic disorders of the elderly. Despite the traditional incorporation of delirium in the spectrum of psychiatric diagnoses, the syndrome usually represents an acute medical illness state with significant risk for mortality and intercurrent morbidity. Its commonness and variability are reflections of many causes and contributors. Nonetheless, most cases of delirium in elderly patients are completely reversible. When a strategy of intense supportive care, coupled with an aggressive diagnostic approach, is adopted, a favorable outcome can be achieved for many patients.

REFERENCES

1. Blass JP, Plum F. Metabolic encephalopathies in older adults. In Katzman R, Terry R. The Neurology of Aging. Philadelphia: F A Davis, 1983:189–220.

2. American Psychiatric Association. Diagnostic and Statistical
    Manual of Mental Disorders, Third Edition, revised. Washing-
    ton DC: American Psychiatric Association, 1987:p 103.
3. Mori E, Yamadori A. Acute confusional state and acute agi-
    tated delirium: Occurrence after infarction in the right middle
    cerebral artery territory. Arch Neurol 1987; 1139–1143.
4. Ross CA, Peyser CE, Shapiro I, Folstein MF. Delirium:
    phenomenologic and etiologic subtypes. Internat Psychogeriatr
    1991; 3:135–147.
5. World Health Organization. ICD-10, Diagnostic Criteria for
    Delirium, Geneva, Switzerland (in press).
6. Geschwind N. Disorders of attention: Frontier in neuro-
    psychology. Philos Trans R Soc London 1982; 298:173–185.
7. Hernández-Peón R. Neurophysiologic aspects of attention. In:
    Fredericks JAM, ed., Handbook of Clinical Neurology, vol. 3.
    Amsterdam: Elsevier, 1969:155–185.
8. Lipowski ZJ. Transient cognitive disorders (delirium, acute
    confusional states) in the elderly. Am J Psychiatry 1983;
    140:1426–1436.
9. Willanger R, Klee A. Metamorphopsia and other visual distur-
    bances with latency occurring in patients with diffuse cerebral
    lesions. Acta Neurol Scand 1966; 42:1–8.
10. Chedru F, Geshwind N. Disorders of higher cortical function
    in confusional states. Cortex 1972; 8:395–411.
11. Chedru F, Geshwind N. Writing disturbances in acute confu-
    sional states. Neuropsychologia 1972; 10:343–353.
12. Weddington WW. The mortality of delirium: An under-
    appreciated problem? Psychosomatics 1982; 23:1232–1235.
13. Bedford PD. General medical aspects of confusional states in
    elderly people. Br Med J, 1959; 2:185–188.
14. Simon A, Cahan RB. The acute brain syndrome in geriatric
    patients. Psychiatric Research Reports 1963; 16:8–21.
15. Hodkinson HM. Mental impairment in the elderly. J R Coll
    Physicians (London) 1973; 7:305–317.
16. Folstein MF, Bassett SS, Romanoski AJ, et al. The epidemiol-
    ogy of delirium in the community for the Eastern Baltimore
    Mental Health Survey. Int Psychogeriatr 1991; 3:169–176.
17. Cameron D, Thomas R, Mulvihil M, et al. Delirium: A test of
    the Diagnostic and Statistical Manual III criteria on medical
    inpatients. J Am Geriatr Soc 1987; 35:1007–1010.

18. Romano J, Engel GL. Delirium: A syndrome of cerebral insufficiency. J Chronic Dis 1959; 9(3):260–277.
19. Mendez, MF. Acute Confusional States. In: Bradley WG, Daroff RB, Fenichel GM, Marsden, CD, eds. Principles of Diagnosis and Management, vol. 1. Stoneham, MA: Butterworth-Heinemann, 1991:31–42.
20. Itil T, Fink M. Anticholinergic drug-induces delirium: Experimental modification, quantitative EEG and behavioral correlations. J Nerv Ment Dis 1966; 143:492–507.
21. Lipowski ZJ. Delirium: Acute Brain Failure in Man. Springfield, IL: Charles C. Thomas, 1980.
22. Honer WG, Prohovnik I, Smith G, et al. Scopolamine reduces frontal cortex perfusion. J Cereb Blood Flow Metab 1988; 8:635–641.
23. Hawley RJ, Major LF, Schulman EA, et al. CSF levels of norephinephrine during alcohol withdrawal. Arch Neurol 1981; 38:29–292.
24. Vestal RE. Drug use in the elderly: A review of problems and special considerations. Drugs 1978; 16:358–382.
25. Hanna JP, Schmidley JW, Braselton WE. Datura delirium. Clin Neuropharmacol 1992; 15:109–113.
26. Hasselgren PO, Fischer JE. Septic encephalopathy: Etiology and management. Intensive Care Med 1986; 12:13–16.
27. Mesulam MM, Waxman SG, Geschwind N, Sabin TD. Acute confusional states with right middle cerebral artery infarctions. J Neurol Neurosurg Psychiatry 1976; 39:84–89.
28. Horenstein S, Chamberlain W, Conomy J. Infarction of the fusiform and calcarine regions: agitated delirium and hemianopia. Trans Am Neurol Assoc 1967; 92:85–89.
29. Medina JL, Rubino FA, Ross E. Agitated delirium caused by infarctions of the hippocampal formation and fusiform and lingual gyri: A case report. Neurology 1974; 24:1181–1183.
30. Devinsky O, Bear D, Volpe BT. Confusional states following posterior cerebral artery infarction. Arch Neurol 1988; 45:160–163.
31. Graff-Radford NR, Eslinger PJ, Damasio AR, Yamada T. Nonhemorrhagic infarction of the thalamus: Behavioral, anatomic, and physiological correlates. Neurology 1984; 34:14–23.
32. Santamaria J, Blessa R, Tolosa ES. Confusional syndrome in thalamic stroke. Neurology 1984; 34:1618.

33. Ehyai A, Fenichel GM. The natural history of acute confusional migraine. Arch Neurol 1978; 35:368–369.
34. Futty DE, Conneally PM, Dyken ML, et al. Cooperative study of hospital frequency and character of transient ischemic attacks. V. symptom analysis. JAMA 1977; 238:2386–2390.
35. Adams JH, Graham DI, Murray LS, Scott G. Diffuse axonal injury due to nonmissile head injury in humans: An analysis of 45 cases. Ann Neurol 1982; 12:557–563.
36. Betts TA. Depression, anxiety and epilepsy. In: Reynalds EH, Trimble MR, eds., Epilepsy and Psychiatry. London: Churchill Livingstone, 1983:60–71.
37. Ellis JM, Lee SI. Acute prolonged confusion in later life as an ictal state. Epilepsia 1978; 19:119–128.
38. Somerville ER, Bruni J. Tonic status epilepticus presenting as confusional state. Ann Neurol 1983; 13:549–551.
39. Terzano MG, Parrino L, Mazzucchi A, Moretti G. Confusional states with periodic lateralized epileptiform discharges (PLED's) Epilepsia 1986; 27:446–457.
40. Spence AM, Sumi SM, Ruff R. Paraneoplastic syndromes that involve the nervous system. Curr Probl Cancer 1983; 8:1–43.
41. Foreman M. Confusion in the hospitalized elderly: Incidence, onset, and associated factors. Research in Nursing and Health 1989; 12:21–29
42. Tueth MJ, Cheong JA. Delirium: Diagnosis and treatment in the older patient. Geriatrics 1993; 48:75–80.
43. Moses H, Kaden I. Neurologic consultations in a general hospital: Spectrum of iatrogenic disease. Am J Med 1986; 81:955–958.
44. Lye M. Disturbances of homeostasis. In: Brocklehurst JC, Tallis RC, Fillit HM, eds.. Textbook of Geriatric Medicine and Gerontology. Edinburgh: Churchill Livingstone; 1992:675–693.
45. Chapmann LF, Wolff HG. The cerebral hemispheres and the highest integrative functions of man. Arch Neurol 1959; 1:357–360.
46. Katzman R, Terry R. Normal aging of the nervous system. In: Katzman R, Terry R., eds., The Neurology of Aging. Philadelphia: FA Davis, 1983:15–49.
47. Huttenlocher PR. Synaptic density in human frontal cortex-

developmental changes and effects of aging. Brain Res 1979; 163:195–205.

48. Spokes EGS. An analysis of factors influencing measurements of dopamine, noradrenaline, glutamate decarboxylase, and choline acetylase in human post-mortem brain tissue. Brain 1979; 102:333–346.

49. Spokes EGS, Garrett NJ, Rossor MN, Iversen LL. Distribution of GABA in post-mortem brain tissue from control, psychotic, and Huntington's chorea subjects. J. Neurol Sci 1980; 48:303–313.

50. Zemcov A, Barclay L, and Blass JP. Regional decline of cerebral blood flow with age in cognitively intact subjects. Neurobiol Aging 1984; 5:1–6.

51. Lenzi GL, Frackowiak RS, Jones T, et al. $CMRO_2$ and CBF by the oxygen-15 inhalation technique: Results in normal volunteers and cerebrovascular patients. Eur Neurol 1981;20:285–290.

52. Shinohara Y, Takagi S, Kobatake K. Effect of aging on CBF and autoregulation in normal subjects and CVD patients. Monogr Neural Sci 1984; 11:210–215.

4

Gait Disturbances and Cervical Spondylosis

Rodger J. Elble
Center for Alzheimer Disease and Related Disorders
Southern Illinois University School of Medicine
Springfield, Illinois

Symmetrical gait disturbances are collectively a very common form of disability in older people and are frequently a source of diagnostic confusion. Bilateral cerebral and rostral brainstem disease and high cervical myelopathy are the most common causes and are reviewed in this chapter.

I. THE BASIC ANATOMY AND PHYSIOLOGY OF POSTURE AND LOCOMOTION

Normal locomotion requires the proper control and integration of limb movement, posture, and balance. Studies of spinalized mammalian quadrupeds have shown that normal locomotion emerges from spinal pattern generators that are under the control of supraspinal motor centers (1,2). The neuronal networks that comprise these spinal pattern generators are poorly defined. The locomotor spinal pattern generators are controlled by two parallel motor pathways, one involving the cerebellum and the other involving mesencephalic and diencephalic nuclei (Figure 1). Observations in humans (3), laboratory primates, (4) and cats (5) suggest that reticulospinal and vestibulospinal pathways are crucially important in the activation of spinal locomotor networks.

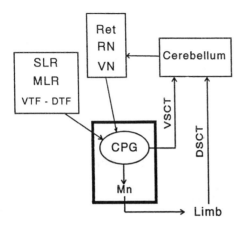

Figure 1 Schematic diagram of the supraspinal control of the spinal locomotor central pattern generator (CPG). Ret = lateral pontomedullary reticular nuclei, RN = red nucleus, VN = lateral vestibular nucleus, SLR = subthalamic locomotor region, MLR = mesencephalic locomotor region, VTF = ventral tegmental field, DTF = dorsal tegmental field, Mn = motoneurons, VSCT = ventral spinocerebellar tract, and DSCT = dorsal spinocerebellar tract.

The cerebellum controls locomotor rhythmicity and phasic coordination of body segments through rubrospinal, lateral pontomedullary reticulospinal, and vestibulospinal (Dieter's nucleus) pathways (6–8). The ventral spinocerebellar pathway carries output from the spinal pattern generators to the cerebellum, and the dorsal spinocerebellar pathway carries sensory feedback from the periphery (Figure 1). With this information, the cerebellum assists in the production of motor activity that is compatible with environmental and musculoskeletal constraints. Damage to the cerebellum or its afferent and efferent pathways causes impaired balance, limb coordination, and rhythmicity of gait. The cerebellar gait is wide based, reeling and lunging because the timing and magnitude of limb movement are incorrect and highly variable from step to step.

The subthalamic locomotor region (SLR), mesencephalic locomotor region (MLR), ventral tegmental field (VTF), and dorsal tegmental field (DTF) are four anatomical loci in the brainstem and diencephalon that appear to participate in the initiation of gait and control of postural tonus (8,9) (Figure 2). The SLR is a poorly defined locus in the lateral hypothalamic area (10). Stimulation of this site in intact cats produces stooped, stealthy locomotion, as in the pursuit of prey. The MLR is in the region of the cholinergic pedunculopontine nucleus of the dorsolateral midbrain, but it is unclear whether the MLR consists of these cholinergic neurons, neighboring noncholinergic neurons, or both. The neighboring noncholinergic neurons have extensive connections with the ipsilateral basal ganglia (11–14). Brief stimulation of the MLR induces rapid walking, followed by running. GABAergic inputs to the MLR from the substantia nigra pars reticulata (SNr) and the globus pallidus interna (GPi) have an inhibitory influence on locomotion (14). Parkinson's disease produces abnormally increased neuronal activity in SNr and GPi that may impair

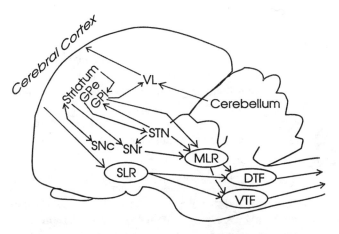

Figure 2   The MLR, SLR, DTF, and VTF are integrated with the basal ganglia, cerebral cortex, and cerebellum. GPe = globus pallidus externa, GPi = globus pallidus interna, SNc = substantia nigra pars compacta, SNr = substantia nigra pars reticulata, STN = subthalamic nucleus, and VL = ventrolateral thalamus.

locomotion through inhibition of the MLR (15). The MLR receives excitatory glutaminergic inputs from the subthalamus and the motor cortex that promote locomotion (14,16).

The MLR and SLR project to the VTF and DTF (8). The VTF corresponds to the rostral nucleus raphe magnus of the caudal midline pons. Stimulation of the VTF increases antigravity muscle tone. The DTF corresponds to the caudal nucleus raphe centralis superior of the caudal midline pons. Stimulation of the DTF decreases antigravity muscle tone. Cholinergic agonists, excitatory amino acid agonists, GABAergic antagonists, and substance P facilitate locomotion when injected into the VTF (17) and inhibit locomotion when injected into the DTF. Therefore, DTF and VTF are probably involved in control of postural tonus during locomotion (7). This integration of MLR, SLR, VTF, and DTF underlies the critically important integration of posture, balance, and movement in the production of normal locomotion.

The motor cortex and other cortical areas influence locomotion by direct projections to the MLR and SLR (6,18) and by indirect projections through the basal ganglia (Figure 2). The sensorimotor cortex also participates with the cerebellum in the control of locomotor rhythmicity and limb coordination. The deep cerebellar nuclei project to the contralateral motor cortex via the ventrolateral thalamus, and the motor cortex projects to the contralateral cerebellum via the pontine and olivary nuclei. Thus, the cerebellum is ideally suited for the feedforward control of posture and movement.

II. BEHAVIORAL STUDIES OF POSTURAL CONTROL

Postural control and balance are requirements of normal locomotion. An investigation of impaired locomotion must therefore include a careful assessment of posture and balance. The line of gravity during normal erect posture is 3–8 cm anterior to the ankles and fluctuates within narrow limits (Figure 3) (19,20). These fluctuations, called postural sway, are reflected in the center of pressure of the feet, as measured

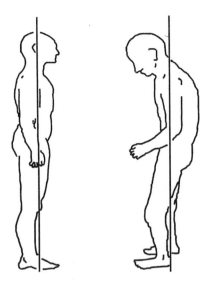

Figure 3 The line of gravity for a normal young adult is 3–8 cm anterior to the ankles. The line of gravity may shift posteriorly with the development of thoracolumbar kyphosis and posterior pelvic rotation.

with floor-mounted force plates, but postural sway is measured more directly with accelerometers, potentiometers, and photogrammetric techniques. It is increased in people over age 65, but this increase is largely due to a variety of pathological conditions, not to age per se (21–23).

Somatosensory (muscle, joint, and cutaneous receptors), vestibular, and visual inputs to the central nervous system are utilized in the control of posture and balance. These sensory inputs are sufficiently redundant that the loss of one is compatible with stable upright stance and routine locomotor tasks. However, the loss or distortion of two sensory modalities usually results in excessive postural sway and loss of balance (24–26). Older people frequently have impaired vision, vestibular function, and somatosensation in the legs and feet. Seemingly healthy older people, compared with young adults, are more likely to fall when subjected to distorted or conflict-ing sensory inputs (27). Thus, the aged nervous system and musculoskeletal system have reduced capacity to deal with novel, conflicting, or greatly reduced sensory feedback.

Modest mechanical perturbations of upright stance (e.g., a sharp nudge to the sternum) produce fairly stereotyped ki-nematic and electromyographic reactions (28–30). Muscles in the legs respond through monosynaptic reflexes to such per-turbations within 45–50 msec, but these short-latency reflexes contribute little to postural control (28). Longer-latency soma-tosensory reflexes at approximately 100 msec produce muscle contractions that are capable of counteracting the effects of postural perturbation and are therefore called functional stretch reflexes. Functional stretch reflexes involve transcortical neu-ral loops and are modulated by vestibular and visual sensory feedback (28,31–37). The coordination of functional stretch reflexes among muscles throughout the limbs and trunk occurs so quickly (within 10–12 msec) and stereotypically that their synergistic activation must be preprogrammed by the nervous system. The functional stretch reflex response to postural per-turbation is delayed or reduced in many older people, and the responses of individual muscles are not as tightly coupled as in younger controls (38,39). Hence, many older people exhibit greater variability in their postural responses to perturbations. Muscle weakness, musculoskeletal deformities, and arthritis impede the ability of older people to respond to postural per-turbations.

Small postural perturbations are counteracted by motion of the body about the ankles. This so-called ankle strategy consists of a distal-to-proximal activation of the ventral or dorsal musculature of the lower extremities and torso in re-sponse to a posterior or anterior perturbation of the body, respectively. The body behaves like a flexible inverted pen-dulum as the functional stretch reflexes produce a counteract-ing torque about the ankles. The ankle strategy of postural control is not adequate for strong postural perturbations and is also insufficient when the base of support is reduced (e.g., on a balance beam) or insecure (e.g., on a slippery surface). The postural response to these more taxing conditions typically includes hip flexion or extension and appropriate arm motion so as to keep the body's center of mass over the base of support provided by the two feet. Of course, perturbations can be so strong that a step or other complex body movement is required to establish an entirely new base of support. These so-called rescue responses require strength and agility that may easily exceed the neurological and musculoskeletal capabilities of older people.

Thus far, only passive, externally imposed postural perturbations have been considered in this review. Self-induced postural perturbations produced by normal volitional movements are a more common threat to postural stability. For example, lifting a heavy suitcase overhead onto a shelf might easily displace the net body-load center of mass beyond the base of support. However, this potentially destabilizing displacement of the center of mass is anticipated by the nervous system, based on prior experience, and a coordinated anticipatory postural response is initiated before the upper extremities begin to move. Thus, postural control and movement are integrated into a coordinated motor act so as to ensure postural stability. The nervous system does not simply react passively (i.e., via reflex) to self-induced postural disturbances. For example, Belen'kii and coworkers (40) found that muscles of the lower extremities and trunk were activated or inactivated 40–50 msec before the deltoid when normal subjects raised an upper extremity during quiet stance. Bouisset and Zattara (41,42) showed that this preparatory muscle activity produced anticipatory accelerations of the body that counteracted the destabilizing accelerations caused by raising the upper extremities (43,44).

Anticipatory postural activity and movement are poorly integrated or delayed in some older people (45,46). Frontal lobe (47) and cerebellar lesions (47,48) delay or reduce the anticipatory activation of postural muscles when the upper extremities are raised. Gurfinkel and El'ner (49) studied 225 patients with frontal lobe lesions and concluded that damage to the supplementary motor cortex suppressed or delayed anticipatory postural activity. The supplementary motor cortex is a major site of projection from the basal ganglia through the ventrolateral thalamus. Therefore, one might predict that basal ganglia pathology would produce similar abnormalities in anticipatory postural activity. Dick and coworkers (50) found that preparatory postural activity in Parkinson's patients was reduced in amplitude but not delayed.

In summary, normal balance and posture are not maintained solely by passive reflex responses to somatosensory, visual, and vestibular inputs to the nervous system. Normal balance requires anticipatory postural adjustments that are an integral part of normal voluntary movement. These anticipatory adjustments are an example of feedforward motor control in which prior experience and current sensory information are used to generate a best-guess postural strategy for preventing instability. Similar integration of postural control and movement occurs in all aspects of locomotion.

III. LOCOMOTION: THE EFFECTS OF NORMAL AGING

There is no generally accepted definition of normal aging (51). Most investigators agree that older people with obvious disease are abnormal. However, many older people have motor, cognitive, and musculoskeletal capacities that deviate significantly from those of young adults, but they do not have identifiable disease. Are these people normal? Some older people compare favorably with young adults and are examples of successful aging. The distinctions between normal aging and successful aging are vague and still debated because the unavoidable consequences of aging are undefined. Most abnormalities of posture and locomotion are due to identifiable disease, not normal aging.

Walking is a cyclical movement with two dimensions: time and length of stride (52,53). The gait cycle is defined arbitrarily as the time between successive heel-floor contacts with the same foot. Consequently, one gait cycle consists of two steps. From right heel-floor contact to left toe-off is a period of double-limb support (stance), which lasts approximately 10% of the total gait cycle. This phase of the cycle is followed by the left swing phase, which is simultaneous with and equal to the right single-limb support phase. The time from left heel-floor contact and right toe-off comprises the second of two double-limb support phases in a gait cycle and is followed by the right swing phase (left single-limb support phase).

Stride length and cadence are generally regarded as the independent variables of walking. The velocity of walking is determined by these variables (velocity = stride length × cadence ÷ 2). The magnitudes of most other kinematic characteristics of gait such as arm swing, toe-floor clearance, hip and knee rotations, and time in double-limb stance are functions of stride length and cadence (54–56). The cyclical patterns of muscle activation also vary with stride length and cadence and are reviewed elsewhere (52,57).

During normal walking, the center of gravity oscillates vertically at a frequency equal to the cadence and horizontally at a frequency of one-half the cadence (52). During a gait cycle, the two maxima in vertical oscillation occur in the middle of right and left single-limb stance, and the two minima of vertical oscillation occur in the middle of the two phases of double-limb stance. The left- and right-most horizontal excursions of the center of gravity occur at the times of mid-left and right single-limb stance. These vertical and horizontal excursions of the center of gravity are optimized in such a way that the center of mass moves forward with the least amount of expended energy (52,58,59). Many characteristics of abnormal gaits are dictated by the principle of energy conservation and by the biomechanical constraints of the body (60).

Most quantitative studies have found that healthy elderly people walk slower than young adults and exhibit a shorter stride and a faster cadence for a given speed of walking (61–68). Therefore, the effects of reduced stride and velocity on an elderly person's pattern of walking must be considered. Increased time in double-limb stance and reduced arm swing, toe-floor clearance, and rotation of the hip and knee are expected to occur when the velocity of walking is reduced (54, 56,69,70–73).

Elble and coworkers (73) used computerized infrared stroboscopic photometry to quantify the kinematic profiles of fast and natural walking in 20 young adults (10 men and 10 women; mean age 30.0 ± 6.1 years) and 20 elderly people (9 men and 11 women; mean age 74.7 ± 6.6 years) who had no history of falling, fear of falling, or abnormal neurological signs other than reduced vibratory sensation in the feet and absent ankle reflexes. The average natural and fast velocities of walking in the elderly were, respectively, 20% and 17% less than in the young. These differences in gait velocity were produced by comparable differences in stride length. Cadence did not differ between the young and old for fast or natural walking. The older people also exhibited comparable reductions in maximum toe displacement, arm swing, and knee flexion, but analysis of covariance revealed that these differences were statistically attributable to the reduced stride of the older people. This dependence of kinematic variables on stride was similar to that reported by Kirtley and coworkers (56) and explains why stride and gait velocity are useful, albeit nonspecific, measures of disability (74–76).

The nonspecific influence of stride on the other kinematic characteristics of gait must be considered in the clinical evaluation of gait disturbances in elderly patients. The need to minimize energy expenditure largely dictates the cadence-stride relationship that is exhibited at a particular velocity of walking (52,77–84). Critchley (85) warned that "an abnormal gait in the aged is frequently the result of disease outside the nervous system." Diseases of the musculoskeletal, circulatory, and respiratory systems are common causes of compensatory reductions in stride length and gait velocity. Increased joint stiffness, reduced muscle strength, and reduced cardiopulmonary reserve force patients to adopt a reduced stride and velocity of walking.

Musculoskeletal stiffness of the limbs, spine, and pelvis makes sitting, standing, turning, and rolling over very difficult. Many older people develop a stooped posture with abnormal lumbothoracic kyphosis, posterior rotation of the pelvis, and excessive flexion at the knees (Figure 3). Normal young adults have great difficulty walking, sitting, standing, turning, and maintaining balance when imitating this posture (86). Even when neurological conditions such as Parkinson's disease are the primary cause of this posture, secondary musculoskeletal changes soon become an important contributing factor (86,87). Patients with a compromised nervous system must then function within the harsh constraints of a compromised musculoskeletal system! This is a particularly disabling situation. The musculoskeletal changes alone are capable of producing greatly impaired balance and mobility and are ample justification for daily posture and range-of-motion exercises.

Age-related neuronal loss could contribute to the "natural" senescence of gait, but there is little direct evidence for this hypothesis. Age-related loss of nigrostriatal dopaminergic input occurs at an estimated rate of 8% per decade of life, which would not be clinically significant in most people before the tenth decade of life (88–90). There is an average 20% reduction in cells of the locus ceruleus by age 85 (91), but this degree of cell loss is not likely to have an appreciable effect on locomotion (92). Age-related cholinergic and noncholinergic cell loss in the dorsolateral midbrain tegmentum has not been demonstrated, but loss of these cells may contribute to the gait disturbances of Parkinson's disease and progressive supranuclear palsy (93–95). Cell loss in the neocortex and cerebellum occurs with aging (96,97) and could contribute to locomotor impairment in the elderly (98,99).

Ventricular size increases significantly after age 60 (100), but the mechanisms and clinical significance of this ventriculomegaly are usually unclear. Fisher (101) suggested that hydrocephalus may play a role in many older people with symmetrical impairment of gait. Fisher (101) and Sudarsky and Ronthal (102) found that the distance across the frontal horns of the lateral ventricles frequently exceeded 38 mm in patients with impaired walking but not in normal elderly. Koller and coworkers (103) also found that enlargement of the ventricular system correlated with the presence of gait impairment. However, the magnitude of ventriculomegaly in most of these elderly people is far below the ventriculomegaly in patients with shunt-responsive hydrocephalus (104) and probably represents central atrophy rather than a disturbance of spinal fluid dynamics.

Type II (fast-twitch) muscle fiber atrophy is a well-documented accompaniment of aging, beginning after age 40 (105, 106). This nonspecific phenomenon is caused by reduced activity, toxins, systemic metabolic disturbances, and endocrine disorders. Healthy active octogenarians lose muscle strength and bulk at a rate far below that exhibited by the general population, indicating that much of the age-related loss of muscle strength is not inevitable (107). Type II muscle atrophy is seen more frequently in elderly people who fall (105, 108) and is reversed by exercise, which improves ambulation (109).

Many older people lose vibratory sensation in the toes and fingers (110,111), but proprioception is well preserved (112). Loss of vibratory sensation is attributable in many older people to a loss of cutaneous sensory receptors and to arthritic joint disease (113,114). Delwaide and Delmotte (115) found that 15% of older people with disturbed ambulation had greatly reduced vibratory sensation in the feet and ankles, but vibratory sensation may be absent in the feet of healthy older people who have no significant abnormality of walking (73). Therefore, the clinical significance of vibratory loss per se is questionable in many older people.

IV. COMMON CLINICAL SYNDROMES OF DISTURBED LOCOMOTION

A. Cautious (Senile) Gait

Impaired ambulation exists in 15–20% of people who are older than 60 years (110,111). Many older people exhibit a guarded or restrained pattern of walking that resembles someone walking on a slippery surface (64,67,116). Stooped posture, reduced arm swing, increased time with both feet on the floor (double-limb stance), loss of the normal heel-toe sequence of foot-floor contact, disturbed coordination of cyclical limb movements, decreased toe-floor clearance, slightly widened base, and reduced hip and knee rotations are observed in most older people with locomotor impairment (117–119). This nonspecific kinematic profile of walking in older people is often called senile gait, particularly when the etiology is unknown. However, many authors prefer the term *cautious gait* because this style of walking is not peculiar to older people (120,121).

Patients with bilateral subdural hematomas (122), Binswanger's disease (123), normal-pressure hydrocephalus (101, 104, 124–129), Parkinson's disease (130,131), and high cervical myelopathy (132) exhibit gait disturbances that are heavily veiled by the characteristics of cautious gait. Consequently, patients with these conditions exhibit similar styles of walking, particularly when the illnesses are mild. Cautious (senile) gait is a nonspecific syndrome of abnormal walking. Its characteristics are largely compensatory effects of reduced stride and velocity, which occur in nearly all neurological gait disturbances. Elble and coworkers (133) compared the gait characteristics in 19 healthy older people with those of 10 elderly patients with a mixture of neurological conditions, including vascular dementia, shunt-responsive normal-pressure hydrocephalus (NPH), dementia of Alzheimer type (DAT), levodopa-resistant parkinsonism, and sensorimotor polyneuropathy. All patients were still ambulatory. Quantitatively, their kinematic characteristics of gait differed greatly from those of elderly controls, far more than the differences between young and older controls. Nevertheless, an analysis of covariance revealed that these differences were statistically attributable to reduced stride.

B. Paraplegia in Flexion and Senile Paraplegia

Paraplegia in flexion is an old neurological concept that encompasses the natural evolution of disturbed posture and locomotion in patients with bilateral cerebral disease. Pathologically enhanced flexor reflexes and hypertonia in the lower extremities are associated with flexion and adduction of the hips, flexion of the knees, and extension of the ankles, which ultimately lead to musculoskeletal contractures (134,135). Patients with paraplegia in flexion usually have severe damage to both frontal lobes. The original descriptions of this syndrome were mainly in patients with advanced vascular degeneration of the centrum semiovale and basal ganglia. However, this syndrome also occurs in patients with advanced primary degenerative dementias (e.g., Alzheimer's disease and Pick's disease), general paresis, multiple sclerosis, posttraumatic encephalopathy, and other acquired encephalopathies not limited to the elderly (136). This syndrome in an elderly patient has been called senile paraplegia (137).

Yakovlev (136) noted that paraplegia in flexion begins with the development of paratonic rigidity (gegenhalten), followed by flexion attitude. Paratonic rigidity is a form of muscular hypertonia in which patients seem to actively resist passive limb motion, despite their sincere attempt to relax. Paratonia is frequently associated with hyperactive tendon reflexes, Babinski signs, emotional apathy, perseveration, poor attention span, and reduced avoidance reaction to pain despite normal sensation. Flexion attitude consists of flexion of the torso, neck, hips, and knees; adduction of the shoulders and thighs; cupping of the hands with thumbs in apposition with the forefingers; and postural instability. Facial masking, drooling, bradykinesia, lethargy, reduced spontaneous movement, and tremor of the lips, tongue, and fingers are common. The gait of these patients is hesitant and unstable and is characterized by short shuffling steps. The repertoire of movement is limited. Interaction with the environment is less purposeful, and negotiation with obstacles is less effective. Pseudobulbar palsy and affect may be present. Damage to the frontal lobes, subcortical gray matter, or both is the responsible pathology in most cases (136).

A relatively mild gait disturbance with the stride-dependent characteristics of cautious gait occurs in the earliest stage of paraplegia in flexion. Stooped unstable posture, paratonic rigidity, and hesitancy evolve as this syndrome progresses. These advanced characteristics depend as much on the stage of illness as on the location of the pathology.

C. Gait Apraxia, Frontal Ataxia, and Start Hesitation

Many neurologists of the 19th and early 20th centuries recognized that frontal lobe lesions were capable of producing contralateral clumsiness (ataxia) of the limbs similar to that produced by lesions of the ipsilateral cerebellum (138,139). This phenomenon is called frontal ataxia, and some patients with bilateral frontal lobe disease exhibit a gait disturbance that is dominated by disturbed balance and posture (frontal dysequilibrium). Other patients with bilateral frontal lobe disease exhibit a very different gait disturbance in which lower limb motion is relatively normal except when attempts are made to stand and walk. Then, the feet appear to stick to the floor, and gait initiation is hesitant and stuttering (start hesitation). The relative preservation of lower limb motion except when standing and walking led to the notion of gait apraxia (140,141).

Patients purported to have gait apraxia rarely, if ever, fulfill Wilson's strict definition of apraxia: "an inability to perform certain subjectively purposive movements or movement-complexes, with conservation of motility, of sensation, and of coordination" (142). This definition is compromised in virtually all discussions of gait apraxia (138,143). Gait apraxia is typically defined as the loss of ability to properly use the lower limbs in the act of walking, which cannot be accounted for, in the examiner's opinion, by demonstrable sensory impairment or motor weakness. Patients with gait apraxia typically exhibit various combinations and degrees of postural instability, retropulsion, hypertonia, perseveration of posture, bradykinesia, reduced spontaneous movement, hyperreflexia, and Babinski signs. The concept of gait apraxia is objectionable because it implies an underlying disturbance of higher cortical function rather than a more basic disturbance of posture, balance, movement, or some combination thereof.

Most published examples of gait apraxia do not differ significantly from the advanced stages of paraplegia in flexion, described by Yakovlev. Some neurological patients exhibit relatively isolated start hesitation when attempting to walk (120,144,145), but some degree of postural instability is nearly always present (146). The initiation of gait is produced by a carefully formulated sequence of postural shifts that propels the body into forward motion (20). When considering the phenomenon of start hesitation, clinicians must remember that normal locomotion requires the proper control and integration of limb movement, posture, and balance. Seemingly insignificant deficits in any of these requirements could severely limit the ability of the nervous system to produce effective locomotion. Moving a lower limb while sitting or recumbent is a much easier task that moving the same limb in an upright stance. Similarly, the ability to adjust to a modest postural perturbation during a quiet stance is not as difficult as controlling posture and balance during walking, turning, starting, and stopping.

V. SPECIFIC CAUSES OF DISTURBED LOCOMOTION

A. Arteriosclerotic Parkinsonism and Binswanger's Disease

Multiple vascular lesions of the frontal lobes and basal ganglia, with or without subcortical white matter degeneration

(Binswanger's disease), can produce motor signs and a gait disturbance that resemble idiopathic Parkinson's disease. This vascular syndrome is referred to as arteriosclerotic parkinsonism and consists of mild generalized weakness, bradykinesia, and hypertonia. The hypertonia is frequently a paratonia (gegenhalten), rather than typical spasticity or parkinsonian rigidity. Patients initially exhibit a cautious gait with shortened stride and slow uncertain steps (147). As the disease progresses, foot-floor clearance is reduced, and posture becomes stooped. There is a tendency to fall backward. The toes may flex excessively as though gripping the floor. Muscle stretch reflexes are usually brisk, and Babinski signs are frequently present. The gait becomes hesitant and halting, and patients may exhibit prominent start hesitation. Turns are made stiffly and with multiple steps. Dejerine and Marie referred to this gait as marche a petit pas.

Thompson and Marsden (123) emphasized the presence of a wide base and noted that festination, reduced arm swing, and facial masking are typically absent. During walking, the upper extremities are frequently abducted, in contrast to the adducted, flexed posture in Parkinson's disease. These features distinguish idiopathic Parkinson's disease from the lower-half parkinsonism produced by vascular disease.

Thompson and Marsden (123) noted that the characteristics of gait in Binswanger's disease are similar to those in many patients with normal-pressure hydrocephalus, bilateral frontal lobe disease, Parkinson's disease, multiple-system atrophy, progressive supranuclear palsy, and cryptogenic senile gait. They proposed that dysfunction of pathways to and from the supplementary motor cortex and mesial motor cortex (leg area) may comprise the critical pathology. The symptoms and signs of arteriosclerotic parkinsonism are largely contained within the syndrome of paraplegia in flexion and are not peculiar to patients with multiple vascular lesions of the frontal lobes and basal ganglia.

Physical therapy is the only treatment for this form of gait disturbance. The prevention of cerebral vascular disease and stroke are therefore critical. The treatment of concomitant musculoskeletal, medical, and psychiatric illnesses may improve motor function (Sections VI and VII of this chapter).

B. Normal-Pressure Hydrocephalus

Many published reports document the variability and nonspecificity of the gait disturbance in late-onset normal-pressure hydrocephalus (101,124–129). Mildly affected patients exhibit a cautious gait or a nonspecific dysequilibrium. More advanced cases exhibit a hesitant, halting pattern of walking or a more severe dysequilibrium.

The gait disturbance of normal-pressure hydrocephalus is frequently referred to as gait apraxia (148), despite the nearly invariable presence of generalized motor dysfunction. Estañol (149) reasoned that the gait disturbance of communicating hydrocephalus is due to a release of proprioceptive supporting reactions. This notion is congruent with the observation that voluntary motion in the lower limbs is relatively normal except when the patients stand up and attempt to walk. This characteristic of lower limb function suggests that a postural disturbance, not apraxia, plays a critical role in this disturbance of gait. The upper extremities are less impaired than the lower extremities (124,126,150). However, mild weakness, clumsiness, postural tremor, paratonia, increased tendon reflexes, and bradykinesia may occur in the upper extremities (128). Impairment of oculomotor control is also possible (149). Therefore, NPH is a generalized disturbance of motor control with many features of paraplegia in flexion (136). The greater impairment of the lower extremities in NPH has been attributed to greater stretching of fibers from the paracentral cerebral cortex (150). This region of the motor-sensory cortex contains neurons that control the lower extremities, and this region also contains the supplementary motor cortex, which is involved in basal ganglia function.

NPH is always included in discussions of dementia and gait disorders because it is treatable. It is a rare condition that is very difficult to diagnose. Vanneste and coworkers (151) recently estimated an annual incidence of only 2.2 per million people. The clinical triad of NPH is a combination of gait disturbance, dementia, and urinary incontinence. This triad is not specific and occurs in vascular dementia, subdural hematoma, and advanced Alzheimer's disease. The radiological finding of hydrocephalus is therefore necessary to make the diagnosis, but it is frequently difficult to distinguish severe central cerebral atrophy from moderate hydrocephalus in older people. Cisternography (152,153), cerebrospinal fluid flow studies (154), and other diagnostic tests are not reliable in predicting those patients who will benefit from ventricular shunting (155–157). The onset of gait disturbance before dementia (158), a known etiology (151,159), and a classic triad of symptoms (104,152) are weak predictors of shunt responsiveness. The prognostic significance of cortical atrophy is controversial (104,159,160). The likelihood of sustained improvement following ventricular shunting is roughly 30%, and there is a comparable incidence of postoperative complications, including seizures, shunt malfunction, intracranial infection, subdural collections, ischemic stroke, extracranial infections, cerebral hemorrhage, and death (104,151,161). Extreme caution is recommended when considering this diagnosis and treatment.

C. Parkinson's Disease

Patients with early Parkinson's disease often exhibit a nonspecific cautious gait. The examination of gait in early Parkinson's disease is diagnostically helpful only when facial masking, reduced arm swing, festination, or characteristic rest tremor is also present. Hesitation, festination, en bloc turning, and flexed posture are usually present in patients with advanced disease (102). Increased time in double-limb stance, increased minimum knee flexion, and reduced gait velocity, cadence, stride length, sagittal rotations of the hips and knees, toe-floor clearance, and arm swing are not specific for Parkinson's disease (130,131) and are probably, in part, compensatory neurological changes.

The gait disturbance of Parkinson's disease is relatively refractory to available treatment modalities. The reason for this is unclear. Disturbed locomotion occurs in the mid to late stages of the disease, so advanced loss of dopaminergic nigrostriatal function is probably an important factor. Advanced loss of neurons in the locus ceruleus may also play a role and could affect cerebellar function. It is also possible that function of SLR, MLR, and related posterior fossa structures is relatively refractory to the loss of dopaminergic and noradrenergic neurons. The difficulty in treating and understanding the locomotor disturbance of Parkinson's disease makes the correction of contributing musculoskeletal, systemic, and psychiatric conditions extremely important, as discussed in Sections VI and VII of this chapter.

D. Progressive Supranuclear Palsy (see also Chapter 7)

Progressive supranuclear palsy (PSP; Steele-Richardson-Olszewski syndrome) is far less common than Parkinson's disease (162) but is frequently discussed as a cause of parkinsonism. However, PSP has pathological and clinical features that are different from those of Parkinson's disease and bilateral cerebral diseases. Widespread pathology in the brainstem and deep cerebellar nuclei produces symmetrical disturbances of gait that recapitulate much of what is known about the anatomy and physiology of locomotion.

PSP was described by Steele, Richardson, and Olszewski in 1964 (163). Cell loss, gliosis, and neurofibrillary tangles are found throughout the basal ganglia, brainstem, and deep cerebellar nuclei. The globus pallidus, subthalamic nucleus, red nucleus, substantia nigra, superior colliculi, dorsolateral midbrain tegmentum (i.e., the MLR), periaqueductal gray matter, pontine tegmentum, and dentate nucleus are most affected, but pathology is found in virtually all subcortical and brainstem nuclei that participate in the control of locomotion (163). Consequently, a prominent disturbance of locomotion is an early manifestation of this disease, even when the classic supranuclear ophthalmoplegia is not present (164,165). The gait disturbance is a variable blend of axial dystonia, truncal instability, short shuffling steps, start hesitation, freezing, and bradykinesia. In some patients, the gait may be so wide based and unsteady as to suggest the diagnosis of olivopontocerebellar degeneration. Other patients may exhibit a gait that is reminiscent of Parkinson's disease except for the preservation of arm swing and the presence of severe axial hypertonia. Rare patients have a syndrome of "pure akinesia," characterized by severe start hesitation and freezing (166). Mildly affected patients often exhibit only a nonspecific unsteadiness and cautious pattern of walking (163). Extension of the neck and the absence of stooped posture are clues that PSP is the underlying etiology.

The motor dysfunction of PSP responds poorly to available medications. The anti-Parkinson medications are generally tried, but the response to these medications is usually disappointing. This is not surprising given the widespread degeneration of central motor pathways.

E. Cervical Spondylosis

Cervical myelopathy affects locomotion in a variety of ways. The gait disturbance of some older patients is dominated by signs of pyramidal tract dysfunction consisting of stiff, scissoring, mechanical movements of the lower extremities and equinovarus posturing of the foot. The upper extremities may also appear stiff and poorly coordinated with the lower extremities. Other patients with cervical myelopathy are predominantly affected by posterior column or spinocerebellar tract dysfunction, causing sensory or cerebellar ataxia (167). However, many older people with cervical spondylotic myelopathy exhibit only a nonspecific cautious pattern of walking.

Cervical spondylosis is the most common cervical spine disease in older people. Narrowing of intervertebral disks and osteophyte formation are common findings in older people, reaching a prevalence of 75% in people older than 60 years (168). Most people are not significantly symptomatic. Radiculopathy is common and painful, but it is not as potentially disabling as compressive myelopathy.

Cervical spondylotic myelopathy is produced directly or indirectly by proliferative degenerative bony changes in the cervical spine. These degenerative changes occur most commonly at the intervertebral levels of C5–6 and C6–7. There is reduced mobility at these levels and associated vertebrolisthesis at C3–4 and C4–5. These factors combine to narrow the spinal canal both statically and dynamically at multiple intervertebral levels.

The high prevalence of spondylotic changes in older people makes the diagnosis surprisingly difficult. Routine spine films are helpful insofar as they reveal the spondylotic changes and the reduced canal diameter. The anteroposterior (AP) diameter of the cervical spinal cord is 9–10 mm. A spinal canal diameter less than 11 mm is suggestive of compressive myelopathy but also occurs in asymptomatic people (168). Some symptomatic patients have AP diameters exceeding 11 mm. Consequently, factors other than spinal stenosis undoubtedly play a role, such as repeated contusion of the cord by vertebral retrolisthesis, transient disk protrusion, and infolding of the ligamenta flava. Secondary cord ischemia also occurs (169,170).

The signs and symptoms of spondylotic myelopathy may develop insidiously or acutely. Neurological deficits can remain stable for several years after an initial phase of deterioration (171). Progression is not inevitable. Acute and subacute progression occasionally occurs, usually in patients with some preexisting disability. In this situation, acute soft-disk herniation must be distinguished from spondylotic cord contusion and vascular compromise. Acute and subacute progression often occur after a minor fall or whiplash injury but may also occur without an obvious precipitating event (172). There may be little or no cervical or radicular pain. Complaints of stiff, sore, and fatigable lower extremities and urinary urgency without incontinence are common. Numb clumsy hands are also common and are associated with loss of sensation for vibration, joint position, and two-point discrimination (173). Hyperreflexia is usually present in the lower extremities, but Babinski signs are frequently absent. Lower motor neuron signs in the upper extremities, Brown-Séquard's syndrome, and spastic tetraparesis or paraparesis are variably seen. None of these signs or symptoms is a reliable predictor of surgical outcome (174). The associated gait disturbance is often flavored heavily with the nonspecific characteristics of cautious gait (132). Stooped posture, stiff lower extremity movement, and steps that are broad-based, shuffling, and ataxic are common features.

Magnetic resonance imaging (MRI) is preferred by most clinicians in the initial diagnostic evaluation of suspected cervical spondylotic myelopathy (174–176). Subsequent myelography or computed tomographic (CT) myelography is occasionally needed. Most experienced clinicians can cite individual cases in which one method proved superior to all others. None is clearly superior in predicting surgical outcome. Fujiwara and coworkers (177) found that a cross-sectional area of the cord less than 30 mm² was a statistically significant predictor of poor surgical outcome, but this measurement accounted for only 30% of the total outcome variance. Central flattening and lateral distortion of the cord were not predictors of surgical outcome or preoperative clinical status. Several authors have suggested that patients with increased T2 cord signal are more likely to benefit from surgery (172,174), and Mehalic and coworkers (174) found that persistence of this abnormality after surgery was associated with a poor surgical outcome.

A sizable list of conditions must be considered when planning the laboratory evaluation of an older patient with cervical myelopathy. Many of these conditions are treatable (Table 1). Cervical spondylotic myelopathy should be distinguished from soft-disk herniation, which responds better to surgery (177,178).

Many anecdotal clinical reports have touted a variety of surgical and nonsurgical approaches to the treatment of cervical spondylotic myelopathy. A success rate of greater than 50% is found in most published reports (178–180). However, most surgical series represent a subpopulation of myelopathic patients referred by primary physicians, and the criteria for surgical referral are rarely described in published reports. The definition of surgical success usually includes the common outcome of an apparently stable neurological deficit. This outcome is difficult to interpret because 30–50% of patients experience little or no progression when treated with a cervical collar or other conservative therapy (171,181,182). Furthermore, patients may deteriorate years after a seemingly successful surgery (183). The advantages and disadvantages of decompressive posterior laminectomy (179,184), anterior

Table 1 Differential Diagnosis of Cervical Myelopathy

Cervical soft-disk herniation
Ossification of the posterior longitudinal ligament
Amyotrophic lateral sclerosis
Demyelinating disease
Primary lateral sclerosis
Subacute combined degeneration of the spinal cord
Intracranial parasagittal meningioma and bifrontal butterfly glioma
Intracranial subdural hematomas
Syringomyelia
Intra- and extramedullary spinal tumors
Epidural abscess
Fractured odontoid and atlantoaxial subluxation
Arteriovenous malformation of the spinal cord

---

diskectomy, and removal of osteophytes (179,180,185), and anterior corpectomy and strut graft arthrodesis (186,187) have been discussed extensively, but no randomized clinical trial has been conducted (188). Many surgeons prefer posterior laminectomy when spinal stenosis exists at more than two levels.

Criteria are needed for selecting those patients who are most likely to benefit from surgery and for selecting the best surgical approach. Previous uncontrolled studies are inconclusive, and a well-designed multicenter controlled trial is needed (188).

VI. FALLS

Lipsitz and coworkers (189) found that recurrent falling was attributable to a primary cause in 73% of elderly patients. Stroke, parkinsonism, visual impairment, orthostatic hypotension, and severe arthritis were the most common causes. Most of these patients had additional contributing medical conditions. Twenty-seven percent of Lipsitz's patients had multiple medical problems that could not be prioritized in the explanation of falls. Impaired vision (39,150), orthopedic problems including foot pathology (68,190,191), cognitive and emotional disorders (192–196), systemic disorders, and medication effects (197,198) should be considered in all patients, including those with an obvious neurological diagnosis. Treatment of these coexisting conditions may improve ambulation, even when the primary neurological condition is not treatable.

Environmental hazards and errors in judgment were responsible for 35–50% of falls in some studies (197) and for very few falls in other studies (189). An experienced occupational therapist, physical therapist, or visiting nurse can reduce falls by performing a comprehensive safety evaluation of the patient's home. The bedroom and bathroom should be searched for loose rugs and clothing, slippery floors and bathtubs, and poor lighting. Handrails, raised toilet seats, adequate lighting, and rubber floormats can be installed. Elimination of electrical cords, clutter, and throwrugs throughout the home and repair of uneven floors and cracked sidewalks are additional considerations. Shoes with slippery soles or high heels should be avoided.

Increased immobility may occur for no apparent reason following a serious fall (194). The pathophysiology of this postfall syndrome is unclear. Fear of additional falls is probably an important factor. Many patients openly express an increased fear of falling. Many falls lead to hospitalization, unnecessary confinement, and bedrest. All of these factors can cause further impairment of walking. Hospitalized and home-bound patients should be ambulated as much as possible. Nurses provide a great service by regularly walking elderly inpatients in the hallways.

VII. DIAGNOSTIC APPROACH TO PATIENTS WITH IMPAIRED MOBILITY

As emphasized throughout this chapter, the gait disturbances of many older patients are heavily veiled by nonspecific stride-dependent characteristics of gait, which comprise the syndrome of cautious or senile gait. This syndrome dominates the characteristics of walking when the underlying neurological illness is mild. Advanced gait disturbances may also lack diagnostic features that permit a specific diagnosis. This is because many features of gait are compensatory and because so many causes of disturbed locomotion impair the frontal lobes, basal ganglia, and brainstem motor nuclei. Associated neurological signs and symptoms are needed to make an accurate diagnosis (Table 2). Despite the diagnostic limitations of gait analysis, a careful clinical assessment of locomotion provides important functional measures of gross motor performance and should be included in the neurological examination of all older people. A comprehensive, performance-oriented evaluation of motor function (Table 3) will often disclose pathology that would otherwise be missed (190,199–202).

Table 2 Signs, Symptoms and Radiologic Findings that Are Helpful in Distinguishing the Neurological Etiologies of Symmetrical Gait Disturbances

	Binswanger's disease	NPH	PD	PSP	Cervical spondylosis
Reduced arm swing			+		
Festination			+		
Rest tremor			+ +		
Numb clumsy hands and Romberg's sign					+ +
Stepwise progression	+ +				
Vertical and horizontal gaze palsies				+ +	
Speech impairment	+		+	+	
Extension of the neck and torso				+ +	
Pyramidal tract signs	+				+
Urinary incontinence	+	+			+
Dementia	+	+		+	
Facial masking			+ +	+	
Spondylotic cervical spine and cord compression					+ +
Hydrocephalus		+ +			
Subcortical white-matter degeneration and microinfarcts	+ +				

+ = suggestive
+ + = relatively diagnostic

The specific treatment of many neurological gait disturbances is limited or nonexistent. Consequently, it is critically important to identify contributing illnesses of systemic, musculoskeletal, and psychiatric origin. These contributing illnesses are often far more treatable than the primary neurologi-

Table 3   Performance-Oriented Measures of Gait and Posture

Posture and balance during quiet stance:
   Curvature of spine
   Head position
   Pelvic tilt
   Flexion of knees and hips
   Romberg test
Sitting and arising from a chair
Initiation of gait
Turning 360 degrees
Step length, width, rhythmicity, and symmetry
Coordination of upper and lower limbs
Foot-floor clearance and contact
Walking path
Gait velocity
Climbing stairs
Bending over and reaching while standing
Rolling over in bed
Walking on heels and toes
Tandem walking
Response to active and passive neck motion while standing
Response to a nudge on chest or back

---

cal disease. Contributing illnesses are particularly common in older people, and a thorough history and physical examination are required to identify these illnesses. A routine neurological examination is not sufficient. Particular attention should be paid to each patient's vision, cognitive function, and musculoskeletal system. Do not overlook foot pathology, depression, hypothyroidism, vestibulopathy (203), peripheral neuropathy, orthostatic hypotension, cardiopulmonary disease, deconditioned skeletal muscles, vitamin B_{12} deficiency, offending medications, and orthopedic deformities of the spine and extremities. Multiple abnormalities of uncertain significance are often found, but as in the treatment of dementia, a compulsive correction of all treatable conditions is necessary and often rewarding.

ACKNOWLEDGMENTS

Supported by grants P30 AG08014 and RO1 AG10837 from the National Institute on Aging.

REFERENCES

1. Brown TG. On the nature of the fundamental activity of the nervous centres, together with an analysis of the conditioning of rhythmic activity in progression, and a theory of evolution of function in the nervous system. J Physiol (London) 1914; 48:18–46.

2. Grillner S. Control of locomotion in bipeds, tetrapods, and fish. In: Brooks VB, ed., Handbook of Physiology: The Nervous System, Motor Control. Baltimore: Williams & Wilkins, 1981:1179–1236.

3. Holmes G. Spinal injuries of warfare. Br. Med J 1915; 2: 815–821.

4. Eidelberg E, Walden JG, Nguyen LH. Locomotor control in macaque monkeys. Brain 1981; 104:647–663.

5. Eidelberg E, Story JL, Walden JG, and Meyer BL. Anatomical correlates of return of locomotor function after partial spinal cord lesions in cats. Exp Brain Res 1981; 42:81–88.

6. Armstrong DM. The supraspinal control of mammalian locomotion. J Physiol (London) 1988; 405:1–37.

7. Kawahara K, Mori S, Tomiyama T, Kanaya T. Discharges in neurons in the midpontine dorsal tegmentum of mesencephalic cat during locomotion. Brain Res 1985; 341:377–380.

8. Mori S. Integration of posture and locomotion in acute decerebrate cats and in awake, freely moving cats. Prog Neurobiol 1987; 28:161–195.

9. Mori S, Sakamoto T, Ohta Y, Takakusaki K, Matsuyama K. Site-specific postural and locomotor changes evoked in awake, freely moving intact cats by stimulating the brainstem. Brain Res 1989; 505:66–74.

10. Marciello M, Sinnamon HM. Locomotor stepping initiated by glutamate injections into the hypothalamus of the anesthetized rat. Behav Neurosci 1990; 104:980–990.

11. Rye DB, Saper CB, Lee HJ, Wainer BH. Pedunculopontine tegmental nucleus of the rat: Cytoarchitecture, cytochemistry, and some extrapyramidal connections of the mesopontine tegmentum. J Comp Neurol 1987; 259:483–528.

12. Rye DB, Lee HJ, Saper CB, Wainer BH. Medullary and spinal efferents of the pedunculopontine tegmental nucleus and adjacent mesopontine tegmentum in the rat. J Comp Neurol 1988; 269:315–341.

13. Garcia-Rill E. The basal ganglia and the locomotor regions. Brain Res Reviews 1986; 11:47–63.

14. Garcia-Rill E, Kinjo N, Atsuta Y, Ishikawa Y, Webber M, Skinner, RD. Posterior midbrain-induced locomotion. Brain Res Bull 1990; 24:499–508.

15. DeLong MR, Wichmann T. Basal ganglia-thalamocortical circuits in parkinsonian signs. Clin Neurosci 1993; 1:18–26.

16. Canteras NS, Shammah-Lagnado SJ, Silva BA, Ricardo JA. Afferent connections of the subthalamic nucleus: A combined retrograde and anterograde horseradish peroxidase study in the rat. Brain Res 1990; 513:43–59.

17. Kinjo N, Atsuta Y, Webber M, Kyle R, Skinner RD, Garcia-Rill E. Medioventral medulla-induced locomotion. Brain Res Bull 1990; 24:509–516.

18. Drew T. Motor cortical cell discharge during voluntary gait modification. Brain Res 1988; 457:181–187.

19. Brenière Y, Do MC, Sanchez J. A biomechanical study of the gait initiation process. J Biophys et Méd Nucl 1981; 5:197–205.

20. Elble RJ, Moody C, Leffler K, Sinha R. The initiation of normal walking. Mov Disord 1994; 9:139–146.

21. Brocklehurst JC, Robertson D, James-Groom P. Clinical correlates of sway in old age—sensory modalities. Age Ageing 1982; 11:1–10.

22. Sinclair AJ, Nayak USL. Age-related changes in postural sway. Compr Ther 1990; 16:44–48.

23. Thyssen HH, Brynskov J, Jansen EC, Münster-Swendsen J. Normal ranges and reproducibility for the quantitative Romberg's test. Acta Neurol Scand 1982; 66:100–104.

24. Horak FB, Nashner LM, Diener NC. Postural strategies associated with somatosensory and vestibular loss. Exp Brain Res 1990; 82:167–177.

25. Dichgans J, Mauritz KH, Allum JHJ, Brandt T. Postural sway in normals and atactic patients: Analysis of the stabilizing and destabilizing effects of vision. Agressologie 1976; 17:15–24.

26. Lestienne F, Soechting J, Berthoz A. Postural readjustments induced by linear motion of visual scenes. Exp Brain Res 1977; 28:363–384.

27. Wolfson L, Whipple R, Derby CA, Amerman P, Murphy T, Tobin JN, Nashner L. A dynamic posturography study of balance in healthy elderly. Neurology 1992; 42:2069–2075.

28. Nashner LM. Adapting reflexes controlling the human posture. Exp Brain Res 1976; 26:59–72.

29. Nashner LM. Fixed patterns of rapid postural responses among leg muscles during stance. Exp Brain Res 1977; 30: 13–24.

30. Nashner LM, Woollacott M, Tuma G. Organization of rapid responses to postural and locomotor-like perturbations of standing man. Exp Brain Res 1979; 36:463–476.

31. Woollacott MH, Shumway-Cook A, Nashner L. Postural reflexes and aging. In: Mortimer JA, Pirozzolo FJ, Maletta GJ, eds., The Aging Motor System. New York: Praeger, 1982: 98–119.

32. Dietz V, Quintern J, Berger W, Schenck E. Cerebral potentials and leg muscle e.m.g. responses associated with stance perturbation. Exp Brain Res 1985; 57:348–354.

33. Nashner LM, McCollum G. The organization of human postural movements: A formal basis and experimental synthesis. Behav Brain Sci 1985; 8:135–172.

34. Nashner LM, Black FO, Wall C. Adaptation to altered support and visual conditions during stance: Patients with vestibular deficits. J Neurosci 1982; 2:536–544.

35. Keshner EA, Allum JHJ, Pfaltz CR. Postural coactivation and adaptation in the sway stabilizing responses of normals and patients with bilateral vestibular deficit. Exp Brain Res 1987; 69:77–92.

36. Nashner L, Berthoz A. Visual contribution to rapid motor responses during postural control. Brain Res 1978; 150:403–407.

37. Aniss AM, Diener H-C, Hore J, Gandevia SC, Burke D. Behavior of human muscle receptors when reliant on proprioceptive feedback during standing. J Neurophysiol 1990; 64: 661–670.

38. Brooke JD, Singh R, Wilson MK, Yoon P, McIlroy WE. Aging of human segmental oligosynaptic reflexes for control of leg movement. Neurobiol Aging 1989; 10:721–725.

39. Stelmach GE, Phillips J, DiFabio RP, Teasdale N. Age, functional postural reflexes, and voluntary sway. J Gerontol 1989; 44:B100–106.

40. Belen'kii VY, Gurfinkel VS, Pal'tsev YI. Elements of control of voluntary movements. Biofizika 1967; 12:135–141.

41. Bouisset S, Zattara M. A sequence of postural movements precedes voluntary movement. Neurosci Lett 1981; 22:263–270.

42. Bouisset S, Zattara M. Biomechanical study of the programming of anticipatory postural adjustments associated with voluntary movement. J Biomech 1987; 20:735–742.

43. Zattara M, Bouisset S. Posturo-kinetic organisation during the early phase of voluntary upper limb movement. 1. Normal subjects. J Neurol Neurosurg Psychiatry 1988; 51:956–965.

44. Cordo PJ, Nashner LM. Properties of postural adjustments associated with rapid arm movements. J Neurophysiol 1982; 47:287–302.

45. Stelmach GE, Populin L, Müller F. Postural muscle onset and voluntary movement in the elderly. Neurosci Lett 1990; 117: 188–193.

46. Inglin B, Woollacott M. Age-related changes in anticipatory postural adjustments associated with arm movements. J Gerontol 1988; 43:M105–M113.

47. Pal'tsev YI, El'ner AM. Preparatory and compensatory period during voluntary movement in patients with involvement of the brain of different localization. Biofizika 1967; 12: 142–147.

48. Traub MM, Rothwell JC, Marsden CD. Anticipatory postural reflexes in Parkinson's disease and other akinetic-rigid syndromes and cerebellar ataxia. Brain 1980; 103:393–412.

49. Gurfinkel VS, El'ner AM. Contribution of the frontal lobe secondary motor area to organization of postural components in human voluntary movement. Neirofiziologiia 1988; 20:7–15.

50. Dick JPR, Rothwell JC, Berardelli A, Thompson PD, Gioux M, Benecke R, Day BL, Marsden CD. Associated postural adjustments in Parkinson's disease. J Neurol Neurosurg Psychiatry 1986; 49:1378–1385.

51. Calne DB, Eisen A, Meneilly G. Normal aging of the nervous system. Ann Neurol 1991; 30:206–207.

52. Inman VT, Ralston HJ, Todd F. Human Walking. Baltimore: Williams and Wilkins, 1981.

53. Winter DA. The Biomechanics and Motor Control of Human Gait. Waterloo, Ontario: University of Waterloo Press, 1987.

54. Murray MP, Kory RC, Clarkson BH, Sepic SB. A comparison of free and fast speed walking patterns of normal men. Am J Phys Med 1966; 45:8–24.

55. Grillner S, Halbertsma J, Nilsson J, Thorstensson A. The adaptation to speed in human locomotion. Brain Res 1979; 165:177–182.

56. Kirtley C, Whittle MW, Jefferson RJ. Influence of walking speed on gait parameters. J Biomed Eng 1985; 7:282–288.

57. Shiavi R. Electromyographic patterns in normal adult locomotion. In: Smidt GL, ed., Gait in Rehabilitation. New York: Churchill Livingstone, 1990:97–119.

58. McMahon TA. Muscles, Reflexes, and Locomotion. Princeton, NJ: Princeton University Press, 1984; chap. 8.

59. Saunders JB de CM, Inman VT, Eberhart HD. The major determinants in normal and pathological gait. J Bone Joint Surg 1953; 35:543–558.

60. Waters R, Yakura J. Energy expenditure of normal and abnormal ambulation. In: Smidt GL, ed., Gait in Rehabilitation. New York: Churchill Livingstone, 1990:65–96.

61. Blanke DJ, Hageman PA. Comparison of gait of young men and elderly men. Phys Ther 1989; 69:144–148.

62. Finley FR, Cody KA, Finizie RV. Locomotion patterns in elderly women. Phys Med Rehabil 1969; 50:140–146.

63. Hageman PA, Blanke DJ. Comparison of gait of young women and elderly women. Phys Ther 1986; 66:1382–1387.

64. Imms FJ, Edholm OG. Studies of gait and mobility in the elderly. Age Ageing 1981; 10:147–156.

65. Jansen EC, Vittas D, Hellberg S, Hansen J. Normal gait of young and old men and women: Ground reaction force measurement on a treadmill. Acta Orthop Scand 1982; 53:193–196.

66. Larish DD, Martin PE, Mungiole M. Characteristic patterns of gait in the healthy old. Ann NY Acad Sci 1988; 515: 18–31.

67. Murray MP, Kory RC, Clarkson BH. Walking patterns in healthy old men. J Gerontol 1969; 24:169–178.

68. Lundgren-Lindquist B, Aniansson A, Rundgren Å. Functional studies in 79-year-olds. III. Walking performance and climbing capacity. Scand J Rehabil Med 1983; 15:125–131.

69. Hirokawa S. Normal gait characteristics under temporal and distance constraints. J Biomed Eng 1989; 11:449–456.

70. Larrson L-E, Odenrick P, Sandlund B, Weitz P, Berg P. The phases of the stride and their interaction in human gait. Scand J Rehabil Med 1980; 12:107–112.

71. Murray MP, Clarkson BH. The vertical pathways of the foot during level walking: I. Range of variability in normal men. J Am Phys Ther Assoc 1966; 46:585–589.

72. Murray MP, Sepic SB, Barnard EJ. Patterns of sagittal rotation of the upper limbs in walking. J Am Phys Ther Assoc 1967; 47:272–284.

73. Elble RJ, Thomas SS, Higgins C, Colliver J. Stride-dependent changes in gait of older people. J Neurol 1991; 238:1–5.

74. Nakamura R, Handa T, Watanabe S, Morohashi I. Walking cycle after stroke. Tohoku J Exp Med 1988; 154:241–244.

75. Smidt GL. Gait assessment and training in clinical practice. In: Smidt GL, ed., Gait in Rehabilitation. New York: Churchill Livingstone, 1990:301–315.

76. Wade DT, Wood VA, Heller A, Maggs J, Hewer RL. Walking after stroke: Measurement and recovery over the first 3 months. Scand J Rehabil Med 1987; 19:25–30.

77. Alexander R McN. Optimization and gaits in the locomotion of vertebrates. Physiol Rev 1989; 69:1199–1227.

78. Cavagna GA, Franzetti P. The determinants of the step frequency in walking in humans. J Physiol (London) 1986; 373: 235–242.

79. Cavagna GA, Thys H, Zamboni A. The sources of external work in level walking and running. J Physiol (London) 1976; 262:639–657.

80. Heglund NC, Taylor CR. Speed, stride frequency and energy cost per stride: How do they change with body size and gait? J Exp Biol 1988; 138:301–318.

81. Nilsson J, Thorstensson A. Adaptability in frequency and amplitude of leg movements during human locomotion at different speeds. Acta Physiol Scand 1987; 129:107–114.
82. Ralston HJ. Energy-speed relation and optimal speed during level walking. Int Z Angew Physiol 1958; 17:277–283.
83. Zarrugh MY, Todd FN, Ralston HJ. Optimization of energy expenditure during level walking. Europ J Appl Physiol 1974; 33:293–306.
84. Buskirk ER, Hodgson JL. Age and aerobic power: The rate of change in men and women. FASEB J 1987; 46:1824–1829.
85. Critchley M. The neurology of old age. Lancet 1931; i: 1221–1230.
86. Schenkman M, Butler RB. A model for multisystem evaluation treatment of individuals with Parkinson's disease. Phys Ther 1989; 69:932–943.
87. Schenkman M, Donovan J, Tsubota J, Kluss M, Stebbins P, Butler RB. Management of individuals with Parkinson's disease: Rationale and case studies. Phys Ther 1989; 69:944–955.
88. De Keyser J, Ebinger G, Vauquelin G. Age-related changes in the human nigrostriatal dopaminergic system. Ann Neurol 1990; 27:157–161.
89. McGeer PL, Itagaki S, Akiyama H, McGeer EG. Comparison of neuronal loss in Parkinson's disease and aging. In: Calne DB, Crippa D, Comi G, Horowski R, Trabucchi M, eds., Parkinsonism and Aging. New York: Raven Press, 1989:25–34.
90. Scherman D, Desnos C, Darchen F, Pollak P, Javoy-Agid F, Agid Y. Striatal dopamine deficiency in Parkinson's disease: Role of aging. Ann Neurol 1989; 26:551–557.
91. Marcyniuk B, Mann DMA, Yates PO. The topography of nerve cell loss from the locus caeruleus in elderly persons. Neurobiol Aging 1989; 10:5–9.
92. Fishman RHB, Feigenbaum JJ, Yanai J, Klawans HL. The relative importance of dopamine and norepinephrine in mediating locomotor activity. Prog Neurobiol 1983; 20:55–88.
93. Hirsch EC, Graybiel AM, Duyckaerts C, Javoy-Agid F. Neuronal loss in the pedunculopontine tegmental nucleus in Parkinson's disease and in progressive supranuclear palsy. Proc Natl Acad Sci 1987; 84:5976–5980.

94. Jellinger K. Neuropathological substrates of Alzheimer's disease and Parkinson's disease. J Neural Transm 1987; 24: 109–129.

95. Jellinger K. The pedunculopontine nucleus in Parkinson's disease, progressive supranuclear palsy and Alzheimer's disease. J Neurol Neurosurg Psychiatry 1988; 51:540–543.

96. Coleman PD, Flood DG. Neuron numbers and dendritic extent in normal aging and Alzheimer's disease. Neurobiol Aging 1987; 8:521–545.

97. Flood DG, Coleman PD. Neuron numbers and sizes in aging brain: Comparisons of human, monkey, and rodent data. Neurobiol Aging 1988; 9:453–463.

98. Scheibel ME, Tomiyasu U, Scheibel AB. The aging human betz cell. Exp Neurol 1977; 56:598–609.

99. Scheibel AB. Falls, motor dysfunction, and correlative neurohistologic changes in the elderly. Clin Geriatr Med 1985; 1: 671–676.

100. Stafford JL, Albert MS, Naeser MA, Sandor T, Garvey AJ. Age-related differences in computed tomographic scan measurements. Arch Neurol 1988; 45:409–415.

101. Fisher CM. Hydrocephalus as a cause of disturbances of gait in the elderly. Neurology 1982; 32:1358–1363.

102. Sudarsky L, Ronthal M. Gait disorders among elderly patients: A survey study of 50 patients. Arch Neurol 1983; 40: 740–743.

103. Koller WC, Wilson RS, Glatt SL, Huckman MS, Fox JH. Senile gait: Correlation with computed tomographic scans. Ann Neurol 1983; 13:343–344.

104. Black P McL. Idiopathic normal-pressure hydrocephalus: Results of shunting in 62 patients. J Neurosurg 1980; 52: 371–377.

105. Aniansson A, Zetterberg C, Hedberg M, Henriksson KG. Impaired muscle function with aging: A background factor in the incidence of fractures of the proximal end of the femur. Clin Orthop 1984; 191:193–201.

106. Bassey EJ, Bendall MJ, Pearson M. Muscle strength in the triceps surae and objectively measured customary walking activity in men and women over 65 years of age. Clin Sci 1988; 74:85–89.

107. Greig CA, Botella J, Young A. The quadriceps strength of

healthy elderly people remeasured after eight years. Muscle Nerve 1993; 16:6–10.

108.   Whipple RH, Wolfson LI, Amerman PM. The relationship of knee and ankle weakness to falls in nursing home residents: An isokinetic study. J Am Geriatr Soc 1987; 35:13–20.

109.   Fiatarone MA, Marks EC, Ryan ND, Meredith CN, Lipsitz LA, Evans WJ. High-intensity strength training in nonagenarians: Effects on skeletal muscle. JAMA 1990; 263:3029–3034.

110.   Newman G, Dovenmuehle RH, Busse EW. Alterations in neurologic status with age. J Am Geriatr Soc 1960; 8:915–917.

111.   Prakash C, Stern G. Neurological signs in the elderly. Age Ageing 1973; 2:24–27.

112.   Kokmen E, Bossemeyer RW, Williams WJ. Quantitative evaluation of joint motion sensation in an aging population. J Gerontol 1978; 33:62–67.

113.   Newman HW, Corbin KB. Quantitative determination of vibratory sensibility. Proc Soc Exp Biol 1936; 35:273–276.

114.   Bolton CF, Winkelmann RK, Dyck PJ. A quantitative study of Meissner's corpuscles in man. Neurology 1966; 16:1–9.

115.   Delwaide PJ, Delmotte PH. Comparison of normal senile gait with parkinsonian gait. In: Calne DB, Crippa D, Comi G, Horowski R, Trabucchi M, eds., Parkinsonism and Aging. New York: Raven Press, 1989:229–237.

116.   Imms FJ, Edholm OG. The assessment of gait and mobility in the elderly. Age Ageing 1979; 8(suppl):261–267.

117.   Spielberg PI. Walking of old people: Cyclographic analysis. In: Bernstein NA, ed., Investigations on the Biodynamics of Walking, Running, and Jumping. Moscow, 1940:72–76.

118.   Tinetti M. Performance-oriented assessment of mobility problems in elderly patients. J Am Geriatr Soc 1986; 34:119–126.

119.   Wolfson L, Whipple R, Amerman P, Tobin JN. Gait assessment in the elderly: A gait abnormality rating scale and its relation to falls. J Gerontol (Med Sci) 1990; 45:M12–M19.

120.   Nutt JG, Marsden CD, Thompson PD. Human walking and higher-level gait disorders, particularly in the elderly. Neurology 1993; 43:268–279.

121.   Koller WC, Glatt SL, Fox JH. Senile gait, a distinct neurologic entity. Clin Geriatr Med 1985; 1:661–668.

122. Goto I, Kuroiwa Y, Kitamura K. The triad of neurological manifestations in bilateral chronic subdural hematoma and normal-pressure hydrocephalus. J Neurosurg Sci 1986; 30: 123–128.

123. Thompson PD, Marsden CD. Gait disorder of subcortical arteriosclerotic encephalopathy: Binswanger's disease. Mov Disord 1987; 2:1–8.

124. Adams RD, Fisher CM, Hakim S, Ojemann RG, Sweet WH. Symptomatic occult hydrocephalus with "normal" cerebrospinal fluid pressure. New Engl J Med 1965; 273:117–126.

125. Fisher CM. The clinical picture of occult hydrocephalus. Clin Neurosurg 1977; 24:270–284.

126. McHugh PR. Occult hydrocephalus. Q J Med 1964; 33: 297–308.

127. Messert B, Wannamaker BB. Reappraisal of the adult occult hydrocephalus syndrome. Neurology 1974; 24:224–231.

128. Sorensen PS, Jansen EC, Gjerris F. Motor disturbances in normal-pressure hydrocephalus. Arch Neurol 1986; 43:34–38.

129. Sudarsky L, Simon S. Gait disorder in late-life hydrocephalus. Arch Neurol 1987; 44:263–267.

130. Knutsson E. An analysis of parkinsonian gait. Brain 1972; 95:475–486.

131. Murray MP, Sepic SB, Gardner GM, Downs WJ. Walking patterns of men with parkinsonism. Am J Phys Med 1978; 57:278–294.

132. Murray PK. Cervical spondylotic myelopathy: A cause of gait disturbance and urinary incontinence in older persons. J Am Geriatr Soc 1984; 32:324–330.

133. Elble RJ, Higgins C, Hughes L. The syndrome of senile gait. J Neurol 1991; 239:71–75.

134. Daniels LE. Paraplegia in flexion. Arch Neurol Psychiatry 1940; 43:736–764.

135. Stewart P. Senile paraplegia. In: Allbutt TC, ed., A System of Medicine. New York: Macmillan, 1910:805–809.

136. Yakovlev PI. Paraplegia in flexion of cerebral origin. J Neuropath Exp Neurol 1954; 13:267–296.

137. Critchley M. On senile disorders of gait, including the so-called "senile paraplegia." Geriatrics 1948; 3:364–370.

138. Meyer JS, Barron DW. Apraxia of gait: A clinico-physiological study. Brain 1960; 83:261–284.

139. Montgomery EB. Signs and symptoms from a cerebral lesion that suggest cerebellar dysfunction. Arch Neurol 1983; 40: 422–423.

140. Gerstmann J, Schilder P. Ber eine besondere Gangstrung bei Stirnhirnerkrankung. Wien Med Wochenschr 1926; 76: 97–102.

141. Van Bogaert MML, Martin P. L'apraxie de la marche et l'atonie statique. Encephale 1929; 24:11–18.

142. Wilson SAK. A contribution to the study of apraxia with a review of the literature. Brain 1908; 31:164–216.

143. Denny-Brown D. The nature of apraxia. J Nerv Ment Dis 1958; 216:9–32.

144. Achiron A, Ziv I, Goren M, Goldberg H, Zoldan Y, Sroka H, Melamed E. Primary progressive freezing gait. Mov Disord 1993; 8:293–297.

145. Atchison PR, Thompson PD, Frackowiak RSJ, Marsden CD. The syndrome of gait ignition failure: A report of six cases. Mov Disord 1993; 8:285–292.

146. Petrovici I. Apraxia of gait and of trunk movements. J Neurol Sci 1968; 7:229–243.

147. Critchley M. Arteriosclerotic parkinsonism. Brain 1929; 52: 23–83.

148. Messert B, Henke TK, Langheim W. Syndrome of akinetic mutism associated with obstructive hydrocephalus. Neurology 1966; 16:635–649.

149. Estañol V. Gait apraxia in communicating hydrocephalus. J Neurol Neurosurg Psychiatry 1981; 44:305–308.

150. Yakovlev PI. Paraplegias of hydrocephalics. Am J Ment Defic 1947; 51:561–576.

151. Vanneste J, Augustijn P, Dirven C, Tan WF, Goedhart ZD. Shunting normal-pressure hydrocephalus: Do the benefits outweigh the risks? A multicenter study and literature review. Neurology 1992; 42:54–59.

152. Benzel EC, Pelletier AL, Levy PG. Communicating hydrocephalus in adults: Prediction of outcome after ventricular shunting procedures. Neurosurgery 1990; 26:655–660.

153. Vanneste J, Augustijn P, Davies GAG, Dirven C, Tan WF. Normal-pressure hydrocephalus. Is cisternography still useful in selecting patients for a shunt? Arch Neurol 1992; 49:366–370.

154. Tans J Th J, Poortvliet DCJ. Reduction of ventricular size after shunting for normal-pressure hydrocephalus related to CSF dynamics before shunting. J Neurol Neurosurg Psychiatry 1988; 51:521–525.

155. Clarfield AM. Normal-pressure hydrocephalus: Saga or swamp? JAMA 1989; 262:2592–2593.

156. Symon L, Hinzpeter T. The enigma of normal-pressure hydrocephalus: Tests to select patients for surgery and to predict shunt function. Clin Neurosurg 1977; 24:285–315.

157. Wolinsky JS, Barnes BD, Margolis MT. Diagnostic tests in normal-pressure hydrocephalus. Neurology 1973; 23:706–713.

158. Graff-Radford NR, Godersky JC. Normal-pressure hydrocephalus. Onset of gait abnormality before dementia predicts good surgical outcome. Arch Neurol 1986; 43:940–942.

159. Thomsen AM, Borgesen SE, Bruhn P, Gjerris F. Prognosis of dementia in normal-pressure hydrocephalus after a shunt operation. Ann Neurol 1986; 20:304–310.

160. Jacobs L, Kinkel W. Computerized axial transverse tomography in normal-pressure hydrocephalus. Neurology 1976; 26:501–507.

161. Hughes CP, Siegel BA, Coxe WS, Gado MH, Grubb RL, Coleman RE, Berg L. Adult idiopathic communicating hydrocephalus with and without shunting. J Neurol Neurosurg Psychiatry 1978; 41:961–971.

162. Golbe LI, Davis PH, Schoenberg BS, Duvoisin RC. Prevalence and natural history of progressive supranuclear palsy. Neurology 1988;38:1031–1034.

163. Steele JC, Richardson JC, Olszewski J. Progressive supranuclear palsy. Arch Neurol 1964; 10:333–359.

164. Davis PH, Bergeron C, McLachlan DR. Atypical presentation of progressive supranuclear palsy. Ann Neurol 1985; 17:337–343.

165. Maher ER, Lees AJ. The clinical features and natural history of the Steele-Richardson-Olszewski syndrome (progressive supranuclear palsy). Neurology 1986; 36:1005–1008.

166. Matsuo H, Takashima H, Kishikawa M, Kinoshita I, Mori M, Tsujihata M, Nagataki S. Pure akinesia: An atypical manifestation of progressive supranuclear palsy. J Neurol Neurosurg Psychiatry 1991; 54:397–400.

167. Hainline B, Tuszynski MH, Posner JB. Ataxia in epidural spinal cord compression. Neurology 1992; 42:2193–2195.
168. Hayashi H, Okada K, Hamada M, Tada K, Ueno R. Etiologic factors of myelopathy: A radiographic evaluation of the aging changes in the cervical spine. Clin Orthop 1987; 214:-200–209.
169. Ono K, Ota H, Tada K, Yamamoto T. Cervical myelopathy secondary to multiple spondylotic protrusions: A clinicopathologic study. Spine 1977; 2:109–125.
170. Robinson RA, Afeiche N, Dunn EJ, Northrup BE. Cervical spondylotic myelopathy: Etiology and treatment concepts. Spine 1977; 2:89–99.
171. Nurick S. The natural history and the results of surgical treatment of the spinal cord disorder associated with cervical spondylosis. Brain 1972; 95:101–108.
172. Wilberger JE, Chedid MK. Acute cervical spondylytic myelopathy. Neurosurgery 1988; 22:145–146.
173. Good DC, Couch JR, Wacasar L. "Numb clumsy hands" and high cervical spondylosis. Surg Neurol 1984; 22:285–291.
174. Mehalic TF, Pezzuti RT, Applebaum BI. Magnetic resonance imaging and cervical spondylotic myelopathy. Neurosurgery 1990; 26:217–227.
175. Masaryk TJ, Modic MT, Geisinger MA, Standefer J, Hardy RW, Boumphrey F, Duchesneau PM. Cervical myelopathy: A comparison of magnetic resonance and myelography. J Comp Assist Tomogr 1986; 10:184–194.
176. Statham PF, Hadley DM, Macpherson P, Johnston RA, Bone I, Teasdale GM. MRI in the management of suspected cervical spondylotic myelopathy. J Neurol Neurosurg Psychiatry 1991; 54:484–489.
177. Fujiwara K, Yonenobu K, Ebara S, Yamashita K, Ono K. The prognosis of surgery for cervical compression myelopathy: An analysis of the factors involved. J Bone Joint Surg 1989; 71-B:393–398.
178. Bertalanffy H, Eggert HR. Clinical long-term results of anterior discectomy without fusion for treatment of cervical radiculopathy and myelopathy. Acta Neurochir (Wien) 1988; 90:127–135.
179. Jeffreys RV. The surgical treatment of cervical myelopathy due to spondylosis and disc degeneration. J Neurol Neurosurg Psychiatry 1986; 49:353–361.

180. Yang KC, Lu XS, Cai QL, Ye LX, Lu WQ. Cervical spondylotic myelopathy treated by anterior multilevel decompression and fusion: Follow-up report of 214 cases. Clin Orthop 1987; 221:161–164.

181. Arnasson O, Carlsson CA, Pellettieri L. Surgical and conservative treatment of cervical spondylotic radiculopathy and myelopathy. Acta Neurochir (Wien) 1987; 84:48–53.

182. LaRocca H. Cervical spondylotic myelopathy: Natural history. Spine 1988; 13:854–855.

183. Goto S, Mochizuki M, Watanabe T, Hiramatu K, Tanno T, Kitahara H, Moriya H. Long-term follow-up study of anterior surgery for cervical spondylotic myelopathy with special reference to the magnetic resonance imaging findings in 52 cases. Clin Orthop 1993; 291:142–153.

184. Epstein JA. The surgical management of cervical spinal stenosis, spondylosis, and myeloradiculopathy by means of the posterior approach. Spine 1988; 13:864–869.

185. Whitecloud TS. Anterior surgery for cervical spondylotic myelopathy: Smith-Robinson, Cloward, and vertebrectomy. Spine 1988; 13:861–863.

186. Kurz LT, Herkowitz HN. Surgical management of myelopathy. Orthop Clin North Am 1992; 23:495–504.

187. Saunders RL, Bernini PM, Shirreffs TG, Reeves AG. Central corpectomy for cervical spondylotic myelopathy: A consecutive series with long-term follow-up evaluation. J Neurosurg 1991; 74:163–170.

188. Rowland LP. Surgical treatment of cervical spondylotic myelopathy: Time for a controlled trial. Neurology 1992; 42:5–13.

189. Lipsitz LA, Jonsson PV, Kelley MM, Koestner JS. Causes and correlates of recurrent falls in ambulatory frail elderly. J Gerontol 1991; 46:M114–122.

190. Collyer MI. Maintaining the elderly patient's mobility. Geriatr Med 1981; 11:27–30.

191. Wyke B. Cervical articular contributions to posture and gait: Their relation to senile disequilibrium. Age Ageing 1979; 8:251–258.

192. Maki BE, Holliday PJ, Topper AK. Fear of falling and postural performance in the elderly. J Gerontol 1991; 46:M123–131.

193. Mossey JM. Social and psychological factors related to falls among the elderly. Clin Geriatr Med 1985; 1:541–552.
194. Murphy J, Isaacs B. The post-fall syndrome. A study of 36 elderly patients. Gerontology 1982; 28:265–270.
195. Sloman L, Berridge M, Homatidis S, Hunter D, Duck T. Gait patterns of depressed patients and normal subjects. Am J Psychiatry 1982; 139:94–97.
196. Visser H. Gait and balance in senile dementia of Alzheimer's type. Age Ageing 1983; 12:296–301.
197. Rubenstein LZ, Robbins AS, Schulman BL, Rosado J, Osterweil D, Josephson KR. Falls and instability in the elderly. J Am Geriatr Soc 1988; 36:266–278.
198. Sudarsky L. Geriatrics: Gait disorders in the elderly. New Engl J Med 1990; 322:1441–1446.
199. Davie JW, Blumental MD, Robinson-Hawkins S. A model of risk of falling for psychogeriatric patients. Arch Gen Psychiatry 1981; 38:463–467.
200. Perry BC. Falls among the elderly: A review of the methods and conclusions of epidemiologic studies. J Am Geriatr Soc 1982; 30:367–371.
201. Prudham D, Evans JG. Factors associated with falls in the elderly: A community study. Age Ageing 1981; 10:141–146.
202. Tinetti ME, Williams TF, Mayewski R. Fall risk index for elderly patients based on number of chronic disabilities. Am J Med 1986; 80:429–434.
203. Fife TD, Baloh RW. Disequilibrium of unknown cause in older people. Ann Neurol 1993; 34:694–702.

5

Myasthenia Gravis in the Elderly

James F. Howard, Jr.
The University of North Carolina at Chapel Hill
Chapel Hill, North Carolina

I. INTRODUCTION

Myasthenia gravis (MG) is the most common primary disorder of neuromuscular transmission. In most cases the cause is an acquired immunologic abnormality, but some cases result from a variety of genetic abnormalities at the neuromuscular junction. Previously a relatively obscure disease of interest primarily to neurologists, acquired MG is now the best characterized and understood autoimmune disease. A wide range of potentially effective treatments are available, many of which have implications for the treatment of other autoimmune disorders. This chapter will focus on acquired MG with emphasis on those aspects that pertain to its diagnosis and management in the elderly. The reader is referred to recent reviews for a more comprehensive discussion of myasthenia gravis in general (1,2). Many of the observations noted in this chapter are drawn from a 20-year collaboration with colleagues since the author's training as a neurological house officer.

II. PATHOPHYSIOLOGY

The neuromuscular junction is composed of the motor nerve terminal, the synaptic cleft, and the highly organized postsynaptic region (end-plate) of the muscle membrane (Fig-

ure 1). The nerve terminal contains 180,000–200,000 synaptic
vesicles and the associated machinery necessary for the synthesis and packaging of the neurotransmitter, acetylcholine
(ACh), into each vesicle. Each quantum (the amount of ACh
contained in a single vesicle) is approximately 10,000 mol-
ecules of ACh. The normal neuromuscular junction releases
ACh from the motor nerve terminal in discrete packages or
quanta by exocytosis. The ACh quanta diffuse across the
synaptic cleft and bind to receptors on the end-plate membrane. This region is highly infolded, thus increasing the
density of acetylcholine receptors (AChR) presented to the
synaptic cleft. Stimulation of the motor nerve releases many
ACh quanta that depolarize the muscle end-plate region, producing an end-plate potential (EPP) that propagates a muscle
action potential (AP) when reaching threshold.

In acquired myasthenia gravis, the postsynaptic muscle
membrane is distorted and simplified, having lost its normal

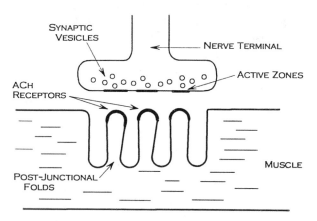

Figure 1   The normal neuromuscular junction. In acquired myasthenia gravis the muscle end-plate membrane is distorted and the
normal folded pattern on the postjunctional membrane is lost. Acetylcholine (ACh) receptors are lost from the crests of the folds and
antibodies (AChR Ab) are attached to multiple epitopes on the postsynaptic membrane.

folded shape (3–5). The concentration of functional AChR on the muscle end-plate membrane is reduced, and antibodies are attached to a number of different determinants on the membrane (6). Acetylcholine is released normally, but its effect on the postsynaptic membrane is reduced (7). The postjunctional membrane is less sensitive to applied ACh, and the probability that any nerve impulse will cause a muscle action potential is reduced.

Several observations support the concept that myasthenia gravis is an immune-mediated disease of the AChR complex. Patients with MG have an increased incidence of other presumed or known immune-mediated diseases, e.g., pernicious anemia and rheumatoid arthritis (8–10). There is a high frequency and similarity of MHC (major histocompatibility complex) antigens in patients with myasthenia gravis and other autoimmune diseases (11,12). Transient neonatal myasthenia gravis, due to the transplacental transfer of maternal immunoglobulin, occurs in 7–12% of infants born to mothers with MG (13,14). Myasthenic weakness can be improved after removal of lymph by thoracic duct drainage and worsened after reinfusion of a high-molecular-weight protein fraction from the lymph (15). Immunosuppressive treatment and plasma exchange produce improvement in most patients with myasthenia gravis (1,16–18). An animal model of myasthenia gravis, experimental autoimmune myasthenia gravis (EAMG), can be produced by immunization with purified AChR protein (19,20). Antibodies against human AChR are found in the serum of most patients with myasthenia gravis and IgG and complement components are attached to the postsynaptic end-plate membrane in myasthenic muscle (5,21). Finally, myasthenic serum or IgG produces a defect of neuromuscular transmission when injected into normal animals (22).

The role of serum antibodies against AChR in the pathophysiology of the disease is not fully understood. Antibody levels do not necessarily correlate with disease severity, and as many as 25% of patients are seronegative (1,23,24). Even seronegative patients improve after plasma exchange, and the neuromuscular abnormality can be transferred to animals by injecting serum from seronegative patients (22). The antibodies responsible for the neuromuscular abnormality may not always be those that are measured, and the serum antibody level may not reflect the amount of antibody attached to the muscle end plate.

III. EPIDEMIOLOGY

The prevalence of acquired myasthenia gravis in the United States is recently estimated to be 14 cases per 100,000 population with approximately 36,000 cases in the United States (25). Others have reported the point prevalence rate to be 1 to 12 per 100,000 (26–29). However, myasthenia gravis is probably underdiagnosed and the prevalence is more likely higher. The most common age at onset is the second and third decades in women and the seventh and eighth decades in men (Figure 2).

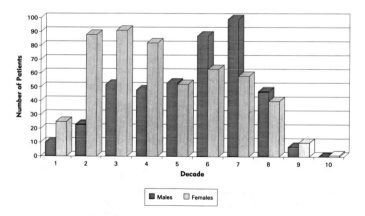

Figure 2 Decade at onset of myasthenic symptoms in 936 patients with acquired myasthenia gravis, demonstrating the preponderance of younger females and older males.

IV. CLINICAL SYMPTOMS

Patients with myasthenia gravis present to the physician complaining of specific muscle weakness and rarely of generalized fatigue (Table 1). Ptosis or diplopia are the initial symptoms of myasthenia gravis in two-thirds of patients; almost all have both symptoms within 2 years. Oropharyngeal muscle weakness—difficulty chewing, swallowing, or talking—is the initial symptom in one-sixth of patients, and isolated limb weakness initially occurs in only 10%. Initial weakness is rarely limited to single muscle groups such as neck or finger extensors or hip flexors.

The severity of weakness fluctuates during the day, usually being least severe in the morning and worse as the day progresses, especially after prolonged use of affected muscles. Ocular symptoms typically become worse while reading, watching television, or driving, especially in bright sunlight, and many patients find that wearing dark glasses reduces their

Table 1 Characteristic Symptoms and Signs in Myasthenia Gravis

Symptoms	Complaints of specific muscle weakness, rarely fatigue
	Initial complaints:
	Ptosis and diplopia in 66%
	Oropharyngeal weakness in 17%
	Limb weakness in 10%
	Fluctuating symptoms during the day
	Improvement with rest
Clinical signs	Variable weakness from examination to examination
	Asymmetrical weakness, particularly of eyelids (ptosis)
	Weakness of eye closure
	Worsening weakness with repetitive testing
	Improvement with short periods of rest

diplopia and also hides drooping eyelids. Jaw muscle weakness typically becomes worse during prolonged chewing, especially with lettuce, tough meats, or chewy candy.

Careful questioning often reveals evidence of previously unrecognized myasthenic features. Friends may have noted a sleepy or sad facial appearance caused by ptosis or facial weakness. There may have been frequent purchases of new eyeglasses to correct blurry vision, avoidance of foods that became difficult to chew or swallow, and cessation of activities that require prolonged use of specific muscles. The course of disease is variable but usually progressive. Weakness is restricted to the ocular muscles in about 10% of cases. The rest have progressive weakness during the first 2 years that involves oropharyngeal and limb muscles. Maximum weakness occurs during the first year in 66% of patients. Previous to the use of corticosteroids for treatment, approximately one-third of patients improved spontaneously, one-third became worse, and one-third died of the disease. Spontaneous improvement frequently occurred early in the course. Symptoms fluctuated over a relatively short period of time and then became progressively severe for several years (active stage) (30).

The active stage is followed by an inactive state in which fluctuations in strength still occur but are attributable to fatigue, intercurrent illness, or other identifiable factors. After 15–20 years, weakness becomes fixed and the most severely involved muscles are frequently atrophic (burned-out stage). Factors that worsen myasthenic symptoms are emotional upset, systemic illness (especially viral respiratory infections), hypothyroidism or hyperthyroidism, pregnancy, menses, increases in body temperature, and drugs affecting neuromuscular transmission.

The unusual distribution and fluctuating weakness of myasthenia gravis often suggests psychiatric illness. Many younger patients, particularly women, have been treated for periods of months to years for psychiatric problems prior to the diagnosis of myasthenia gravis (31). Conversely, ptosis and

diplopia suggest increased intracranial pressure and often lead
to unnecessary cranial imaging studies or arteriography (32).

V. CLINICAL SIGNS

The examination must be modified to demonstrate variable
weakness in specific muscle groups when examining patients
with known or suspected myasthenia gravis (Table 1).
Strength should be assessed repetitively during maximum effort and again after brief periods of rest. Performance on such
tests fluctuates in diseases other than myasthenia gravis, especially if testing causes pain. The strength fluctuations of
myasthenia gravis are best shown by tests of ocular and oropharyngeal muscle function because these are less likely to be
affected by other factors. It is easiest to classify myasthenic
patients on the basis of the distribution and severity of their
weakness (Table 2).

A. Ocular Muscles

Most patients with MG have weakness of ocular muscles.
Asymmetrical weakness of several muscles in both eyes is
typical. The pattern of weakness is not characteristic of lesions
of one or more nerves, and the pupillary responses are nor-

Table 2 Patient Classification Scheme for Myasthenia Gravis

Disease class	Distribution and severity of weakness
0	Clinical remission
I	Restricted ocular weakness
II	Mild generalized weakness usually with ocular muscle weakness
III	Predominantly oropharyngeal weakness usually with mild generalized involvement
IV	Moderate generalized weakness
V	Severe generalized weakness (respirator dependent)

mal. Weakness is most frequent and most severe in the medial rectus muscles and the inferior rectus muscle is the least involved. Ptosis is usually asymmetrical and varies during sustained activity. To compensate for ptosis, the frontalis muscle may be chronically contracted, producing a worried or surprised look. This finding may be the only visible evidence of facial weakness. The strength of eye closure is usually diminished in patients with myasthenia gravis and may be the only weakness that remains after treatment.

B. Oropharnygeal Muscles

Oropharyngeal muscle weakness causes changes in the voice, difficulty chewing and swallowing, inadequate maintenance of the upper airway, and altered facial appearance. The voice may be nasal or dysarthric, especially after prolonged talking. This can be shown by asking the patient to repeat the phrase "puh-kuh-tuh." Liquids may escape through the nose when swallowing because of palatal muscle weakness. Weakness of the laryngeal muscles causes hoarseness. This can also be shown by asking the patient to make a high-pitched "eeeee" sound. Difficulty chewing and swallowing is detected by a history of frequent choking or clearing of the throat or coughing after eating. Jaw weakness can be shown by manually opening the jaw against resistance, which is not possible in normal people, but a more important sign of jaw weakness is that the patient holds the jaw closed with the thumb under the chin, the middle finger curled under the bottom lip, and the index finger extended up the cheek, producing an attentive appearance. The loss of normal smiling may make the patient appear depressed. The characteristic myasthenic snarl results from the inability to turn the corners of the mouth upward.

C. Limb Muscles

Any trunk or limb muscle can be affected, but some are more often affected than others. Neck flexors are usually weaker than neck extensors, and the deltoids, triceps, and extensors of the wrist and fingers are frequently weaker than other limb muscles.

VI. DIFFERENTIAL DIAGNOSIS

While the differential diagnosis of MG may be extensive given the variability of presentation, practically speaking the clinical signs and symptoms of MG are characteristic and the experienced neurologist will not have difficulty making the diagnosis. There are situations in which patients with asthenia (33), conversion reactions (34), or chronic fatigue syndrome (35) will have symptoms suggestive of MG, but no true weakness can be found. In other situations, the presenting signs and symptoms will determine the degree of evaluation necessary to exclude other causes. The daily fluctuations in symptoms and signs and the asymmetry of eyelid and eye muscle weakness exclude disorders of the cranial nerves and brainstem. The few, uncommon myopathies associated with ophthalmoplegia (thyroid ophthalmopathy, oculo-cranio-somatic neuromuscular disease with ragged red fibers and oculopharyngeal dystrophy) have no fluctuation in their physical findings and minimal, if any, response to intravenous edrophonium. Thyroid eye disease may be the most problematic for the clinician as it may coexist with MG. Careful electrophysiological testing and ultrasound of the orbit may be necessary to distinguish the two.

Several other primary disorders of the neuromuscular junction may mimic myasthenia gravis. Botulism, a presynaptic disorder of ACh release, is caused by the toxin *Clostridium botulinum* (36). These patients will have involvement of pupillary function, and will not demonstrate the daily fluctuations in symptoms and signs typical of MG. The Lambert-Eaton myasthenic syndrome (LEMS) is also a presynaptic disorder of ACh release (1,37). This disorder is cause by an antibody directed against voltage-gated calcium channels on the presynaptic nerve terminal. Although there are similarities between MG and LEMS, the clinical features of the two conditions are usually distinct. The weakness in LEMS is rarely severe (i.e., class V) and in most cases the differential diagnosis would include inflammatory myopathy, cachexia, or a motor neuropathy due to paraneoplastic neuromuscular disease. Unlike patients with MG, patients will have autonomic disturbances and a reduction in muscle stretch reflexes. In some patients the clinical and electrodiagnostic features overlap with those of MG (38–40). The distinction between these two diseases is clear when small-cell carcinoma of the lung or AChR antibodies are present.

VII. THE THYMUS GLAND

Thymus gland abnormalities are clearly associated with myasthenia gravis. It is still uncertain whether the role of the thymus in the pathogenesis of myasthenia gravis is primary or secondary. Ten percent of patients with myasthenia gravis have a thymic tumor and 70% have hyperplastic changes (germinal centers) that indicate an active immune response. Because the thymus is the central organ for immunological self-tolerance, it is reasonable to suspect that thymic abnormalities mediate the breakdown in tolerance that causes an immune-mediated attack on AChR in myasthenia gravis. The thymus gland contains all the necessary elements for the pathogenesis of myasthenia gravis: myoid cells that express the AChR antigen, antigen-presenting cells, and immunocompetent T cells. Thymus tissue from patients with myasthenia gravis produces AChR antibodies when implanted into immunodeficient mice (41).

Most thymic tumors in patients with myasthenia gravis are benign, well differentiated, and encapsulated, and can be removed completely at surgery. It is unlikely that thymomas result from chronic thymic hyperactivity because myasthenia gravis can develop years after thymoma removal and the HLA haplotypes that predominate in patients with thymic hyperplasia are different from those with thymomas.

In this author's experience, patients with thymoma usually have more severe disease, higher levels of AChR antibodies, and more severe EMG abnormalities than patients without thymoma. Almost 20% of our patients with myasthenia gravis whose symptoms began between the ages of 30 and 60 years have thymoma; the frequency is much lower when symptom onset is after age 60.

VIII.   DIAGNOSTIC PROCEDURES

A.   Edrophonium (Tensilon) Test

Weakness caused by abnormal neuromuscular transmission characteristically improves after intravenous administration of edrophonium chloride, an acetylcholinesterase (AChE) inhibitor. With the exception of the ocular and pharyngeal muscles, the examiner must rely on the patient to exert maximum effort before and after drug administration to assess its effect. For this reason, the test is most reliable when the patient has ptosis or nasal speech.

Improved strength after edrophonium chloride administration is not unique to myasthenia gravis. It may also be seen in motor neuron disease where neuromuscular transmission is abnormal because of rapidly progressive denervation (42). Improved eye movements can be seen in patients with lesions of the oculomotor nerves.

The ideal dose of edrophonium chloride cannot be predetermined. A single fixed dose, such as 10 mg, may be too much in some patients and cause increased weakness. An incremental dosing schedule is recommended. Two milligrams are injected intravenously and the response is monitored for 60 seconds. Subsequent injections are 3 mg and 5 mg. If improvement is seen within 60 seconds after any dose, no further injections are given. Ten milligrams of edrophonium does not weaken normal muscle, and the occurrence of weakness after edrophonium indicates an abnormality of neuromuscular transmission. The total dose of edrophonium chloride in children is 0.15 mg/kg administered incrementally. Subcutaneous administration can be used in newborns and infants, but the response may be delayed for 2–5 minutes. An Ambu bag and oral suctioning equipment should be available when giving edrophonium since some people are supersensitive to even small dosages and may stop breathing or have excessive secretions that may interfere with respiration.

Some clinicians administer edrophonium in a blinded or double-blinded fashion to improve objectivity. This method has questionable value and is not needed when the endpoint is well defined, such as relief of ptosis.

Not all patients will respond to intravenous edrophonium chloride. Some of these patients may respond to intramuscular neostigmine, because of the longer duration of action. Intramuscular neostigmine is particularly useful in infants and children whose response to intravenous edrophonium chloride may be too brief for adequate observation. In some patients, a therapeutic trial of daily oral pyridostigmine may produce improvement that cannot be appreciated after a single dose of edrophonium chloride or neostigmine.

Techniques that show a more objective effect of cholinesterase inhibitors on ocular muscles are EMG of the ocular muscles, tonometry, oculography, and Lancaster red-green tests of ocular motility (43–45). These tests increase sensitivity to detect a neuromuscular abnormality, but are nonspecific and cannot be recommended.

B. Acetylcholine Receptor Antibodies

Seventy-six percent of our patients with acquired generalized myasthenia and 54% with ocular myasthenia have serum antibodies that bind human AChR. The serum concentration of AChR antibody varies widely among patients with similar degrees of weakness and is not an indicator of the severity of disease in individual patients (1). Approximately 10% of patients who do not have binding antibodies have other antibodies that modulate the turnover of AChR in tissue culture. The concentration of binding antibodies may be low at symptom onset and become elevated later. Repeat studies are appropriate when initial values are normal. AChR-binding antibody concentrations are sometimes increased in patients with systemic lupus erythematosus, inflammatory neuropathy, amyotrophic lateral sclerosis, rheumatoid arthritis who are taking D-penicillamine, thymoma without myasthenia gravis, and in normal relatives of patients with myasthenia gravis. False positive may occur when blood is drawn within 48 hours of a surgical procedure involving the use of general anesthesia and muscle relaxants. In general, an elevated concentration of AChR-binding antibodies in a patient with compatible clinical features confirms the diagnosis of myasthenia gravis, but normal antibody concentrations do not exclude the diagnosis.

Nearly one-quarter of patients with acquired immune-mediated myasthenia gravis do not have detectable serum antibodies against AChR-Ab (1). Seronegative patients are more likely to be male and to have milder disease, ocular myasthenia gravis, fewer thymomas, less frequent thymic hyperplasia, and more frequent thymic atrophy. In seronegative patients, the diagnosis is based on the clinical presentation, the response to AChE inhibitors, and electrodiagnostic findings. Genetic myasthenia must be considered in all childhood-onset seronegative myasthenia gravis. The treatment of seronegative, acquired myasthenia gravis is the same as for seropositive patients. The absence of AChR antibodies does not necessarily mean that an unsatisfactory response to immunosuppression, plasma exchange, or thymectomy is expected.

C. Electrodiagnosis

The basis of the clinical electrodiagnostic abnormalities in patients with MG is the failure of the muscle fiber to depolarize sufficiently enough for the EPP to reach AP threshold (46). The resulting impulse blocking accounts for the decremental responses seen on repetitive nerve stimulation (RNS) studies and the impulse blocking seen with single-fiber EMG

(SFEMG). In addition, the time variability of when the EPP reaches AP threshold accounts for the neuromuscular jitter seen in the latter technique. Besides their diagnostic utility, serial measurements can be useful in following the course of disease and in assessing the effect of treatment (47,48).

1. *Needle EMG*

It is necessary to perform needle electrode EMG examinations in patients suspected of MG to exclude diseases that may mimic or coexist with MG such as inflammatory (49), thyroid (50), ocular myopathies (51) or peripheral neuropathies (52). In the absence of other neuromuscular disorders, the EMG examination may demonstrate motor unit action potentials that vary in their configuration with consecutive discharges.

2. *Repetitive nerve stimulation*

The RNS test is the most frequently used electrodiagnostic test of neuromuscular transmission (46). Abnormal results from RNS studies are not diagnostic of MG, and abnormalities may be detected by this technique in patients with multiple sclerosis (53), motor neuron disease (54), peripheral neuropathy (55), radiculopathy (56), primary muscle membrane disease (57), as well as other disorders of neuromuscular transmission (58, 59). The amplitude of the compound muscle action potential (CMAP) elicited by nerve stimulation is normal or only slightly reduced. The amplitude of the fourth or fifth response to a train of low-frequency nerve stimuli falls at least 10% from the initial value (Figure 3A). This decrementing response to RNS is seen more often in proximal muscles, such as the facial and trapezius muscles, than in hand muscles. We have found a significant decrement to RNS in either a hand or shoulder muscle in 70% of patients with generalized myasthenia but in less than 50% of patients with ocular MG (46).

3. *Single-fiber EMG*

Neuromuscular jitter, the variation in the time interval between pairs of muscle fiber action potentials (APs), is a sensitive measure of the safety factor of neuromuscular transmis-

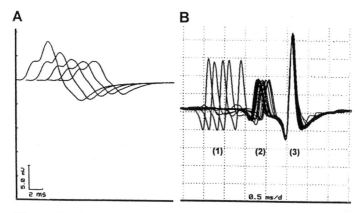

Figure 3   The characteristic electrodiagnostic features found in patients with myasthenia gravis demonstrating the abnormalities of neuromuscular transmission. **A.** The typical abnormal decrement seen on repetitive nerve stimulation (RNS) study. Note the normal compound muscle action potential amplitude (first response) and the greater than 10% decrement between the 1st and 5th responses. **B.** Single-fiber EMG (SFEMG) recordings from the extensor digitorum communis muscle of a myasthenic patient. Note the triggered potential (#3), increased neuromuscular jitter (potential #2), and increased jitter with impulse blocking (potential #1).

sion. It is increased whenever the ratio between the AP threshold and the end-plate potential is greater than normal. SFEMG is the most sensitive clinical test of neuromuscular transmission and shows increased jitter in some muscles in almost all patients with myasthenia gravis (46,60). When neuromuscular transmission is sufficiently impaired, nerve impulses fail to elicit muscle APs and SFEMG demonstrates intermittent impulse blocking (Figure 3B). When blocking occurs in many end-plates in a muscle there is clinical weakness. Jitter varies among different end-plates in a muscle, even among several end-plates within one muscle and from muscle to muscle. It is greatest in weak, proximal muscles. However, SFEMG can demonstrate abnormal neuromuscular transmission (as increased jitter) in muscles that are clinically normal and have no decrement to repetitive nerve stimulation. Patients with mild or purely ocular muscle weakness may have increased jitter only in facial muscles.

Increased jitter is a nonspecific sign of abnormal neuromuscular transmission and can be seen in other motor unit diseases (61). Therefore, increased jitter requires conventional needle EMG to exclude neuronopathy, neuropathy, and myopathy. Normal jitter in a weak muscle excludes abnormal neuromuscular transmission as the cause of weakness (60).

D. Comparison of Diagnostic Techniques

Intravenous edrophonium chloride is often diagnostic in patients with ptosis or ophthalmoparesis, but is less useful when other muscles are weak. Elevated serum concentrations of AChR-binding antibodies virtually assure the diagnosis of myasthenia gravis, but normal concentrations do not exclude the diagnosis (1). Repetitive nerve stimulation confirms impaired neuromuscular transmission but is not specific to myasthenia gravis and is frequently normal in patients with mild or purely ocular disease (46,60). The measurement of jitter by SFEMG is the most sensitive clinical test of neuromuscular transmission and is abnormal in nearly all patients with myasthenia gravis if the appropriate muscles are examined (46,60). A normal test in a weak muscle excludes the diagnosis of myasthenia gravis, but an abnormal test can occur when other motor unit disorders cause defects in neuromuscular transmission.

IX. TREATMENT

A controlled clinical trial has never been reported for any medical or surgical modality used to treat MG. All recommended regimens are empirical and experts disagree on treatments of choice. Treatment decisions must be individualized and based on knowledge of the natural history of disease and the predicted response to a specific form of therapy (62). Treatment goals will be different for each patient and must be established according to the severity of disease, the patient's age and sex, and the degree of functional impairment. The response to any form of treatment is difficult to assess because the severity of symptoms fluctuates. Spontaneous improvement, even remissions, occur without specific therapy, especially during the early stages of the disease.

A. Cholinesterase Inhibitors

Acetylcholinesterase inhibitors (AChE) (Table 3) retard the enzymatic hydrolysis of ACh at cholinergic synapses so that ACh accumulates at the neuromuscular junction and its duration of effect is prolonged (63). Acetylcholinesterase inhibitors may produce significant improvement in some patients and little to none in others (1,62). These drugs produce a differential response, that is, different muscles respond differ-

Table 3 Acetylcholinesterase Inhibitors in Myasthenia Gravis

Advantages	Produce *symptomatic* improvement in most patients
	No proven chronic side effects
	Physician familiarity
Disadvantages	Differential response
	Prone to over- and underdosage
	Frequent side effects, even at therapeutic levels
	Never makes strength normal
	Requires close medical supervision
	Usually become less effective with time
Major role	As a diagnostic test
	Early *symptomatic* treatment in most patients
	May be satisfactory chronic treatment in some patients
	Adjunctive therapy in the majority of patients undergoing more definitive therapy

ently; with any dose, certain muscles get stronger, others do not change, and still others become weaker. Strength rarely returns to normal. Pyridostigmine bromide (Mestinon) and neostigmine bromide (Prostigmin) are the most commonly used AChE inhibitors. Pyridostigmine is generally preferred because it has a lower frequency of gastrointestinal side effects. The initial oral dose in adults is 30–60 mg every 6–8 hours. The equivalent dose of neostigmine is 7.5–15 mg. Equivalent dosages of these drugs are listed in Table 4. Pyridostigmine is available as a syrup (60 mg/5 ml) for nasogastric tube administration in patients with impaired swallowing. A timed-release tablet of pyridostigmine (Mestinon Timespan, 180 mg) has been recommended as a bedtime dose for patients who are too weak to swallow in the morning. However, its absorption is erratic, leading to possible overdosage and underdosage, and it may be preferable for the patient to awaken at the appropriate dosing interval and take the regular tablet. Neostigmine and pyridostigmine can be administered by nasal spray or nebulizer to patients who cannot tolerate or swallow oral medications.

Table 4 Equivalent Doses of Acetylcholinesterase Inhibitors

	Route and dose (mg)			
	Oral	Intramuscular	Syrup	Intravenous
Neostigmine bromide (Prostigmin)	15			
Neostigmine methylsulfate (Prostigmin)		0.5	0.5	
Pyridostigmine bromide (Mestinon)	60	2.0	0.7	60 mg/5 ml
Mestinon Timespan	90–180			
Ambenonium chloride (Mytelase)	7.5			

Note: These dosages are approximations only. The appropriate dosages should be determined for each patient based on the clinical response.

No fixed dosage schedule will suit all patients. The need for ACh inhibitors varies from day to day and during the same day in response to emotional stress, infection, menstruation, and hot weather. The drug schedule should be titrated to produce an optimal response in muscles causing the greatest disability. Patients with oropharyngeal weakness need doses timed to provide optimal strength during meals. Ideally, the effect of each dose should last until time for the next, without significant underdosing or overdosing at any time. In practice, this is not possible. Attempts to eliminate all weakness by increasing the dose or shortening the interval cause overdosage at the time of peak effect. Our goal is to keep the dose low enough to provide definite improvement 30–45 minutes later, and for the effect to wear off before the next one is given. This minimizes the possibility that the dose will be increased to the point of causing cholinergic weakness.

The practice of giving edrophonium at the time when pyridostigmine has its maximal effect, to determine if the patient will respond to greater dosages of AChE inhibitors, is dangerous. Acute overdosage may cause cholinergic weakness of respiratory muscles and apnea and muscarinic toxicity with bronchorrhea.

Adverse effects of AChE inhibitors may result from ACh accumulation at muscarinic receptors on smooth muscle and autonomic glands and at nicotinic receptors of skeletal muscle (Table 5). Gastrointestinal complaints are common: queasiness, loose stools, nausea, vomiting, abdominal cramps, and diarrhea. Increased bronchial and oral secretions are a serious problem in patients with swallowing or respiratory insufficiency. Central nervous system side effects are rarely seen with the doses used to treat MG. Symptoms of muscarinic overdosage may indicate that nicotinic overdosage (weakness) is also occurring. Gastrointestinal side effects can be controlled with atropine, glycopyrrolate, loperamide, propantheline, and diphenoxylate. Some of these drugs can produce weakness at high dosage. Bromism, presenting as acute psychosis, is a rare complication in patients taking large amounts

Table 5 Side Effects of Acetylcholinesterase Inhibitors

Nicotinic receptors	
Skeletal muscle	Muscle fasciculations
	Muscle weakness
Muscarinic receptors	
Smooth muscle	Abdominal queasiness, cramps
	Loose stools, diarrhea
	Nausea, vomiting
Autonomic glands	Increased salivation, lacrimation
	and bronchial secretions
Central nervous system	Anxiety, irritability, insomnia
(rare)	Mental clouding, coma
	Seizures

of pyridostigmine bromide. Some patients are allergic to bromide and develop a rash even at modest doses.

B. Corticosteroids

Marked improvement or complete relief of symptoms occurs in more than 75% of patients treated with prednisone, and some improvement occurs in most of the rest (Table 6) (18, 64,65). Much of the improvement occurs in the first 6–8 weeks, but strength may increase to total remission in the months that follow. The best responses occur in patients with recent onset of symptoms, but patients with chronic disease may also respond. The severity of disease does not predict the ultimate improvement. Patients with thymoma have an excellent response to prednisone before or after removal of the tumor.

The most predictable response to prednisone occurs when treatment begins with a daily dose of 1.5–2 mg/kg/day (18). This dose is given until sustained improvement occurs, which is usually within 2 weeks, and is then switched to an alternate daily schedule beginning with 100–120 mg. This dose is gradually decreased over many months to the lowest dose neces-

Table 6 Corticosteroids in Myasthenia Gravis

Advantages	Produce rapid improvement in most patients
	Produce total remission or marked improvement in 90% of patients (high-dose, daily steroids)
	Predictable time of response
	Relatively simple drug schedule
	Reduce the morbidity and mortality of subsequent thymectomy
Disadvantages	Steroid side effects
	Exacerbation of weakness after initiation
	Requires chronic administration for maximum benefit
Major role	As initial definitive therapy, producing rapid, virtually complete improvement in the majority of patients
	As secondary treatment, producing improvement in most patients who fail to respond to thymectomy or other immunosuppressive therapy

sary to maintain improvement, which is usually less than 20 mg every other day. The rate of decrease must be individualized: patients who have a prompt, complete response to prednisone can reduce the alternate-day dose by 20 mg each month until the dose is 60 mg, then by 10 mg each month until the dose is 20 mg every other day, then by 5 mg every 3 months to a minimal dose of 10 mg every other day. Most patients who respond well to prednisone become weak if the drug is stopped but maintain strength on very low dosages (5–10 mg qod). For this reason, we do not reduce the dose further. Others recommend discontinuing prednisone if the patient is doing well after 2 years. In our experience, weakness ultimately returns if this is done.

About one-half of patients become weaker temporarily after starting prednisone, usually within the first 7–10 days, and lasting for up to 6 days (18). This worsening can usually be managed with AChE inhibitors. In patients with oropharyngeal weakness or respiratory insufficiency, we use plasma exchange before beginning prednisone to prevent or reduce the severity of steroid-induced exacerbations and produce a more rapid response. Because initial high-dose prednisone may exacerbate weakness, patients with oropharyngeal or respiratory involvement should be hospitalized to start treatment. Once improvement begins, further exacerbations are unusual. Treatment can be started at low dose to minimize exacerbations; the dose is then slowly increased until improvement occurs (66). Exacerbations may also occur with this approach and the response is less predictable.

The preceding prednisone regimen can be used for both generalized and purely ocular myasthenia. An alternative approach in treating ocular myasthenia is to begin with 5 or 10 mg of daily prednisone and increase the dose 5 mg every 3–4 weeks until improvement begins. The dose is then kept constant until maximum improvement is achieved, and then tapered over 4–6 months to a maintenance dose of 5–10 mg every other day.

The major disadvantages of chronic corticosteroid therapy are the side effects (18). Hypercorticism occurs in about half of patients treated with the suggested regimen. The severity and frequency of adverse reactions increase when high daily doses are continued for more than one month. Fortunately, this is rarely necessary, especially if plasma exchange is begun at the same time as prednisone. Most side effects begin resolving as prednisone is tapered and become minimal at doses less than 20 mg every other day. Side effects are minimized when patients take supplemental calcium. Postmenopausal women should also take supplementary vitamin D (67). Patients with peptic ulcer disease or symptoms of gastritis need H_2 antagonists or frequent antacids. Prednisone should not be given to people with tuberculosis. Prednisone may be given with azathioprine if either drug is ineffective alone (see below).

C. Immunosuppressive Drugs

Azathioprine improves myasthenic symptoms in most patients, but the effect is delayed 4–8 months (Table 7) (17,62,68). The initial dose is 50 mg/day, which is increased in 50 mg/day increments every 7 days to a total of 150–200 mg/day. Once improvement begins, it is maintained for as long as the drug is given, but symptoms recur 2–3 months after the drug is discontinued or the dose is reduced below therapeutic levels (69). Patients who fail corticosteroids may respond to azathioprine and the reverse is also true. Some respond better to treatment with both drugs than to either alone. Because the response to azathioprine is delayed, both drugs may be started simultaneously with the intent of rapidly tapering prednisone when azathioprine becomes effective.

Approximately one-third of patients have mild dose-dependent side effects that may require dose reductions but do not require stopping treatment (Cui L, Sanders DB, Howard JF, unpublished data) (70–72). Gastrointestinal irritation can be minimized by using divided doses after meals or by dose reduction. Leukopenia and even pancytopenia can occur any time during treatment. The blood count must be monitored every week during the first month, each month for a year, and

Table 7 Immunosuppressive Drugs in Myasthenia Gravis

Advantages	Produce marked, sustained improvement in most patients
Disadvantages	May be long delay before improvement
	Serious side effects
Major role	As initial definitive therapy in patients with late-onset myasthenia gravis or in whom corticosteroids are contraindicated
	As secondary treatment in patients who fail to respond to corticosteroids or thymectomy
	In combination with prednisone to enhance the response or to permit more rapid reduction of prednisone dose

every 3–6 months thereafter. If the peripheral white blood count falls below 3500 cells/cu mm, the dose should be temporarily reduced and then gradually increased after the white blood count rises above 3500 cells/cu mm. Counts below 1000 WBC/cu mm require that the drug be temporarily discontinued. Serum transaminase concentrations may be slightly elevated, but clinical liver toxicity is rare. Treatment should be discontinued if transaminase concentrations exceed twice the upper limit of normal and the drug should be restarted at lower doses when normal values are obtained. Because azathioprine is potentially mutagenic, females of child-bearing age should practice adequate contraception. A severe allergic reaction, with flu-like symptoms and rash, may occur within 2 weeks after starting treatment, which requires that the drug be stopped.

Cyclosporine inhibits predominantly T-lymphocyte-dependent immune responses and is sometimes beneficial in treating myasthenia gravis (73–75). Treatment is begun with 5–6 mg/kg/day, in two divided doses taken 12 hours apart. Serum concentrations of cyclosporine and creatinine should be measured monthly, and the dose should be adjusted to produce a trough serum cyclosporine concentration of 75–150 ng/ml and a serum creatinine concentration less than 150% of pretreatment values. The needed dose decreases after tissue saturation is achieved. We usually give 10–20 mg prednisone every other day with cyclosporine to maximize the response.

Most patients with myasthenia gravis improve 1–2 months after starting cyclosporine and improvement is maintained as long as therapeutic doses are given. Maximum improvement is achieved 6 months or longer after starting treatment. After achieving the maximal response, the dose is gradually reduced to the minimum that maintains improvement. Renal toxicity and hypertension, the important adverse reactions of cyclosporine, are usually avoided or managed using the regimen provided. Many drugs interfere with cyclosporine metabolism and should be avoided or used with caution (76).

Cyclophosphamide has been used intravenously and orally for the treatment of myasthenia gravis (77). The intravenous dose is 200 mg/day for 5 days and the oral dose is 150–200 mg/day to a total of 5–10 grams as required to relieve symptoms. More than half of patients become asymptomatic after one year. Side effects are common; alopecia is most frequent. Leukopenia, nausea, vomiting, anorexia, hemorrhagic cystitis, and discoloration of the nails and skin occur less frequently.

Life-threatening infections are an important risk in the immunosuppressed and most commonly occurs in patients with invasive thymoma. However, disseminated cytomegalovirus (CMV) (78) and *Pneumocystis carinii* (PCP) (Howard JF, personal observation) have occurred in patients taking multiple immunosuppressive drugs. The long-term risk of malignancy is not established, but there are no reports of an increased incidence of malignancy in patients with myasthenia gravis receiving immunosuppression.

D. Thymectomy

Thymectomy is recommended for most patients with myasthenia gravis (Table 8) (79). Most reports do not correlate the severity of weakness before surgery and the timing or

Table 8 Thymectomy in Myasthenia Gravis

Advantages	May produce long-lasting improvement in most patients
	No known chronic side effects
	Excludes or removes thymomas
Disadvantages	Frequent long delay before improvement
	Total remission is rare
	Operative morbidity and mortality
Major role	Potentially beneficial in all patients with a life expectancy of more than 10 years or in whom a thymoma is suspected

degree of improvement after thymectomy. The maximal favorable response generally occurs 2–5 years after surgery, presumably due to the presence of circulating memory cells. However, the response is relatively unpredictable and significant impairment may continue for months or years after surgery. Sometimes, improvement is only appreciated in retrospect. The best responses to thymectomy are in young people early in the course of their disease, but improvement can occur even after 30 years of symptoms. In our experience, patients with disease onset after the age of 60 rarely show substantial improvement from thymectomy. Patients with thymomas do not respond as well to thymectomy as do patients without thymoma.

The preferred surgical approach is through a sternotomy with exploration of the anterior mediastinum (80–82). Transcervical and endoscopic approaches have less postoperative morbidity, but do not allow sufficient exposure for total thymic removal (83,84). In our experience, the operative morbidity from transthoracic thymectomy is minimal when patients are optimally prepared with plasma exchange or immunosuppression and skilled postoperative management is provided. Extubation is usually accomplished in the operating room and patients may be discharged home as early as the third or fourth postoperative day.

Repeat thymectomy provides significant improvement in some patients with chronic, refractory disease (85,86) and should be considered when there is concern that all thymic tissue was not removed at prior surgery and when a good response to the original surgery is followed by later relapse.

E. Plasma Exchange

Plasma exchange is used as a short-term intervention for patients with sudden worsening of myasthenic symptoms for any reason, to rapidly improve strength before surgery, and as a chronic intermittent treatment for patients who are refractory to all other treatments (Table 9). The need for plasma ex-

Table 9 Plasma Exchange in Myasthenia Gravis

Advantages	Produces rapid improvement in most patients
	No known chronic side effects
Disadvantages	Expensive
	Requires concomitant immunosuppression, corticosteroids, or thymectomy for long-lasting benefit
Major role	Adjunctive therapy, most useful in:
	Patients who have failed to respond to other forms of treatment
	Producing rapid improvement before thymectomy or other surgery or in myasthenic crisis
	Initiating improvement that may be maintained by other forms of immunotherapy

change and its frequency of use are determined by the clinical response in the individual patient.

Almost all patients with acquired myasthenia gravis improve temporarily following plasma exchange (16). A typical protocol of plasma exchange is to remove 2–3 liters of plasma three times a week until improvement plateaus, usually after five or six exchanges. Improvement begins within 48 hours of the first exchange. Maximum improvement may be reached after the first exchange or as late as the fourteenth. Improvement lasts for weeks or months and then the effect is lost unless the exchange is followed by thymectomy or immunosuppressive therapy. Most patients who respond to the first plasma exchange will respond again to subsequent courses. Repeated exchanges do not have a cumulative benefit.

Adverse reactions to plasma exchange include transitory hypotension and cardiac arrhythmias, nausea, lightheadedness, chills, visual obscurations, and pedal edema (16). Other reactions occur in specific situations: thromboses, thrombophlebitis, and subacute bacterial endocarditis when arteriovenous shunts or grafts are placed for vascular access; an influenza-like illness in patients with reduced immunoglobulin levels; and severe bacterial and systemic cytomegalovirus infections in patients being treated with cyclophosphamide (62,87).

F. Intravenous Immune Globulin

Many patients will have significant improvement in strength high-dose (2 grams/kg infused over 2–5 days) IVIG (88–90). The most likely mechanisms of action are downregulation of antibodies directed against AChR and the introduction of anti-idiotypic antibodies (91). The indications for IVIG are similar to those for plasma exchange. With further experience, IVIG may prove to be an effective alternative to plasma exchange, especially in patients with poor vascular access. Improvement occurs in 50–100% of patients, usually beginning within 1 week and lasting for several weeks or months (Table 10) (89).

The common side effects of IVIG are related to the rate of infusion, and include headaches, chills, and fever. These reactions can be reduced by giving acetaminophen or aspirin with Benadryl before each infusion. Severe reactions such as alopecia, aseptic meningitis, leukopenia, and retinal necrosis are rare and reported in patients receiving IVIG for diseases

Table 10 Intravenous Immunoglobulin in Myasthenia Gravis

Advantages	Produces fairly rapid improvement (slower than plasma exchange) in most patients
Disadvantages	Expensive
	Requires concomitant immunosuppression, corticosteroids, or thymectomy for long-lasting benefit
	Potentially serious side effects
Major role	Adjunctive therapy, most useful in patients who have failed to respond to other forms of treatment
	May be used as chronic maintenance therapy

other than myasthenia gravis (92–94). Renal failure may occur in patients with impaired renal function (95,96). Vascu-
lar-like headaches are often sufficiently severe to limit the use
of IVIG, but we find that the headaches can sometimes be
managed by giving intravenous dihydroergotamine before and
immediately after the IVIG infusion (Howard, JF, personal
observation). IVIG is contraindicated in patients with selective IgA deficiency as they may develop anaphylaxis to the
IgA in immune globulin preparations. Immunoglobulin levels
are obtained in all patients prior to starting IVIG therapy in
order to detect such conditions. Human immunodeficiency
virus is not known to be transmitted by IVIG; transmission of
hepatitis C by IVIG has been reported in Europe but not in
the United States (97).

G. Miscellaneous Treatments

Ephedrine can be useful when AChE inhibitors alone are not
effective (98). Many myasthenic patients complain of increased weakness when their serum potassium level is low or
at low-normal values (62,99). Replacement therapy to maintain a serum potassium level in the mid-4.0 range is often
reported by the patient to be helpful. Splenectomy, splenic
radiation, and total body irradiation have been used with partial or transient success in a small number of patients who
failed all other forms of immunotherapy (100,101). The amin-
opyridines facilitate neurotransmitter release at central and
peripheral synapses. They produce significant and sometimes
dramatic improvement in acquired myasthenia gravis, especially when used in combination with pyridostigmine (102,
103). Confusion and seizures are the side effects that limit the
use of 4-aminopyridine; 3,4-diaminopyridine has less central
toxicity but is not commercially available.

Guanidine hydrochloride also facilitates the release of
ACh at the neuromuscular junction and can produce transient
improvement in patients with MG. However, because of the
serious side effects that occur with chronic administration, its
use cannot be recommended.

X. CAVEATS FOR THE ELDERLY MYASTHENIC
     PATIENT

Numerous age-related changes of the peripheral nerve, neu-romuscular junction, and muscle have been described in ani-mal models and humans. In the elderly, these include some slowing of conduction velocity (104), a reduction in the num-ber of functioning motor units (105), and some change in the morphology of the neuromuscular junction (106). Quantitative measures of muscle strength have shown a modest reduction in peak strength with aging (107). There is no known role of these observations in the development, severity, and distribu-tion of weakness in patients with myasthenia gravis.

A. Demographics

Previous studies showed that women were more often affected than men (108). As Figure 4 shows, the previously reported female preponderance has changed and now males are more often affected than females. Further, as the population has aged in the last 40 years, the average age at onset has in-creased correspondingly (Figure 5). The reasons for these observations remain unclear.

B. Diagnosis

The diagnostic approach for the patient suspected of MG is the same regardless of age. Edrophonium tests must be per-formed carefully in the elderly. There are anecdotal reports of the precipitation of atrial arrhythmias and syncope in pa-tients receiving a bolus of this drug. The electrodiagnostic findings must be interpreted in light of any underlying abnor-mality such as neuropathy or radiculopathy. Decremental re-sponses with repetitive nerve stimulation have been demon-strated in patients with cervical radiculopathy and neuropathy and SFEMG recordings may be abnormal in patients with axonal neuropathy (see above). Previous reports that serum AChR antibodies occur in high frequency in elderly nonmyas-

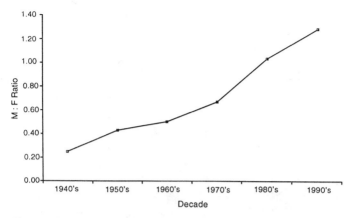

Figure 4 The changing male-to-female ratio in 936 patients with acquired myasthenia gravis. Prior to the 1980s there was a female preponderance and over the last 12 years a male preponderance.

thenic Japanese (109) have not been demonstrated by others (110,111). The reasons for this are not clear and may be related to genetic or environmental differences between the populations. It is our feeling that the presence of antibody to the acetylcholine receptor is diagnostic of MG.

C. Association of Myasthenia Gravis with Other Diseases

There are numerous reports of associations of MG with other immune-mediated diseases (112), especially hyperthyroidism (113), rheumatoid arthritis (114), and systemic lupus erythematosus (115). Twenty percent of our myasthenic patients have another disease: 7% have diabetes mellitus before corticosteroid treatment, 6% have thyroid disease, 3% have nonthymus neoplasm, and less than 2% have rheumatoid arthritis. In addition, many elderly patients will have diseases that may impact on the management of their MG because of a predisposition to treatment-induced side effects. Careful

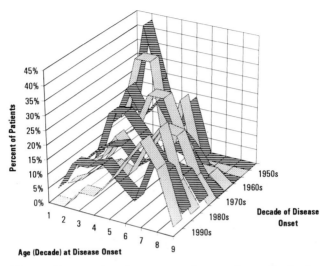

Figure 5 The changing pattern of age and sex distributions of acquired myasthenia gravis (MG) in 10-year intervals from the 1950s through 1994 (y-axis). Stippled ribbons represent males; diagonal ribbons represent females. Age at disease onset is by decade (e.g., 1 = birth through 10 years, 2 = age 11 through age 20, etc.). The z-axis represents the percent of patients of a given sex for a given 10-year interval (x-axis). For example, the first stippled and diagonal ribbons represent the percent of male and female patients acquiring MG in decades in the 1990s.

thought must be given to the treatment goals and the potential risks.

D. Treatment of Associated Diseases

The effect of concomitant diseases and their treatment (see below) on myasthenic symptoms is an important consideration. Thyroid disease should be vigorously treated since both hypo- and hyperthyroidism can adversely affect myasthenic weakness. Intercurrent infections require immediate attention because they exacerbate myasthenia gravis and can be life-threatening in patients who are immunosuppressed.

E. Adverse Drug Reactions

Patients with disorders of neuromuscular transmission may experience worsening of their strength following the administration of a variety of therapeutic agents (116). In all instances there is a further reduction in the safety factor of neuromuscular transmission. With the exception of D-penicillamine, there are no drugs absolutely contraindicated in patients with MG. Although it is desirable to avoid certain drugs, in some cases they must be used to manage other conditions. In such instances they must be used with caution, and a thorough knowledge by the physician of the deleterious side effects can minimize their potential danger (Table 11). Competitive neuromuscular blocking agents, such as pancuronium and *d*-tubocurarine, have an exaggerated and prolonged response in patients with MG. Depolarizing blocking agents such as succinylcholine have similar effects on myasthenic weakness. Many antibiotics, particularly the aminoglycosides

Table 11   Drug Alert for Patients with Myasthenia Gravis

- D-penicillamine should never be used in myasthenic patients.
- The following drugs produce worsening of myasthenic weakness in most patients who receive them. Use with caution and monitor patient for exacerbation of myasthenic symptoms.
  - Neuromuscular blocking agents: e.g., pancuronium, *d*-tubocurarine, or succinylcholine
  - Quinine, quinidine, or procainamide
  - Antibiotics, particularly the aminoglycosides (gentamicin, kanamycin, neomycin, or streptomycin) and erythromycin
  - Beta-blockers: e.g., propranolol, nadolol, and timolol and betalol eyedrops
  - Calcium channel blockers
  - Local anesthetics (in large dosages)
- Many other drugs are reported to exacerbate the weakness in some patients with myasthenia gravis (116). All patients with myasthenia gravis should be observed for increased weakness whenever a new medication is started.

and erythromycin, may also potentiate myasthenic weakness (117). If corticosteroids are needed to treat concomitant illness, the potential adverse and beneficial effects on myasthenia gravis must be anticipated and explained to the patient.

Glaucoma, coronary artery or peripheral vascular disease, and hypertension are common in the aging myasthenic population. Treatment of these disorders is problematic for the patient with MG (116). Unwittingly, these patients are often given beta- (118,119) or calcium-channel blockers (120) or quinidine (121) by their physicians, not recognizing that these drugs have the potential for markedly worsening myasthenic weakness. Alternative treatments should be used, but if these drugs must be prescribed, patients must be monitored closely for any change in their clinical examination.

F. Treatment

As with any patient with MG, the treatment plan must be individualized according to the patient's needs, underlying illness, reliability, etc. Careful attention must be paid to the complications of myasthenic treatment modalities and their interactions with other medical problems and vice versa. For example, diuretic-induced hypokalemia, resulting from treatment of hypertension, may aggravate myasthenic weakness. The hypokalemia may be accentuated in patients receiving prednisone as treatment for their MG. Treatment with intravenous immunoglobulin has the potential for precipitating or worsening congestive heart failure due to the osmotic actions of a high protein load. The following protocols have been established to treat patients with myasthenia gravis.

1.   *Ocular myasthenia*

Most patients are initially treated with AChE inhibitors. If the response is unsatisfactory, prednisone is added. Many of these patients will respond to low-dose daily or alternate-day prednisone. The development of weakness in muscles other than the ocular or periocular muscles moves them to the generalized MG treatment protocol.

2. *Generalized myasthenia, onset after age 60*

Life expectancy and concurrent illness are important considerations in developing a treatment plan in this population. Whereas younger patients are treated with thymectomy with or without immunosuppressive therapy, the initial treatment in the elderly patient is usually AChE inhibitors for symptomatic treatment. If the response is unsatisfactory, azathioprine is begun in patients who can tolerate a delay before responding. If treatment with azathioprine is unsatisfactory, high-dose daily prednisone can be added. It is preferable not to start with prednisone because of the possibility of osteoporosis. Cyclosporine can also be used as long as the patient does not have significant hypertension or renal disease. High-dose daily prednisone is used as the first drug, with or without plasma exchange, in patients who need a rapid response. Azathioprine is added to prednisone if the response to prednisone alone is not satisfactory or unacceptable weakness develops as the prednisone dose is reduced.

3. *Thymoma*

Thymectomy is indicated in all patients with thymoma. Patients should be pretreated with immunosuppressive drugs, with or without plasma exchange, until maximal improvement is attained. Postoperative radiation is used if tumor resection is incomplete or if the tumor has spread beyond the tumor capsule. Medical treatment is then the same as for patients without thymoma. Elderly patients with small tumors, who are not good candidates for surgery because of other health problems, can be managed medically while monitoring tumor size radiologically.

G. Other Considerations

Annual immunization against influenza is recommended for all patients with myasthenia gravis, and immunization against pneumococcus is recommended before starting prednisone or other immunosuppressive drugs. Immunization after the patient has been on significant dosages of prednisone or other immunosuppressive drugs raises the possibility that the immunization will not be effective.

H. Special Situations

1. *Myasthenic and cholinergic crisis*

Myasthenic crisis is respiratory failure from worsening myasthenia. Patients in myasthenic crisis who previously had well-compensated respiratory function usually have a definable precipitating event, such as infection, surgery, or the rapid tapering or discontinuation of their immunosuppressive therapy.

Cholinergic crisis is respiratory failure from an overdosage of AChE inhibitors. It was more common before the introduction of immunosuppressive therapy when very large dosages of AChE inhibitors were used. Respiratory failure of any cause is a medical emergency and requires prompt intubation and ventilatory support.

In theory, it should be easy to determine if a patient is weak because of too little or too much AChE inhibitor, but in practice this is often very difficult. Administration of edrophonium chloride should distinguish overdose from underdose, but its use in crisis is dangerous unless the patient is already intubated and ventilated, and an apprehensive patient cannot fully cooperate with the test. Further, edrophonium chloride may make some muscles stronger and others weaker. The safest approach to crisis is to admit the patient to an intensive care unit, discontinue all AChE inhibitors, and ventilate the patient. AChE inhibitors should be resumed at low doses and slowly increased as needed.

2. *Anesthetic management*

The stress of surgery and some drugs used perioperatively may worsen myasthenic weakness. As a rule, local or spinal anesthesia is preferred over inhalation anesthesia. However, local anesthetics, which also have neuromuscular blocking properties, are not without risk, particularly in the patient with generalized weakness. Neuromuscular blocking agents should not be used and, if necessary, used sparingly. Adequate muscle relaxation can usually be produced by inhalation anesthetic agents alone. The required dose of depolarizing blocking agents may be greater than needed in nonmyasthenic patients, but low doses of nondepolarizing agents cause pronounced and long-lasting blockade that require prolonged postoperative-assisted respiration.

Dental procedures requiring local anesthetic can be safely performed by using short-acting preparations in conjunction with a vasoconstrictive agent, e.g., Carbocaine. Interligamentous injections are preferred, thus minimizing the systemic absorption of the anesthetic agent and reducing the chance of exacerbating myasthenic weakness.

3. *Penicillamine-induced myasthenia gravis*

D-penicillamine is used to treat rheumatoid arthritis, Wilson's disease, and cystinuria. Patients treated with D-penicillamine for several months may develop a myasthenic syndrome that disappears when the drug is stopped (122,123). D-penicillamine-induced myasthenia is usually mild and often restricted to the ocular muscles. The diagnosis is often difficult because weakness may not be recognized when there is severe arthritis. The diagnosis is established by the response to AChE inhibitors, characteristic electrodiagnostic abnormalities, and the presence of serum AChR antibodies (124).

Animal studies indicate that D-penicillamine has no direct effect on neuromuscular transmission (125). The likely mechanism of action is that D-penicillamine stimulates or enhances an immunologic reaction against the neuromuscular junction. The myasthenic response induced by D-penicillamine usually remits within one year after the drug is stopped. AChE inhibitors usually relieve the symptoms. If myasthenic symptoms persist after D-penicillamine is stopped, the patient should be treated for acquired myasthenia gravis.

XI. GENETIC MYASTHENIC SYNDROMES

There are several genetic disorders of neuromuscular transmission that fall under the rubric of congenital myasthenia. Genetic forms of myasthenia are not immune mediated. They are a heterogeneous group of disorders caused by several different abnormalities of neuromuscular transmission (2). Some have characteristic physiological or histological features. Symptoms are typically present at birth or early childhood, but can be delayed until young adult life. They do not present in the elderly adult patient. Abnormal neuromuscular transmission is confirmed by the response to edrophonium chloride, characteristic EMG findings, or both. The onset of myasthenic symptoms at birth is always genetic with the exception of the transient neonatal form of MG. All genetic forms of myasthenia are known or presumed to be transmitted by autosomal-recessive inheritance (although there is a 2:1 male preponderance) except the slow-channel syndrome, which is transmitted by autosomal-dominant inheritance. Myasthenia that begins in infancy or childhood may be genetic or acquired.

ACKNOWLEDGMENT

The author wishes to acknowledge Donald B. Sanders, M.D., for his continuing collaboration over the last 20 years in the field of myasthenia gravis and with whom much of the data have been collected during our tenures at the University of North Carolina at Chapel Hill, Duke University, and the University of Virginia.

REFERENCES

1. Sanders DB, Howard JF. Disorders of neuromuscular transmission. In: Bradley WG, Daroff RB, Fenichel GM, Marsden CD, eds., Neurology in Clinical Practice. Boston: Butterworth, 1991; 1819–1842.

2. Engel AG. The investigation of congenital myasthenic syndromes. Annals of the New York Academy of Sciences 1993; 681:425–434.

3. Santa T, Engel AG, Lambert EH. Histometric study of neuromuscular junction ultrastructure. I. Myasthenia gravis. Neurology 1972; 22:71–82.

4. Engel AG. Morphologic and immunopathologic findings in myasthenia gravis and in congenital myasthenic syndromes. Journal of Neurology, Neurosurgery, and Psychiatry 1980; 43:577–589.

5. Engel AG, Lambert EH, Howard FM. Immune complexes (IgG and C3) at the motor endplate in myasthenia gravis: Ultrastructural and light microscopic localization and electrophysiologic correlation. Mayo Clinic Proceedings 1977; 52: 267–280.

6. Engel AG, Lindstrom JM, Lambert EH, Lennon VA. Ultrastructural localization of the acetylcholine receptor in myasthenia gravis and its experimental autoimmune model. Neurology 1977; 27:307–315.

7. Albuquerque EX, Rash JE, Mayer RF, Satterfield JF. An electrophysiological and morphological study of the neuromuscular junction in patients with myasthenia gravis. Experimental Neurology 1976; 51:536–563.

8. Simpson JA. Myasthenia gravis as an autoimmune disease: Clinical aspects. Annals of the New York Academy of Sciences 1966; 135:506–516.

9. Simpson JA. Myasthenia gravis: A new hypothesis. Scottish Medical Journal 1960; 5:419–436.

10. Howard FM, Silverstein MN, Mulder DW. The coexistence of myasthenia gravis and pernicious anemia. American Journal of the Medical Sciences 1965; 71:518–526.

11. Demaine A, Willcox N, Welsh K, Newsom-Davis J. Associations of the autoimmune myasthenias with genetic markers in the immunoglobulin heavy chain region. Annals of the New York Academy of Sciences 1988; 540:266–268.

12. Apolostolski S, Susakovic N, Lavrnic S, Stolic I, Trikic R. HLA antigens and immunoglobulin allotypes in myasthenia gravis. Neurology 1987; 36:41–49.

13. Wise GA, McQuillen MP. Transient neonatal myasthenia. Clinical and electromyographic study. Archives of Neurology 1970; 22:556–565.

14. Morel E, Bach JF, Briard ML, Aubry JP. Neonatal myasthenia gravis. Anti-acetylcholine receptor antibodies in the amniotic fluid. Journal of Neuroimmunology 1984; 6:313–317.

15. Bergstrom K, Franksson C, Matell G, et al. Drainage of thoracic duct lymph in twelve patients with myasthenia gravis. European Neurology 1975; 73:19–30.

16. Howard JF. Treatment of myasthenia gravis with plasma exchange. Seminars in Neurology 1982; 2:273–279.

17. Howard JF. Nonsteroidal immunosuppressive therapy for myasthenia gravis. Seminars in Neurology 1982; 2:265–270.

18. Sanders DB, Howard JF, Johns TR, Campa JF. High-dose daily prednisone in the treatment of myasthenia gravis. In: Dau PC, ed., Plasmapheresis and the Immunobiology of Myasthenia Gravis. Boston: Houghton-Mifflin Publishers, 1979; 289–306.

19. Tarrab-Hazdai R, Aharonov A, Silman I, Fuchs S, Abramsky O. Experimental autoimmune myasthenia induced in monkeys by purified acetycholine receptor. Nature 1975; 256:128–130.

20. Lennon VA, Lindstrom JM, Seybold ME. Experimental autoimmune myasthenia gravis: A model of myasthenia gravis in rats and guinea pigs. J Exp Med 1975; 141(6):1365–1375.

21. Sahashi K, Engel AG, Lambert EH, Howard FM. Ultrastructural localization of the terminal and lytic ninth complement component (C9) at the motor endplate in myasthenia gravis. Journal of Neuropathology and Experimental Neurology 1980; 39:160–172.

22. Howard JF, Sanders DB. Passive transfer of human myasthenia gravis to rats. I. Electrophysiology of the developing neuromuscular block. Neurology (Minneapolis) 1978; 28:346 (Abstract).

23. Brenner T, Wirguin I, Abramsky O. Anti-acetylcholine receptor antibody measurement in myasthenia gravis. Journal of Neurology, Neurosurgery and Psychiatry 1993; 56:115–116.

24. Soliven BC, Lange DJ, Penn AS, et al. Seronegative myasthenia gravis. Neurology 1988; 38:514–517.

25. Phillips LH,II, Torner JC, Anderson MS, Cox GM. The epidemiology of myasthenia gravis in central and western Virginia. Neurology 1992; 42:1888–1893.

26. Cohen MS. Epidemiology of myasthenia gravis. Monogr Allergy 1987; 21:246–251.

27. Cornelio F. Surveillance of myasthenia gravis through a multicenter survey. Italian Collaborative Group on MG (ICGMG). Muscle and Nerve 1986; 9:154.

28. Storm-Mathisen A. Epidemiology of myasthenia gravis in Norway. Acta Neurologica Scandinavica 1984;70:274–284.

29. Kurtzke J. Epidemiology of myasthenia gravis. In: Schoenberg BS, ed., Advances in Neurology. New York: Raven Press, 1978;545–564.

30. Grob D. Clinical manifestations of myasthenia gravis. In: Albuquerque EX, Eldefrawi AT, eds., Myasthenia Gravis. London: Chapman and Hall, Ltd, 1983;319–345.

31. Burgess KE. The onset, early treatment, diagnosis and psychosocial effects of myasthenia gravis. Master's Thesis, School of Nursing, University of North Carolina at Chapel Hill, 1983 (unpublished).

32. Herishanu Y, Abrmasky O, Feldman S. Myasthenia gravis in the elderly. Journal of the American Geriatric Society 1976; 24:228–231.

33. Johns RJ, McQuillen MP. Syndromes simulating myasthenia gravis: Asthenia with anticholinesterase tolerance. Annals of the New York Academy of Sciences 1966; 135:385–397.

34. Fullerton DT, Munsat TL. Psychogenic weakness simulating myasthenia. Journal of Nervous and Mental Disease 1966; 142:78–86.

35. Schwab RS, Perlo VP. Syndromes simulating myasthenia gravis. Annals of the New York Academy of Sciences 1966; 135:350–365.

36. Cherington M. Botulism. Seminars in Neurology 1990; 10: 27–31.

37. Lambert EH, Elmqvist D. Quantal components of end-plate potentials in the myasthenia syndrome. Annals of the New York Academy of Sciences 1971; 183:183–199.

38. Taphoorn MJ, Van Duijn H, Wolters EC. A neuromuscular transmission disorder: Combined myasthenia gravis and Lambert-Eaton syndrome in one patient. J Neurol Neurosurg Psychiatry 1988; 51:880–882.

39. Tsujihata M, Takashima H, Satoh A, Mori M, Nagataki S. Myasthenia gravis with features of the Eaton-Lambert syndrome. Clin Neurol 1986; 26:128–132.

40. Fettel MR, Shin HS, Penn AS. Combined Eaton-Lambert syndrome and myasthenia gravis. Neurology 1978; 28:398.

41. Schönbeck S, Padberg F, Hohlfeld R, Wekerle H. Transplantation of thymic autoimmune microenvironment to severe combined immunodeficiency mice. A new model of myasthenia gravis. Journal of Clinical Investigation 1992; 90: 245–250.

42. Oh SJ, Cho HK. Edrophonium responsiveness not necessarily diagnostic of myasthenia gravis. Muscle and Nerve 1990; 13:187–191.

43. Jacobson DM. Edrophonium tonography in suspected ocular myasthenia. Case report. Arch Ophthalmol 1987; 105: 1174–1175.

44. Retzlaff JA, Kearns TP, Howard FM, Cronin ML. Lancaster red-green test in the evaluation of edrophonium effect in myasthenia gravis. American Journal of Ophthalmology 1969; 67:13–21.

45. Sollberger CE, Meienberg O, Ludin HP. The contribution of oculography to early diagnosis of myasthenia gravis. A study of saccadic eye movements using the infrared reflection method in 22 cases. Eur Arch Psychiatry Neurol Sci 1986; 236:102–108.

46. Howard JF, Sanders DB, Massey JM. The electrodiagnosis of myasthenia gravis and the Lambert-Eaton myasthenic syndrome. Neurologic Clinics 1994; 12(2):305–330.

47. Howard JF, Sanders DB. Serial single-fiber EMG studies in myasthenic patients treated with corticosteroids and plasma exchange. Muscle and Nerve 1981; 4:254 (Abstract).

48. Sanders DB, Howard JF. Serial studies in myasthenia gravis: The effects of treatment on jitter. Muscle and Nerve 1982; 5:551 (Abstract).

49. Johns TR, Miller JQ, Campa JF. The syndrome of myasthenia and polymyositis with comments on therapy. Annals of the New York Academy of Sciences 1971; 183:64–71.

50. Aarli JA, Thunold S, Heimann P. Thyroiditis in myasthenia gravis. Acta Neurologica Scandinavica 1978; 58:121–127.

51. Ross RT. Ocular myopathy sensitive to curare. Brain 1963; 86:67–74.

52. Steidl RM, Oswald AJ, Kottke FJ. Myasthenic syndrome with associated neuropathy. Archives of Neurology 1962; 6: 451–459.

53. Patten BM, Hart A, Lovelace R. Multiple sclerosis associated

with defects in neuromuscular transmission. Journal of Neurology, Neurosurgery and Psychiatry 1972; 35:385–394.

54. Bernstein LP, Antel JP. Motor neuron disease: Decremental responses to repetitive nerve stimulation. Neurology 1981; 31:202–204.

55. Lambert EH. Defects of neuromuscular transmission in syndromes other than myasthenia gravis. Annals of the New York Academy of Sciences 1966; 135:367–384.

56. Gilchrist JM, Sanders DB. Myasthenic U-shaped decrement in multifocal cervical radiculopathy. Muscle and Nerve 1989; 12:64–66.

57. Streib EW. Successful treatment with tocainide of recessive generalized congenital myotonia. Annals of Neurology 1986; 19:501–504.

58. Gutmann L, Bodensteiner J, Gutierrez A. Electrodiagnosis of botulism. Journal of Pediatrics 1992; 121:835.

59. Eaton LM, Lambert EH. Electromyography and electric stimulation of nerves in diseases of motor unit. Journal of American Medical Association 1957; 163:1117–1124.

60. Sanders DB, Howard JF. AAEE mini-monograph #25: Single-fiber electromyography in myasthenia gravis. Muscle and Nerve 1986; 9:809–819.

61. Stålberg EV, Trontelj JV. Single Fiber Electromyography, 2nd ed. New York: Raven Press, 1994.

62. Howard JF, Sanders DB. The management of patients with myasthenia gravis. In: Albuquerque EX, Eldefrawi AT, eds., Myasthenia Gravis. London: Chapman and Hall, LTD, 1983; 457–489.

63. Johns TR. The use of cholinesterase inhibitors. Seminars in Neurology 1982; 2:298–302.

64. Johns TR. Treatment of myasthenia gravis: Long-term administration of corticosteroids with remarks on thymectomy. Advances in Neurology 1977; 17:99–122.

65. Pascuzzi RM, Coslett B, Johns TR. Long-term corticosteroid treatment of myasthenia gravis: Report of 116 patients. Annals of Neurology 1984; 15:291–298.

66. Seybold ME, Drachman DB. Gradually increasing doses of prednisone in myasthenia gravis. Reducing the hazards of treatment. New England Journal of Medicine 1974; 290: 81–84.

67. Sambrook P, Birmingham J, Kelly P, et al. Prevention of corticosteroid osteoporosis—A comparison of calcium, calcitriol, and calcitonin. New England Journal of Medicine 1993; 328:1747–1752.

68. Matell G. Immunosuppressive drugs: Azathioprine in the treatment of myasthenia gravis. Annals of the New York Academy of Sciences 1987; 505:589–594.

69. Hertel G, Mertens HG, Reuther P, Ricker K. The treatment of myasthenia gravis with azathioprine. In: Dau PC, ed., Plasmapheresis and the Immunobiology of Myasthenia Gravis. Boston: Houghton-Mifflin, 1979; 315–328.

70. Levy RJ, Kissel JT, Mendell JR, Griggs RC. The incidence of azathioprine toxicity in neuromuscular disease. Neurology (Cleveland) 1984; 34(suppl):91.

71. Watts GF, Corston R. Hypersensitivity to azathioprine in myasthenia gravis. Postgraduate Medical Journal 1984; 60: 362–363.

72. Hohlfeld R, Michels M, Heininger K, Besinger U, Toyka KV. Azathioprine toxicity during long-term immunosuppression of generalized myasthenia gravis. Neurology 1988; 38: 258–261.

73. Tindall RSA, Rollins JA, Phillips JT, Greenlee RG, Wells L, Belendiuk G. Preliminary results of a double-blind, randomized, placebo-controlled trial of cyclosporine in myasthenia gravis. New England Journal of Medicine 1987; 316: 719–724.

74. Nyberg-Hansen R, Gjerstad L. Myasthenia gravis treated with ciclosporin. Acta Neurologica Scandinavica 1988; 77: 307–313.

75. Goulon M, Elkharrat D, Lokiec F, Gajdos P. Results of a one-year open trial of cyclosporine in ten patients with severe myasthenia gravis. Transplant Proc 1988; 20:211–217.

76. Faulds D, Goa KL, Benfield P. Cyclosporin: A review of its pharmacodynamic and pharmacokinetic properties, and therapeutic use in immunoregulatory disorders. Drugs 1993; 45: 953–1040.

77. Perez MC, Buot WL, Mercado-Danguilan C, Bagabaldo ZG, Renales LD. Stable remissions in myasthenia gravis. Neurology 1981; 31:32–37.

78. Sargent D, Mease E, Howard JF. The diagnosis of viral

pneumonitis in a compromised host: Is an aggressive approach warranted? North Carolina Medical Journal 1985; 46: 245–246.

79. Lanska DJ. Indications for thymectomy in myasthenia gravis. Neurology 1990; 40:1828–1829.

80. Jaretzki A. Thymectomy for myasthenia gravis. Annals of Thoracic Surgery 1990; 49:688.

81. Jaretzki A, Wolff M. Maximal thymectomy for myasthenia gravis. Surgical anatomy and operative technique. J Thorac Cardiovasc Surg 1988; 96:711–716.

82. Jaretzki A, Penn AS, Younger DS, et al. Maximal thymectomy for myasthenia gravis. Results. J Thorac Cardiovasc Surg 1988; 95:747–757.

83. Cooper JD, Al-Jilaihawa AN, Pearson FG, Humphrey JG, Humphrey HE. An improved technique to facilitate transcervical thymectomy for myasthenia gravis. Annals of Thoracic Surgery 1988; 45:242–247.

84. Whyte RI, Kaplan DK, Deegan SP, Donnelly RJ. Cervical thymectomy in the treatment of myasthenia gravis. J R Coll Surg Edinb 1989; 34:74–78.

85. Miller RG, Filler-Katz A, Kiprov D, Roan R. Repeat thymectomy in chronic refractory myasthenia gravis. Neurology 1991; 41:923–924.

86. Yamanaka N, Araki S. Rethymectomy for intractable myasthenia gravis. Rinsho Shinkeigaku 1990; 30:563–566.

87. Dau PC. Plasmapheresis in myasthenia gravis. Progress in Clinical and Biological Research 1982; 88:265–285.

88. Arsura EL, Bick A, Brunner NG, Grob D. Effects of repeated doses of intravenous immunoglobulin in myasthenia gravis. Am J Med Sci 1988; 295:438–443.

89. Cook L, Howard JF, Folds JD. Immediate effects of intravenous IgG administration on peripheral blood B and T cells and polymorphonuclear cells in patients with myasthenia gravis. J Clin Immunol 1988; 8:23–31.

90. Soueidan SA, Dalakas MC. Treatment of autoimmune neuromuscular diseases with high-dose intravenous immune globulin. Pediatr Res 1993; 33:S95–100.

91. Cosi V, Lombardi M, Piccolo G, Erbetta A. Treatment of myasthenia gravis with high-dose intravenous immunoglobulin. Acta Neurologica Scandinavica 1991; 84:81–84.

92. Ayliffe W, Haeney M, Roberts SC, Lavin M. Uveitis afer antineutrophil cytoplasmic antibody contamination of immuno-globulin replacement therapy. Lancet 1992; 339:558–559.

93. Casteels-Van Daele M, Wijndaele L, Brock P, Kruger M, Gillis P. Aseptic meningitis associated with high dose intrave-nous immunoglobulin therapy. Journal of Neurology, Neuro-surgery and Psychiatry 1992; 55:980–981.

94. Vera-Ramirez M, Charlet M, Parry GJ. Recurrent aseptic meningitis complicating intravenous immunoglobulin therapy for chronic inflammatory demyelinating polyradiculoneuro-pathy. Neurology 1992; 42:1636–1637.

95. Tan E, Hajinazarian M, Bay W, Neff J, Mendell JR. Acute renal failure resulting from intravenous immunoglobulin ther-apy. Arch Neurol 1993; 50:137–139.

96. Phillips AO. Renal failure and intravenous immunoglobulin. Clinical Nephrology 1992; 37:217.

97. Thorton CA, Ballow M. Safety of intravenous immunoglobu-lin. Arch Neurol 1993; 50:135–136.

98. Edgeworth H. The effect of ephedrine in the treatment of myasthenia gravis: Second report. JAMA 1933; 100:1401.

99. Cumings JN. The role of potassium in myasthenia gravis. Journal of Neurology and Psychiatry 1940; 3:115.

100. Engel WK, Dalakas MC, Lichter AS. Intractable myasthenia gravis (MG) can respond to splenic radiation (SR). Neurology (Minneapolis) 1980; 30:389.

101. Hofmann WE, Reuther P, Schalke B, Mertens HG. Splen-ectomy in myasthenia gravis: A therapeutic concept? Journal of Neurology 1985; 232:215–218.

102. Lundh H, Milsson O, Rosen I. Effects of 4-aminopyridine in myasthenia gravis. Journal of Neurology, Neurosurgery, and Psychiatry 1979; 42:171–175.

103. Murray NMF, Newsom-Davis J. Treatment with oral 4-aminopyridine in disorders of neuromuscular transmission. Neurology 1981; 315:265–271.

104. Kaeser HE. Nerve conduction velocity measurements. In: Vinken PJ, Bruyn AW, eds., Handbook of Clinical Neurol-ogy. Amsterdam: North Holland Publishing Company, 1970; 116–196.

105. Campbell MJ, McComas AJ, Petito F. Physiological changes in aging muscles. Journal of Neurology, Neurosurgery and Psychiatry 1973; 36:174–182.

106. Courtney J, Steinbach JH. Age changes in neuromuscular junction morphology and acetylcholine receptor distribution on rat skeletal muscle fibres. Journal of Physiology 1981; 320: 435–447.

107. Larsson L, Grimby G, Karlsson J. Muscle strength and speed of movement in relation to age and muscle morphology. Journal of Applied Physiology 1979; 46:451–456.

108. Grob D, Brunner NG, Namba T. The natural history of myasthenia gravis and effect of therapeutic measures. Annals of the New York Academy of Sciences 1981; 377:652–669.

109. Tanaka M, Miyatake T. Anti-acetylcholine receptor antibody in aged individuals and in patients with Down's syndrome. Journal of Neuroimmunology 1983; 4:17–24.

110. Lindstrom JM, Seybold ME, Lennon VA, Whittingham S, Duane D. Antibody to acetylcholine receptor in myasthenia gravis. Neurology 1976; 26:1054–1059.

111. Robb SA, Vincent A, McGregor MA, McGregor AM, Newsom-Davis JM. Acetylcholine receptor antibodies in the elderly and in Down's syndrome. Journal of Neuroimmunology 1985; 9:139–146.

112. Shoenfeld Y, Ben-Yehuda O, Messinger Y, et al. Autoimmune diseases other than lupus share common anti-DNA idiotypes. Immunol Lett 1988; 17:285–291.

113. Takamori M, Gutmann L, Crosby TW, Martin JD. Myasthenic syndromes in hypothyroidism. Arch Neurol 1972; 26: 326–335.

114. Namba T, Grob D. Familial occurrence of myasthenia gravis and rheumatoid arthritis. Arch Int Med 1970; 125:1056–1058.

115. Chan M, Britton M. Comparative clinical features in patients with myasthenia gravis with systemic lupus erythematosus. J Rheumatol 1980; 7(6):838–842.

116. Howard JF. Adverse drug effects on neuromuscular transmission. Semin Neurol 1990; 10:89–102.

117. Pittinger C, Adamson R. Antibiotic blockade of neuromuscular function. Annual Review of Pharmacology 1972; 12: 109–184.

118. Coppeto JR. Timolol-associated myasthenia gravis. American Journal of Ophthalmology 1984; 98:244–245.

119. Herishanu Y, Rosenberg P. Beta-blockers and myasthenia gravis. Annals of Internal Medicine 1975; 83:834–835.

120. Lee SC, Ho ST. Acute effects of verapamil on neuromuscu-

lar transmission in patients with myasthenia gravis. Proc Natl Sci Counc Repub China [B] 1987; 11:307–312.

121. Shy ME, Lange DJ, Howard JF, Gold AP, Lovelace RE, Penn AS. Quinidine exacerbating myasthenia gravis: A case report and intracellular recordings. Annals of Neurology 1985; 18:120 (Abstract).

122. Kuncl RW, Pestronk A, Drachman DB, Rechthand E. The pathophysiology of penicillamine-induced myasthenia gravis. Annals of Neurology 1986; 20:740–744.

123. Edvard Smith CI, Hammarstrom L, Matell G, Nilsson BY. Role of penicillamine for the induction of myasthenia gravis. European Neurology 1983; 22:272–282.

124. Fawcett PR, McLachlan SM, Nicholson LVB, Argov Z, Mastaglia FL. D-penicillamine-associated myasthenia gavis: Immunological and electrophysiological studies. Muscle and Nerve 1982; 5:328–334.

125. Aldrich MS, Kim YI, Sanders DB. Effects of D-penicillamine on neuromuscular transmission in rats. Muscle and Nerve 1979; 2:180–185.

6

Myopathic Disorders

David Lacomis
University of Pittsburgh School of Medicine
Pittsburgh, Pennsylvania

David A. Chad
University of Massachusetts Medical Center
Worcester, Massachusetts

I. INTRODUCTION

Muscle weakness, a common symptom in the elderly, may have many causes, one of which is myopathy—a disturbance in the structure or function (or both) of muscle tissue. Yet, for several reasons, it may be difficult to establish that weakness in the elderly patient stems from a myopathy per se. First, aging alone is associated with a loss of muscle bulk and strength, and even the finest athletes cannot escape this humbling process (1,2). Thus, some might misinterpret true myopathic weakness as part of growing old. Second, chronic medical and physical conditions—arthritis, cardiovascular and cerebrovascular diseases, and rheumatologic disorders—become increasingly more common with aging (3) and may also simulate myopathic weakness. Third, clinicians may choose to forgo an evaluation of weak elderly patients because they may be considered too frail, and the work-up is therefore deemed too complicated or invasive. The result may be that a treatable, myopathic process is overlooked.

In the first half of this chapter, we present an overview of normal muscle anatomy and physiology and address the changes that occur with "normal" aging. A broad overview of the disorders of muscle is then followed by a discussion of the clinical approach to the weak elderly patient suspected of having a myopathy. Myopathic disorders affecting the elderly as well as the histopathologic spectrum of muscle pathology that one encounters in this population are discussed in detail.

II. ANATOMY AND PHYSIOLOGY OF THE NORMAL ADULT MOTOR UNIT

A. The Motor Unit

Skeletal muscle must be studied in the context of its motor unit (MU), which consists of an anterior horn cell (AHC) or motor neuron, a motor axon, and the group of muscle fibers innervated by the motor axon. Depending on the degree of motor control and the type of work required of a particular muscle, MUs may be small (consisting of relatively few muscle fibers as in ocular muscles) or large (consisting of hundreds to about a thousand fibers as in limb muscles).

The AHC determines the fiber type of all myofibers in the MU. These "types" are named based on their physiology and histochemical staining properties. Type 1 fibers are slow twitch and fatigue resistant. They stain lightly with myosin ATPase (pH 9.4) and are rich in oxidative enzymes and poor in glycolytic activity. Due to a high concentration of myoglobin, they appear red (in animals). Type 2 fibers, especially the 2B subtype, are fast twitch and fatigue rapidly. They stain darkly with myosin ATPase and have little oxidative, but abundant glycolytic, enzyme activity. They are low in myoglobin and appear white (in animals). While individual animal muscles may be comprised of a single fiber type, each human muscle contains a random arrangement of both fiber types. Type 1 fibers generally outnumber type 2 fibers, especially in the deltoid and gastrocnemius muscles of humans.

In addition to dictating fiber type, the AHC and motor nerve also exert a trophic influence on muscle fibers (4,5).

Acetylcholine and neural proteins are thought to be important in maintaining the health of the muscle. Muscle may help maintain itself by regular contraction against resistance, and it may also have a trophic influence on its motor nerve and AHC (6,7).

B. Normal Muscle: Morphology

Muscle fibers are approximately 15 mm in diameter at birth and enlarge to an adult mean diameter of 50 mm (8). Muscle fibers are polygonal in shape and are bundled into fascicles (Figure 1). Connective tissue invests individual fibers and forms the border of the endomysial compartment. Capillaries also border myofibers. Fascicles are separated by denser perimysial connective tissue and blood vessels. Groups of fascicles are then surrounded by adipose tissue, blood vessels, and loose connective tissue forming the epimysium.

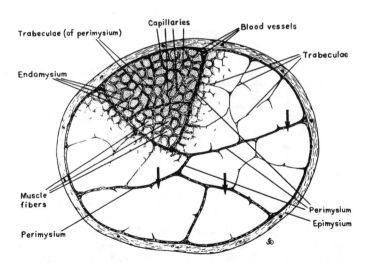

Figure 1   Schematic diagram of the connective tissue sheaths of muscle. Muscle fibers are bundled into fascicles (arrows) bordered by perimysial connective tissue. (From Ref. (8), with permission.)

Nuclei number in the hundreds per cell and are positioned eccentrically. Satellite cells capable of aiding in regeneration are also present at the periphery of the cell beneath the basement membrane. The cytoplasm or sarcoplasm contains the contractile apparatus, lipid and glycogen stores, and organelles such as mitochondria.

Paraffin-embedded longitudinal sections or ultrastructural studies disclose the cross-striations characteristic of skeletal muscle and indicative of the contractile apparatus. Each muscle fiber consists of 50–100 myofibrils. The sarcomere (unit of a myofibril) is the region from Z band to Z band (Figure 2). Within the sarcomere, thick myosin alternates with thin actin filaments. Thin filaments attach at the Z band and form the I (lighter isotropic) band. The thick filaments are located within the A (darker, anisotropic) band, and thin fila-

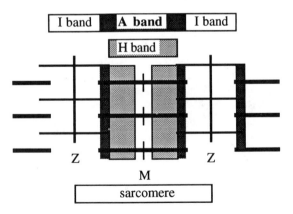

Figure 2 Schematic diagram of a sarcomere. The sarcomere is the unit of a myofibril occupying the region between Z bands. Myosin filaments (thick horizontal lines) alternate with actin filaments (thin horizontal lines). The A band is composed of thick plus thin filaments; the I band, of thin filaments only; and the H band, of thick filaments only. The M line is composed of transverse projections linking thick filaments at the center of the H band.

ments also extend into this region except at the H band where there is no overlap of thick and thin filaments.

C. Normal Muscle: Physiology

In the resting muscle, small fluctuations in membrane potential occur at the end-plate region (9). These fluctuations are called miniature end-plate potentials (MEPPs), and they are produced by the spontaneous release of packets (quanta) of acetylcholine (ACh) from the motor nerve ending. The arrival of an action potential at the axon terminal triggers an influx of calcium ions and the release of hundreds of quanta of ACh all at the same time, producing an end-plate potential (EPP) which, if substantial enough, causes the postsynaptic membrane to depolarize. The action potential then propagates throughout the muscle fiber bidirectionally at a rate of 3–5 m/sec along the transverse tubules (at the junction of the A and I bands). When the action potential comes in contact with the terminal cisternae, it gains access to the contractile apparatus. In another calcium-dependent, ATP-requiring process, cross-bridges are formed between thick and thin filaments. Sliding of the thin against thick filaments leads to muscle contraction.

III. ANATOMY AND PHYSIOLOGY OF THE ELDERLY ADULT

A. The Motor Unit

With advancing age (after 60 years), MUs decrease in number and increase in size, suggesting that reinnervation from collateral sprouting—although limited in the elderly (10)—has occurred (11,12). In humans, there may be as much as a 50–75% decrease in MUs (11,13). It has been inferred that these changes are due to a loss of AHCs (11), although there is limited human pathologic evidence that supports this inference, and some animal studies are contradictory. Supportive evidence includes several studies. Using a manual AHC counting technique during autopsy, patients (who were not evaluated antemortem) showed a decline (mean of 25%) in AHCs in the lumbosacral spinal cord between their 2nd and 10th decades (14). Most of the AHC loss occurred after age 60 (14). It is also known that anterior roots (15) and motor axons are reduced in number with aging (16), again suggesting loss or dysfunction of AHCs. On the other hand, Gutman did not find loss of AHCs with aging in an animal model (17).

Based on the morphologic changes observed in aging rat as well as human muscle (especially the atrophy and loss of type 2 fibers described below), it has been further suggested that with aging there may be selective denervation of fast (type 2) fibers followed by collateral sprouting from nerves that then convert the denervated myofibers to type 1 (18). Such a process could contribute to the loss of fine motor control and perhaps adversely affect overall strength. Other age-related changes of the neural component of the MU in humans include slowing of nerve conduction velocity (19,20); a decrease in the numbers of myelinated and unmyelinated fibers per nerve (21); and, in rats, a reduction in slow axonal transport (22).

The clinical significance of the changes in the nerve component of the MU is uncertain since histologic and electrophysiologic features typical of denervation and reinnervation are not prominent in the healthy elderly (23), although relatively mild neurogenic histologic changes (mostly grouping of type 1 fibers consistent with denervation and reinnervation) have been described (24–27). In many of these small studies, however, patients were not evaluated neurologically or electrophysiologically prior to the histologic studies, nor were confounding variables—such as underlying diabetes mellitus or spinal stenosis—always controlled. Furthermore, atrophy (but not loss) of type 2 fibers is commonly seen in non-neurogenic conditions that affect the elderly such as disuse, polymyalgia rheumatica, endocrinopathies, and corticosteroid therapy (28). Supporting the notion that other variables have a role in producing morphologic changes, aging rodents raised in pathogen-free conditions are less likely to exhibit changes in muscle morphology than their counterparts raised in the customary laboratory setting (29).

B. Muscle Morphology

With aging, muscle mass declines by 25–33% (26,30). After age 65–70, most human studies have disclosed atrophy (26) and sometimes loss of type 2 fibers (31). Active as well as sedentary humans develop type 2 atrophy (32,33), but the degree of atrophy is less in most active elderly (33). Type 1 fibers may consequently encompass a greater surface area (32,33) and increase in proportion to type 2 fibers (31).

With aging, the regenerative process of injured human and rodent muscle may also be impaired (34–36). It is uncertain whether this impairment affects type 1 and 2 fibers differently. The increased action of free radicals may be an important factor in age-related impairment of muscle repair following injury (36).

Many of the noted alterations in aging muscle could reflect, in part, the changes in the neural elements of the MU described above. On the other hand, it has also been suggested that the muscle changes could occur first and lead to the modifications of AHCs (23).

C. Muscle Physiology: Energy Production

Intramuscular glycogen is the substrate utilized for brief, high-intensity work, while lipids and free fatty acids are oxidized at rest and during prolonged, low-intensity work. Substrate utilization and delivery are dependent on oxygen and blood supply, cardiovascular and pulmonary performance, and cellular transport systems. With aging, most researchers have found that aerobic endurance and exercise-related oxygen utilization decline (37). Some of the decline may be due to inactivity; the remainder could be due to aging of the motor unit and decreases in stroke volume or muscle oxygen extraction (38). Results of studies of anaerobic metabolism are often not in agreement, but some groups have found that there is a buildup of lactic acid (therefore less efficient anaerobic metabolism) with aging (39). Glucose utilization itself does not change, but some alterations in the glycolytic enzymes have been identified. The observed loss of type 2, glycogen-rich fibers with a resultant predominance of type 1 fibers may be only partly responsible for the change in glycolytic enzymes (40).

In slow-twitch muscles of rats, mitochondrial enzyme activity is reduced, but there is a shift toward a relative increase in oxidation in fast-twitch fibers (41). This reduction in oxidative metabolism in type 1 fibers is probably due to a reversible (by increasing activity) decrease in mitochondrial protein production, not an abnormality in mitochondrial function (42). Whether or not any of these "metabolic" changes are clinically relevant to loss of strength and bulk is yet to be determined (23).

D. Muscle Physiology: Strength and Endurance

From ages 30 to 80, there is a gradual, 30% decline in arm strength (43) and a 40% decrease in leg strength (30,43). Both isometric (i.e., static: the muscle does not shorten during contraction) and isotonic (i.e., dynamic: the muscle shortens against a constant load) strength are affected (23). The degree of weakness parallels the reduction in muscle mass. Some authors note a strong correlation (30), whereas others feel that only about a third of the loss of strength may be attributed to loss of muscle bulk (43,44). In animal models, for example, when maximum power is corrected for muscle mass, muscles in old mice still generate 20% less power compared to those from younger mice (43). Therefore, factors in addition to muscle atrophy must play a role in causing the loss of strength. These factors may include decreased energy production, deconditioning, changes in the trophic interactions between nerve and muscle, and perhaps a defective contractile apparatus.

Endurance, measured as aerobic work capacity, also seems to decline with age (as noted above) for uncertain reasons. The contributing role of cardiovascular factors is not yet clear and these factors are difficult to control in humans, due partly to the increase in atherosclerosis with aging.

Physical conditioning appears to delay or blunt the age-related decay in strength and in aerobic work capacity (38). Healthy, active humans can maintain strength from their 7th to 8th or even 9th decades (45). Work capacity, oxygen utilization (46,47), and the size of muscle fibers (48) can also increase in elderly who engage in exercise programs. On the other hand, at least in animals, nutritional status does not seem to alter muscle composition or strength (49).

E. Summary

The loss of muscle bulk and strength that occurs with aging is partly related to a decrease in the number of functioning motor units and a loss of AHCs (Table 1). From disease models such as poliomyelitis, however, we know that up to 60% of AHCs may be lost before clinical weakness occurs (50). In amyotrophic lateral sclerosis (ALS), the loss of AHCs parallels loss of strength, and a 15–50% loss of AHCs correlates with mild to moderate weakness (51). The degree of drop-out in motor fibers is much greater than the associated loss of muscle bulk in these patients (52).

Table 1 Changes Occurring During Normal Aging of Muscle and the Motor Unit

Motor unit increases in size
Loss of anterior horn cells
Loss of muscle bulk and strength[a]
Atrophy of type 2 myofibers[a]
Decrease in muscle energy production[a]
Impaired muscle regenerative capability

[a]Improved or blunted by physical conditioning.

Although this age-related AHC degeneration is the proposed primary cause of the loss of MUs and perhaps leads to selective denervation of fast-twitch fibers, it remains uncertain which elements of the MU are affected first (neural or muscle). It is unlikely that the degree of MU or AHC loss present in normal aging would be reflected in nonquantitative measures of strength assessment, because manual muscle testing may not detect up to 43% of losses in leg strength and 26% of losses in arm strength when compared to quantitative testing (53). Therefore, the degree of weakness associated with aging should not be detectable at the "bedside."

It is also unclear to what degree the process of aging in muscle is degenerative and irreversible vs. "metabolic" or activity-related and thus amenable to postponement or treatment. Human data regarding normal aging of muscle are often difficult to interpret and sometimes contradictory given the difficulties of quantitating strength, controlling variables such as general health, nutritional status, and activity levels; and obtaining histologic samples of the PNS over time. Therefore, until we gain more knowledge about these underlying processes with well-controlled, longitudinal human studies, physical conditioning appears to be our greatest ally in maintaining the integrity of the aging motor unit.

IV. DISORDERS OF MUSCLE

A. General Clinical Features and Approach to the Patient

With few exceptions—such as myotonic dystrophy, distal dystrophy (of Welander), and inclusion body myositis—the distribution of weakness in most myopathies is *proximal,* involving neck, limb girdle, humeral and femoral musculature. After a myopathy has been present for many years there may be some degree of muscle thinning, but true muscle atrophy and fasciculations—signs of neurogenic disorders—do not occur in myopathic conditions. Common symptoms include difficulty rising from a chair (Figure 3), climbing stairs, walking, and using the arms above the head. Elevating the head from a supine position may be difficult because of neck flexor muscle weakness. Some myopathies have unusual or atypical distributions of muscle weakness like the mitochondrial (ocular muscles), idiopathic inflammatory (pharyngeal muscles), and

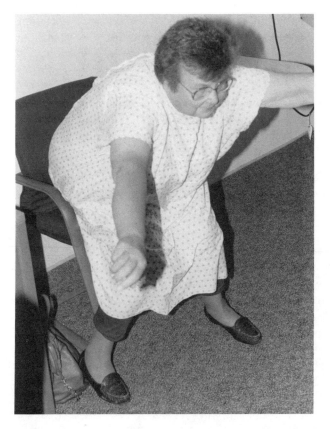

Figure 3 Because of severe pelvifemoral muscle weakness, this woman with the myopathy of Cushing's syndrome has a wide stance as she attempts to rise from a chair.

glycogen storage (respiratory muscles) myopathies, which may suggest a neurogenic or neuromuscular junction disorder. Tendon reflexes are usually normal or reduced initially, but they may become attenuated as the disease progresses and muscles become thinned and severely weakened. While myalgias may accompany some inflammatory and metabolic myopathies, the sensory examination per se is normal.

When a myopathy is suspected, it is necessary to elicit careful family, occupational, and toxin exposure (including prescribed drug) histories. One should also pose questions geared toward uncovering an endocrinopathy or other associated systemic conditons like cancer or collagen-vascular disorders.

A laboratory screen is usually the next step in the evaluation. The serum creatine kinase (CK) is usually elevated if there is muscle necrosis (inflammatory or toxic myopathies, dystrophies, and some inherited myopathies) or a muscle membrane "leak" (perhaps in hypothyroidism, for example). The CK is also elevated after trauma and very strenuous exercise, with neuroleptic malignant syndrome and malignant hyperthermia, and with motor neuron diseases (mild elevation). Most nonnecrotizing myopathies, such as corticosteroid myopathy, are associated with a normal CK. Serum aldolase measurement is not of any further diagnostic help, because the CK is more specific for muscle.

It is also prudent to check the ESR, electrolytes, phosphorus, calcium, CBC, liver enzymes, and thyroid function studies. In patients with a suspicious body habitus or any clinical features of Cushing's syndrome, a 24-hour urine-free cortisol should be obtained or a dexamethasone suppression performed (54). Based on the presence of abnormalities on the laboratory screen (viewed in conjunction with the clinical history and physical examination), a specific work-up may be undertaken. For example, an elevation in calcium and a reduction in phosphorus would prompt an evaluation for hyperparathyroidism.

If a definite diagnosis has not yet been reached, an EMG can provide valuable information especially when combined *with* the CK *and* clinical data. The nerve conduction studies (NCS) and needle EMG are useful extensions of the clinical examination in confirming the diagnosis of all disorders of the lower motor neuron and muscle (55). In most muscle diseases and occasionally with early neurogenic processes and disorders of neuromuscular transmission, motor unit potentials (MUPs) tend to be low in amplitude and short in duration. In myopathies, these changes occur because of random loss of muscle fibers, and the MUPs may also be polyphasic due to desynchronization of the muscle action potentials or regeneration of myofibers. Polyphasic MUPs are also seen in neurogenic disorders, probably because of axonal sprouting into denervated myofibers. In contrast to most neurogenic disorders, early recruitment of MUPs occurs with minimal muscle activation in myopathies due to the need to summon more fibers than normal to perform the required work. Fibrillation potentials are present if there is muscle necrosis, inflammation, denervation of the muscle fiber, or irritability of the muscle membrane. In the setting of longstanding neurogenic processes (after collateral sprouting), MUPs are reduced in number, high in amplitude, and long in duration. Chronic inflammatory myopathies may sometimes share such EMG features (56).

Muscle biopsy is often necessary to confirm the diagnosis of a myopathy and should be performed especially when a treatable disorder is suspected. It is also important to identify the myopathies that are known to be resistant to immunological treatments but that resemble clinically the treatable disorders, thereby avoiding potentially dangerous and unwarranted immunosuppressive therapy. Occasionally, muscle biopsy is helpful in confirming the diagnosis of hereditary disorders, but evaluation of family members and genetic and biochemical studies may sometimes obviate the need for muscle biopsy. This trend is likely to continue and expand in the future.

The histologic features of a myopathy include an abnormal variation in the size of myofibers; myofiber necrosis, regeneration, and inflammation; internalization of nuclei; moth-eaten appearance of fibers; fiber splitting; and an increase in connective tissue (8). None of these features alone is diagnostic of myopathy; the recognition of the pattern of change is most important. Histologic features of individual myopathies will be discussed later in the chapter.

B. The Myopathies: Classification

Muscle diseases may be divided into the inherited and acquired disorders (Table 2). Among the inherited conditions are the muscular dystrophies, which tend to be chronic and slowly progressive. They generally begin in childhood or adolescence, and as time passes, cause progressive loss of strength. Some, such as Duchenne-type muscular dystrophy, lead to profound weakness and a wheelchair-bound existence; others, such as myotonic and facioscapulohumeral dystrophy, may cause relatively mild weakness and may not require a wheelchair. Congenital myopathies are also inherited conditions that are generally recognized at birth; in most patients weakness is slowly progressive and does not result in an inability to walk. Much progress has been made in the last decade with regard to defining the genetic abnormalities in many of these myopathies. Most of them begin in childhood or adolesence and are discussed in this section, but several have a predilection for older adults and will be discussed later in the chapter. The metabolic myopathies are also inherited and include disorders associated with defects in glycogen, lipid, and mitochondrial metabolism. They vary greatly in their clinical features, usually presenting in childhood, but onset in adulthood, even in later life, may occur.

In contrast to the slow progression and long natural history beginning in childhood of most inherited conditons, the acquired diseases of muscle have a much quicker tempo and

Table 2 Classification of Myopathies and Relative Frequency of Onset at Varying Ages

Relative frequency of occurrence in myopathy	Childhood	Young adults	Elderly
Inherited myopathies			
X-Linked dystrophies			
Duchenne muscular dystrophy	+ + +	–	–
Becker muscular dystrophy	+ + +	+ +	–
Emery-Dreifuss muscular dystrophy	+ + +	–	–
Autosomal dystrophies			
Facioscapulohumeral dystrophy	+ + +	+ +	–
Myotonic dystrophy	+ + +	+ +	+
Limb-Girdle dystrophy	+ + +	+ +	–
Oculopharyngeal dystrophy	–	+	+ + +
Distal dystrophy	–	+ +	+ +
Congenital myopathies	+ + +	–[a]	–[a]
Metabolic myopathies			
Mitochondrial myopathies	+ + +	+ +	+
Glycogen storage myopathies	+ + +	+ +	–[a]
Lipid storage myopathies	+ + +	+	–
Acquired myopathies			
Polymyositis	–[a]	+ + +	+ + +
Dermatomyositis	+ +	+ + +	+ +
Inclusion body myositis	–	+	+ + +
Sarcoid myopathy	+	+ +	+ +
Infectious myopathies	+ +	+ +	+ +
Toxic & endocrine myopathies	+	+ + +	+ + +

+ + + Common, + + Uncommon, + Rare, – Absent.
[a]Very rare exceptions.

a predilection for the elderly. With regard to rate of onset, poly- and dermatomyositis usually produce weakness over a period of weeks to months while inclusion-body myositis has a more chronic course, measured in years. Endocrine and toxic myopathies tend to present with the acute to subacute onset of weakness.

1. *Inherited myopathies*
   a. **X-linked muscular dystrophies**
   1. Duchenne's muscular dystrophy
      Clinical features. Duchenne's muscular dystrophy (DMD) is the best known of the muscular dystrophies (57). The incidence of DMD is 20–30 per 100,000 male births; one-third of cases arise from spontaneous mutations (vide infra).

      Patients may present between ages 2 and 5 with a delay in walking, toe-walking, a clumsy (waddling) gait, difficulty climbing stairs, and an inability to keep up physically with peers. Calf pseudohypertrophy, increased lumbar lordosis, and a Gower's sign are additional features. There is also a mild lowering of IQ.

      The proximal lower- and upper-extremity weakness is progressive. Patients usually become wheelchair-bound by about age 12 and then develop contractures and scoliosis. DMD males usually die in their 20s from respiratory compromise or from cardiomyopathy.

      Laboratory features. The CK is highly elevated (3000–30,000 U/L) from the first year of life on, but it decreases by age 10. The EMG reveals typical myopathic MUPs with fibrillation potentials. The EKG usually discloses tall right-sided R waves and deep precordial Q waves. Muscle biopsy specimens disclose absence or near absence of dystrophin (58) (by direct antibody staining or via Western blot).

      Pathogenesis. In both DMD and Becker's muscular dystrophy (BMD), the abnormal gene locus is huge and is present on Xp21. This gene normally codes for the membrane-associated, cytoskeletal protein dystrophin (59). This gene spans about 2.4 million base pairs. At least 60% of patients with DMD harbor a recognized deletion (usually out of frame) at several "hot spots" (58). Translocations and reduplications also occur. In DMD, dystrophin is usually completely absent.

Treatment. Prednisone (0.75 mg/kg/day) has been shown to improve strength and slow the progression of muscle weakness and atrophy and to prolong ambulation (60); however, it has not found widespread use because it does not *halt* progression of DMD, and side effects are often prominent.

2. Becker's muscular dystrophy. Becker's muscular dystrophy (61), an allelic, usually more benign variant of DMD, is also associated with an abnormality in dystrophin. Usually, only 10–30% of the normal amount of dystrophin is present. An in-frame deletion is the type of mutation most often detected. The incidence is 3–6 per 100,000 male births. Onset is later than DMD (5–15 years) and the disorder is more slowly progressive. Mild cases may first be detected in adults. On the other hand, molecular studies have taught us that some patients with BMD are clinically indistinguishable from those with DMD early on. In general, however, patients with BMD usually walk until 16–27 years of age and some do so for much longer. The average age at death is 42 years.

3. Emery-Dreifuss muscular dystrophy. This disorder is a rare, X-linked dystrophy (62) with the abnormal gene locus at Xq28 (63). The abnormal gene product has not yet been identified. The major features include slowly progressive humeroperoneal weakness and atrophy followed by contractures of the elbows, heels, and posterior neck (producing a rigid spine). The primary systemic feature is significant cardiac conduction abnormalities that frequently require pacemaker placement to prevent sudden death. The CK is usually elevated, but the range is broad.

b. Autosomally inherited dystrophies

1. Facioscapulohumeral dystrophy. This dystrophy is autosomal dominant (AD) in inheritance with the genetic abnormality mapping to chromosome 4q35 (64). There is strong penetrance but varying expressivity. The incidence is 3–10 per million, but this incidence is probably underestimated due to the frequent presence of mild undetected cases. Major features include slowly progressive facial (sparing extraocular muscles)

and shoulder girdle (periscapular) weakness that spreads to the hip and anterior tibialis muscles, beginning at about age 10.

2. Limb-girdle dystrophy. In the past, the diagnosis of limb-girdle dystrophy (LGD) (65) has served as a generic grouping or "wastebasket" for patients whose proximal weakness could not be more specifically designated. Cases of Becker's dystrophy, DMD carriers, SCARMD (severe autosomal-recessive dystrophy associated with an abnormality in dystrophin-associated glycoproteins), metabolic myopathies, acquired myopathies like inclusion-body myositis, and the spinal muscular atrophies were frequently allocated to this category. In the 1990s genetic studies have been under way that are likely to stratify more accurately this heterogeneous collection of disorders. In general, the patients with heredofamilial forms of LGD have a variable onset of slowly progressive proximal weakness, elevated CK, and myopathic features on EMG and muscle biopsy. We must await further genetic studies to characterize these patients better.

3. Myotonic muscular dystrophy. Myotonic dystrophy (MyD) is a complex, multisystem AD disorder that is the most common adult form of muscular dystrophy. Its incidence is 1 in 8000 (66).

Clinical features. The onset of symptoms ranges from childhood to adult ages (66). Patients usually present with myotonia (often called cramps or stiffness by the patient), weakness (involving foot dorsiflexors or distal upper-extremity muscles, especially extensors), or extramuscular manifestations of the disorder. Patients often do not seem to recognize that they even have a disorder. Abnormal facies are common. There is frontal balding (men and sometimes women), a long narrow jaw, and ptosis. Patients may also develop dysphagia and dysarthria with nasal speech. There is wasting of neck and temporalis muscles. In the limbs, symmetric distal weakness precedes proximal weakness. Myotonia can be demonstrated in grip (delayed release following contraction) and with percussion of the thenar eminences, forearm extensor compartment, or tongue. Tendon reflexes may be reduced.

Congenital onset may occur in infants of affected mothers. This form is more severe with resultant hypotonia, bulbar weakness (difficulty feeding, swallowing, and breathing), mental retardation, and often clubfoot. In affected infants, the CTG repeat size (vide infra) tends to be large, but the explanation for the maternal transmission of this severe form of MyD is not well understood (66).

Systemic features. Cardiac conduction defects (67) and early-onset colored cataracts are common. The gallbladder and GI smooth muscle may be involved, leading to cholecystitis and constipation. There may also be testicular atrophy and uterine hypotonia. Immunoglobulin G levels tend to be low. Insulin resistance occurs, and overall, IQs are lower than expected. Patients with MyD may be more sensitive to anesthesia (66).

Laboratory features. The CK is usually mildly elevated or normal. In nerve conduction studies, motor amplitudes are low or normal. The needle EMG reveals waxing and waning (myotonic) discharges in addition to myopathic MUPs. Histologically, muscle contains a marked excess of internalized nuclei with variation in fiber size. Nuclear clumps, ring fibers, and abnormal muscle spindles are commonly seen (66).

Pathogenesis and treatment. MyD has been associated with abnormal expansion of the unstable trinucleotide repeat CTG located on the untranslated 3′ end on chromosome 19 (68). Normals have approximately 5–27 copies of this repeated DNA segment while MyD patients have >50 copies. This segment codes for a protein kinase. The repeat generally expands from generation to generation (correlating with worsening severity), but reverse mutations have also been identified (69).

Conservative measures are undertaken for management of weakness, including physical therapy and orthotics. Yearly EKGs should be obtained to evaluate for progressive atrioventricular blocks and QRS widening (67). A cardiac pacemaker is sometimes required. Myotonia may be treated safely with phenytoin.

There are other inherited disorders associated with clinical and electrical myotonia including myotonia congenita, paramyotonia congenita, and hyperkalemic periodic paralysis (70). These disorders are rare and usually occur in childhood.

4. Congenital myopathies. The myopathies in this class have been defined by their pathologic characteristics; the subtypes are not easily distinguished from one another clinically (71). These disorders usually present with hypotonia at birth or shortly thereafter; however, some patients come to medical attention much later. There may be delayed motor milestones, clumsy gait, proximal weakness, hyporeflexia, mild dysmorphic features (such as a high-arched palate and long narrow face), and scoliosis. The body habitus is usually thin, hip dislocation may occur, and some patients are mentally retarded. These disorders are usually static or slowly progressive, but malignant forms do occur. The CK is usually normal while the EMG may show myopathic features.

5. Metabolic myopathies. The inherited metabolic myopathies include the disorders of glycogen and lipid metabolism and abnormalities of mitochondrial function. Any disturbance in the biochemical pathways that supports normal concentrations of ATP in muscle will cause *exercise intolerance,* which leads to true *fatigue* (muscle will no longer perform) and sometimes *pain* during exercise.

With regard to glycogen storage diseases there are basically two modes of clinical presentation: progressive muscle weakness exemplified by acid maltase deficiency; and aches, cramps, and pains typified by McArdle's disease (72). Acid maltase deficiency may manifest for the first time in adolescence or mid-adult life as proximal muscle weakness and may mimic an acquired myopathy (73). Other features of this disorder include respiratory muscle involvement, high CK, an abnormal EMG characterized by fibrillation potentials and myotonic discharges. Usually, McArdles's disease begins in childhood or early adolescence with attacks of muscle cramps, contractures, pain, and sometimes myoglobinuria, but it may also manifest in adult life as slowly progressive muscle weakness. A key diagnostic feature is the absence of a rise in serum venous lactate during the ischemic exercise test.

There are two main lipid myopathies caused by deficiencies of carnitine and carnitine palmityl transferase (CPT) (74). The myopathic form of carnitine deficiency presents usually in adolescent males with progressive limb-girdle weakness, elevated CK, and myopathic EMG. CPT deficiency is found mainly in young adult men and is characterized by bouts of transient weakness with myoglobinuria (but no contractures) after strenuous exercise. Toxins, infections, and rarely dystrophinopathies and mitochondrial disorders are also associated with myoglobinuria.

Mitochondrial myopathies may occur from defects in energy substrate utilization, oxidation and phosphorylation coupling, and respiratory chain function. Most patients present with progressive external ophthalmoplegia (PEO) and varying degrees of limb-girdle weakness, but a variety of extramuscular manifestations—heart block, retinitis pigmentosa, optic neuropathy, elevated CSF protein, sensorineural hearing loss, and peripheral neuropathy—can also occur (75). Ragged red fibers (RRFs) are the hallmark histologic feature of mitochondrial muscle disorders. Occasionally, mitochondrial myopathies present with proximal weakness or exertional myalgias with or without ocular involvement (76). Patients with PEO and other mitochondrial myopathies tend to be young with 61% of patients being less than 20 at onset of symptoms, but the age range is broader (birth to 68 years). Ten percent of patients present after age 50 (76).

2. *Acquired myopathies*

   a. **Idiopathic inflammatory myopathies.** Polymyositis, dermatomyositis, (77–81) and inclusion body myositis (IBM) are immunologically mediated inflammatory myopathies. Since IBM more commonly affects the elderly, it is discussed later in the chapter.

   b. **Polymyositis and dermatomyositis.** The incidence of these disorders is 2–5 per million. Females are affected more frequently than males. The incidence of PM peaks in the fifth decade, while DM peaks in childhood as well as the fifth decade.

These disorders are associated with HLA B8, DR3, and other haplotypes.

1. Clinical features. In both disorders, there is subacute to chronic (rarely acute) onset of progressive proximal weakness. Neck flexors are commonly involved; extraocular, facial, and respiratory muscles are almost always spared. When weakness is severe, distal muscles may be involved. There may be myalgias (occasionally) and dysphagia.

Patients with DM have a rash. It may be a butterfly facial rash with heliotrope discoloration over the eyelids, or there may be a rash over the knuckles along with periungual hyperemia and telangectasias. In childhood DM, subcutaneous calcifications may occur.

Potential visceral involvement includes the heart (cardiomyopathy), lungs (interstitial lung disese), esophagus, and stomach (ulcers). Connective tissues diseases occur in about 20% of cases. DM is especially associated with systemic sclerosis and mixed connective tissue disease, but not usually rheumatoid arthritis or systemic lupus erythematosus. There is probably about a 10–15% association with malignancy (82) except perhaps in childhood DM and when DM and PM are associated with connective tissue diseases (CTDs).

Ultimately, PM is a diagnosis of exclusion. Diagnosis is based on clinical features, and as noted below, an elevated CK, myopathic EMG, and pathologic evidence of muscle inflammation and necrosis. Other causes of such a syndrome, for example, a parasitic myopathy, must be excluded.

2. Laboratory features. The CK is elevated (as much as 100-fold) in at least 75% of patients. The ESR is elevated in 50%. There are many antibody associations: for example, anti-Jo1 (subunit of histidine RNA synthetase) in interstitial lung disease, anti-DNA, nucleolar antihistone antibody in childhood DM, and PM-Scl antibody system in scleroderma.

The EMG reveals myopathic MUPs with increased insertional and spontaneous activity in at least 80% of patients. Histologic examination of muscle reveals myofiber regeneration, degeneration, atrophy, and inflammation (see below). In childhood DM and 50% of adult DM, there is perifascicular atrophy in addition to capillary necrosis and inclusions compatible with a microangiopathic vasculopathy with muscle ischemia.

The immunopathology of DM (79) reveals mononuclear cell inflammation, mostly B cells in perivascular and epimysial sites. There is deposition of the C5b-9 membrane attack complex (MAC) in capillaries with loss of capillaries and presumed muscle ischemia. In PM, inflammation is also mononuclear with mostly CD8+ T cells in endomysial more than perivascular locations. Invasion of nonnecrotic fibers is a classic feature of PM (and IBM).

3. Treatment and prognosis. Due to a lack of controlled trials and the possibility of spontaneous remission, most treatments remain empiric. The first line of treatment in weak patients is corticosteroids (anecdotally effective). Approximately 60–100 mg of prednisone may be used once daily in the morning for 6–8 weeks followed by a slow conversion to alternate-day therapy in which the alternate-day dose is reduced by approximately 5–10 mg every 2 weeks. The rate of tapering is individualized and should be slower if weakness has not improved or if the CK remains high. If side effects occur, the rate of tapering may need to be increased. When the dose is about 40 mg every other day, we taper slower.

Supplemental calcium (1–1.5 g/day) and vitamin D (one dose of 50,000 IU twice a week) are administered in an attempt (unproven) to prevent osteoporosis. A recent study suggests that one should consider using calcitriol and calcium (83) to deter corticosteroid-induced bone loss (as least in the spine). Patients must be monitored for hypercalcemia. Estrogen therapy should also be considered in postmenopausal women (84).

If patients develop dyspepsia, we add antacids or an H_2 receptor blocker. A calcium carbonate-containing antacid (if the dyspepsia is mild) may be ideal because it also provides calcium supplementation. Blood pressure, glucose, potassium, and bone density should be monitored. One should be vigilant of infections and the development of cataracts.

Approximately two-thirds will improve on corticosteroids alone and have no substantial functional deficits in follow-up at 3 years (78). The 5-year mortality (in patients without cancer) is about 20–25% by retrospective analysis (85) and as low as 11% prospectively (86). Prognosis is worse if dysphagia or severe weakness is present. Most patients require low-maintainence doses of prednisone for years, but prednisone therapy may not affect mortality rate (85). One must also monitor patients for corticosteroid myopathy, a diagnosis that is difficult to establish in this setting. A lack of CK elevation and an absence of fibrillation potential activity on EMG despite progression of weakness favor steroid myopathy and warrant a trial of corticosteroid tapering with close follow-up.

Cytotoxic agents such as azathioprine (2–3 mg/kg/day) and methotrexate (7.5–25 mg orally, weekly) are used either in patients who do not respond to high-dose prednisone (after about 3 months) or in conjunction with prednisone in patients with severe disease or in whom there is a relative contraindication to high-dose corticosteroid therapy. Benefits take more than 6 months or so to be realized (87). Intravenous IV immunoglobulin (IV Ig) may also be of some benefit in patients with DM (88); plasma exchange does not appear to be beneficial (89).

c.   Other inflammatory myopathies

1.   Sarcoid myopathy.   Sarcoid myopathy is discussed in the section on myopathies in the elderly.

2.   HIV-related myopathy.   This is a heterogeneous disorder that can affect untreated asymptomatic HIV-infected patients or those with ARC or AIDS. Symptoms include subacute onset of proximal weakness, myalgias, and weight loss (90).

3. Pyomyositis. Ordinarily, skeletal muscle is resistant to infection. Rarely, bacterial invasion with abscess formation (pyomyositis) occurs. Most cases occur in the tropics, although we have seen two cases in Massachusetts. Most infections are caused by staphylococcus in the setting of bacteremia and tend to be focal and painful. Diffuse weakness may rarely occur, mimicking polymyositis (91).

Parasites such as *Trichinella spiralis* (trichinosis) and *Taenia solium* (cysticercosis) may produce a myositis, and the protozoan *Toxoplasma gondii* (toxoplasmosis) occasionally invades muscle. Rarely, fungi and tuberculosis may infect muscle, usually in the setting of systemic illness or local extension of a suppurative process.

d. Endocrine myopathies

1. Corticosteroid excess states. Both endogenous (Cushing's syndrome [CS]) and iatrogenic hypercortisolism may cause a myopathy.

Clinical features. Fifty to 90% of patients with CS complain of weakness (92) and about 7–10% of patients treated with corticosteroids develop weakness (93). Weakness generally develops weeks to months after institution of corticosteroid treatment or after the onset of CS. Progression is insidious, and proximal muscles are primarily affected, first in the lower extremities, then the upper extremities. Myalgias may occur. Facial and extraocular muscles are spared. Higher doses of corticosteroids (>40 mg of prednisone per day [94]), especially fluorinated agents (triamcinolone, betamethasone, and dexamethasone), are more likely to induce myopathy (95).

Rarely, patients with critical illnesses, especially status asthmaticus, undergoing treatment with high-dose intravenous corticosteroids, paralytic agents, and other drugs develop acute generalized weakness sometimes accompanied by rhabdomyolysis (96,97). The process appears to be a toxic myopathy that may affect myosin thick filaments in some patients.

Laboratory features. In the usual corticosteroid myopathies, the CK is normal. In iatrogenic hypercortisolism, the EMG may be normal or reveal myopathic MUPs without fibrillation potentials. In CS, myopathic MUPs are usually noted, and we have observed the occasional increase in insertional and spontaneous activity (98). Muscle pathology in all varieties reveals predominantly atrophy of type 2 fibers.

Pathogenesis. Muscle weakness may be due to glucocorticoid-induced inhibition of protein synthesis with impairment in the function of ribosomes. Accelerated protein catabolism, changes in amino acid export from muscle, and alteration of carbohydrate metabolism are all likely to play a role (99). Steroid hormones also regulate protein expression (including muscle proteins) at the molecular level, possibly leading to these metabolic changes. Type 2 myofibers, preferentially affected in corticosteroid myopathies, contain less mitochondria and are more dependent on glycolytic metabolism. Their atrophy seems to contribute to loss of strength.

Treatment. With iatrogenic hypercortisolism, the corticosteroid should be discontinued if possible, and patients then recover over weeks to months. If the drug cannot be stopped, the lowest tolerable dose should be administered on an alternate-day schedule. A nonfluorinated agent is preferable to one that is fluorinated. Physical therapy is also beneficial. In CS, the underlying cause (adrenal or pituitary tumor, oat cell carcinoma of the lung, etc.) must be treated.

2. Hypothyroid myopathy

Clinical features. About 25% of patients with hypothyroidism have objective proximal weakness with or without myalgias (100,101). Patients usually develop hypothyroidism—and thus the myopathy—in middle adulthood (mean of 57 years), and women are affected more frequently than men.

The weakness is proximal in distribution and occurs at any time during the course of the endocrinopathy. Rarely, respiratory muscles are involved (102), and exceptionally, rhabdomyolysis occurs (103). There may be sluggish (hung-up) reflexes, myoedema (indentation of muscle following direct percussion), and rarely, an increase in muscle bulk (100). The triad of *muscle hypertrophy*, *weakness*, and *creatine kinase (CK) elevation* (see below) has been named the Kocher-

Debré-Sémélaigne syndrome (D-S) in infants; and in adults, the Hoffman syndrome.

Laboratory and pathologic findings. The serum CK is usually elevated (sometimes greater than 10-fold) (104) even if weakness is absent. The EMG may be normal, but increased insertional activity and myopathic MUPs are often detected (105). Myoedema, when studied by EMG, is electrically silent.

Muscle pathology reveals a large number of nonspecific findings; most common is myofiber atrophy (type 2 or type 1 or both) (104,106).

Pathogenesis and treatment. The cause is uncertain, but impairments in glycogenolysis and mitochondrial oxidation (99), increased protein turnover, changes in calcium ion transport, and regulation of muscle Na-K ATPase may all play a role. Thyroid hormone (or the deficiency thereof) may induce such changes at the molecular level (107,108). Thyroid hormone is also known to influence fast and slow myosin isotype patterns (favoring type 1 over type 2 fibers in hypothyroidism and type 2 over type 1 in hyperthyroidism) (109), but the clinical importance of this alteration is uncertain.

The myopathy almost always improves over weeks to months after thyroid hormone replacement is initiated. Pathologic changes in muscle, however, may persist after clinical recovery occurs.

3. Hyperthyroid myopathy

Clinical features. Sixty to eighty percent of patients with hyperthyroidism have muscle weakness with or without atrophy and myalgias (110,111). Women are affected more often than men (reflecting the gender predilection of hyperthyroidism), and the myopathy is more likely to occur after age 40 and if the hyperthyroidism is longstanding.

The weakness is usually predominantly proximal in distribution, beginning several weeks after the clinical onset of the hyperthyroidism. Some patients have distal as well as proximal involvement. Bulbar weakness is rare. Reflexes are normal or increased.

Laboratory features. The CK is usually normal. The EMG generally reveals myopathic MUPs with normal insertional activity (110–113). Histologic examination of muscle reveals atrophy of type 2 fibers predominantly, although mild nonspecific myopathic changes have been described.

Pathogenesis and treatment. The pathogenesis is unknown (99). Increases in protein catabolism and the basal metabolic rate (with increased insulin resistance) leading to glycogen depletion may be important. Muscle membrane excitability may be reduced. A previously suspected defect in mitochondrial metabolism has not been proven.

The myopathy improves with treatment of the underlying disorder.

4. Hyperparathyroid myopathy

Clinical features. At least 25% (and up to 88%) (113) of patients with primary hyperparathyroidism insidiously develop proximal weakness (affecting the lower more than upper extremities) and fatigue along with myalgias, arthralgias, and hyperreflexia. Patients with secondary hyperparathyroidism may also be affected, but they usually have peripheral nerve involvement as well (99).

Laboratory features. The serum calcium, alkaline phosphatase, and parathyroid hormone (PTH) are elevated. The CK is normal (113). The EMG usually reveals mixed myopathic and neurogenic changes, but nerve conduction studies are normal (113,114). Muscle biopsies reveal atrophy, primarily of type 2 fibers, but type 1 fibers may also be involved (113).

Pathogenesis and treatment. The cause is unknown, but alterations in parathyroid hormone and vitamin D may be important in inducing weakness (99). Patients usually regain strength within weeks of successful treatment of the endocrinopathy.

Acromegaly is occasionally associated with a mild myopathy with proximal weakness, normal CK, and minimal histologic or electromyographic abnormalities (115,116).

Osteomalacia may cause a painful myopathy with hyper-reflexia. The CK is normal, but there is hyperphosphatemia, elevated alkaline phosphatase, a borderline low calcium, increased parathyroid hormone, and evidence of vitamin D malabsorption (117). The EMG is usually normal, and muscle histology reveals atrophy of type 2 fibers. X-rays reveal Looser's zones (pseudofractures) especially in the pelvis.

    e. Toxic myopathies. Numerous toxins (especially drugs) lead to a subacute to chronic myopathy that is usually reversible (118). Some of these toxins are more likely to produce myopathy when their clearance is reduced, such as in renal insufficiency.

    Alcohol produces a chronic myopathy, sometimes with episodes of rhabdomyolysis. Emetine may cause a reversible myopathy with distinctive histologic appearance of disrupted myofibrillar architecture (118). *Chloroquine* causes an inflammatory myopathy with vacuolar degeneration (119). *Colchicine* induces an axonal neuropathy and a myopathy with vacuolar degeneration (120). *Cholesterol-lowering agents* also lead to muscle necrosis (121). *Penicillamine* rarely causes myositis. *Zidovudine* (AZT) is associated with a myopathy with abnormal mitochondria in AIDS patients (122). Many other drugs have been reported to produce a toxic myopathy including chlorpromazine, imipramine, procainamide, amiodarone, doxorubicin, and organophosphates (118). In general, with these disorders, the EMG reveals fibrillation potentials and myopathic MUPs and the CK is elevated when muscle necrosis is present.

V. MYOPATHY IN THE ELDERLY

As we described earlier, there is loss of muscle bulk and strength with aging, but this loss is usually measurable only by standardized instrumentation, such as myometry. Furthermore, the loss of bulk and strength is partly reversible by exercise. Therefore, the healthy active elderly should not have detectable muscle weakness on routine examination (with manual muscle testing). Even those affected by chronic nonneuromuscular conditions leading to disuse (deconditioning), for example, should have only mild weakness at most. If the clinician detects obvious muscle weakness in an elderly patient (as in a younger patient), a pathologic state should be considered.

A. Initial Approach to the Elderly Patient with Weakness

Once the elderly patient is found to have weakness and a pathologic state is suspected, the process of neurologic localization begins. In some elderly patients with coexisting medical conditions that may simulate myopathic weakness this process may be more difficult.

In the elderly, we generally follow the standard approach to evaluating weakness as discussed previously, but we are especially attentive to neurological disorders (nonmyopathic as well as myopathic conditions) that have a predilection for this segment of the population.

The history is most helpful in uncovering nonneurologic (and often nonprogressive) causes of weakness such as disuse, or medical conditions such as polymyalgia rheumatica or arthritis that may give the patient the feeling of weakness. *Polymyalgia rheumatica* usually occurs after age 50 (123). Patients complain of proximal muscle pain and stiffness. There may be weight loss, fever, elevation in ESR, anemia, and arthralgias. Some patients also have temporal arteritis. Although patients may complain of weakness, strength and laboratory studies (CK and EMG) are normal. Muscle histology is marked by type 2 fiber atrophy without inflammation or myofiber necrosis.

We also seek historical evidence of CNS (especially stroke) and spinal cord (especially cervical spondylosis) diseases that may be the cause of weakness. In such patients, upper motor neuron signs are present. They include hyperreflexia, Babinski signs, and weakness in antigravity muscles—extensors in the upper extremities; hip flexors, hamstrings, and foot dorsiflexors in the lower extremities. Patients with Parkinson's disease may also complain of weakness and stiffness, but their neurologic findings point toward an extrapyramidal syndrome.

The combination of upper motor neuron and lower motor neuron signs (weakness, atrophy, fasciculations, and sometimes hyporeflexia) is the hallmark of amyotrophic lateral sclerosis (ALS). The presence of increased reflexes in a weak atrophic limb is a powerful clinical clue that this disease is present. Bulbar and respiratory muscle involvement are also common.

Regarding disorders affecting the lower motor neuron, we consider diseases of peripheral nerves—primarily manifested by distal weakness, sensory loss, and areflexia—as well as neuromuscular junction diseases such as myasthenia gravis or Lambert-Eaton myasthenic syndrome (LEMS). Myasthenia gravis is more likely to develop in elderly than in younger adult men (124). Patients with myasthenia gravis may have diurnal variation in weakness with involvement of extraocular, bulbar, respiratory, or limb muscles. LEMS is often paraneoplastic in origin and may present a diagnostic challenge. Patients with LEMS often have proximal weakness and hyporeflexia that may improve with exercise (125)—a phenomenon referred to as postactivation facilitation. Autonomic symptoms, such as dry mouth, are common. There may be mild ptosis; significant facial, ocular, or bulbar muscle weakness is uncommon.

After excluding nonmyopathic causes of weakness, and if an unconfirmed type of myopathy is still suspected on clinical grounds, we then perform the laboratory screen shown in the algorithm (Figure 4). As mentioned previously, in patients with a suspicious body habitus or any clinical features of Cushing's syndrome, we also obtain a 24-hour urinary-free cortisol. Based on the presence of any detected serologic abnormalities, a specific work-up may be undertaken at this point.

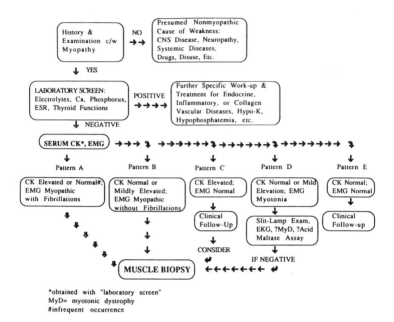

Figure 4 Algorithm for the evaluation of weak elderly patients with a suspected myopathy.

If a definite diagnosis has not yet been reached, we perform an EMG and combine this information with the CK. In the elderly, at least five patterns of EMG and CK changes may be recognized (Figure 4 and Table 3). If both CK and EMG are normal (pattern E), the yield of muscle biopsy is likely to be low; therefore, we generally follow the patient clinically and reconsider the diagnosis. If the CK is elevated and the EMG is normal (pattern C), we may follow the patient, or if weak, obtain a muscle biopsy, because EMG and CK, although useful clinical tools, are not specific or 100% sensitive for any muscle diseases including the inflammatory myopathies (81). If the EMG is consistent with a myopathy and there is fibrillation potential activity (suggestive of inflammation or muscle necrosis), *and* the CK is increased or nor-

Table 3 Classification of Myopathies Affecting the Elderly: Typical CK and EMG Patterns[a]

Myopathy	CK/EMG Pattern
Acquired	
Idiopathic inflammatory	
polymyositis, dermatomyositis	A
Inclusion-body myositis	A[b]
Sarcoidosis	A or B
Toxic	
corticosteroids	B
most drugs and other toxins	A or B
Endocrine	
hypothyroidism	A or B
hyperthyroidism	B
Cushing's syndrome	B
parathyroid diseases, osteomalacia	B
acromegaly	B
Infectious	
viral, bacterial, parasitic	A
Late-onset rod body	A or B
Inherited dystrophies	
oculopharyngeal	A or B
Myotonic[c]	D
distal (Welander)	B
Metabolic	
mitochondrial[c]	B
acid maltase[c]	D
McArdle's disease[c]	B or C

[a]See text and algorithm (Fig. 4) for description of patterns.
[b]CK may be normal; EMG may reveal mixed myopathic and neurogenic features.
[c]Usually presents during early or middle adulthood; elderly onset is rare.
Source: Adapted, with permission, from Ref. 152.

mal (pattern A); or, if the CK is elevated or normal *and* the EMG is myopathic without fibrillation potential activity (pattern B), we obtain a muscle biopsy. There is generally a high correlation (77–90%) between the EMG and histologic changes of a myopathy in selected patients (fully evaluated by neuromuscular specialists) (126,127).

If the EMG reveals myotonic discharges and the CK is normal or mildly elevated (pattern D), we undertake a workup for myotonic dystrophy (ophthalmologic slit-lamp, cardiac, family, or genetic examinations) or sometimes acid maltase deficiency (white blood cell enzyme assay or muscle biopsy). We also consider other muscle diseases associated with electrical myotonia that may occur in the elderly including hypothyroidism and inflammatory myopathies (128).

B. Accuracy of Diagnosis and Spectrum of Myopathology

Based on our experiences in evaluating muscle pathology referred by generalists as well as specialists from community and tertiary hospitals (Table 4), we tell our elderly patients that muscle biopsy confirms the clinical suspicion of myopathy about 40% of the time, and in the majority of these instances a specific diagnosis is rendered and most of the myopathies will be treatable (129). Another important role of the muscle biopsy is to exclude disorders that do not respond to immunosuppression, so that unwarranted use of these agents is avoided—especially in the elderly, who are particularly vulnerable to their toxic side effects. The degree of accuracy of diagnosing myopathy in the elderly is comparable to what is achieved in younger adults aged 30–50 years (129).

The muscle biopsy is more likely (at least 90% of the time) to confirm the clinical suspicion of myopathy when the patient has clinical features of an inflammatory myopathy and the EMG reveals fibrillation potentials and myopathic MUPs (80,81).

We believe that the algorithmic approach described herein increases the yield of muscle biopsy specimens that disclose features of a myopathy, but a prospective analysis of this method has not yet been performed.

Table 4   The Histopathologic Spectrum of Muscle
Biopsies Taken from 77 Elderly Patients (65+ yr)
Suspected of Having a Myopathy

Pathologic diagnosis	No. (%)
Myopathy	32 (42)
Inflammatory myopathy	19
Polymyositis	12
Dermatomyositis	1
IBM	6
Nonspecific myopathy	5
Oculopharyngeal dystrophy	4
Chloroquine myopathy	1
Ocular myopathy	1
Pyomyositis	1
Adult rod body myopathy	1
Neurogenic atrophy	13 (17)
Type 2 fiber atrophy	17 (22)
Normal/mild nonspecific changes	15 (19)
Total	77

Source: Adapted, with permission, from Neurology 1993;
43:825.

About half of the muscle biopsies (from elderly patients
suspected of having a myopathy) that have been referred to
our institution do not confirm the presence of a myopathy
(Table 4). In some instances, this is likely to be a false negative result. From previous studies of inflammatory myopathy,
for example, 5–26% of biopsies are negative even though the
clinical, laboratory, and electrophysiologic features are compatible with the disorder (80,81). In a significant number of
elderly patients (compared to younger adults), muscle histology discloses type 2 atrophy or neurogenic changes. As discussed above, such changes (especially type 2 atrophy) may
be part of normal aging, but in many patients, they are more
likely to reflect underlying disorders that indeed simulate myopathy and complicate the diagnosis (Table 5).

Table 5 Disorders that May Simulate Myopathy in the Elderly

Neurogenic disorders
    Amyotrophic lateral sclerosis
    Polyradiculopathy
    Chronic polyneuropathy
Disorders of the neuromuscular junction
    Myasthenia gravis
    Lambert-Eaton syndrome
Systemic disorders
    Polyarteritis nodosa
    Cachexia of malignancy
    Weakness in the wake of infection

C. Clinical Spectrum of Myopathy in the Elderly

As in all age groups, the elderly are susceptible to both hereditary and acquired myopathies (Table 4). However, it is unusual for inherited myopathies to be first diagnosed after age 65. The most notable exception is oculopharyngeal muscular dystrophy (OPD).

1. *Oculopharyngeal muscular dystrophy*

    a. Clinical features. OPD is a rare AD disorder (chromosomal location unknown) that affects predominantly French-Canadian and Spanish-American peoples. Affected family members generally develop progressive ptosis and dysphagia during their 5th to 6th decades (75,130). Ophthalmoparesis is also common, and facial and mild proximal limb weakness occurs later in the course of the illness.

    b. Laboratory features. The CK is typically normal, and the EMG reveals myopathic MUPs predominantly in weakened muscles. Although insertional activity may be normal, we have observed the presence of musical trains of positive waves, myotonic discharges, and mild fibrillation potential activity in our patients. Muscle biopsy (Figure 5) reveals

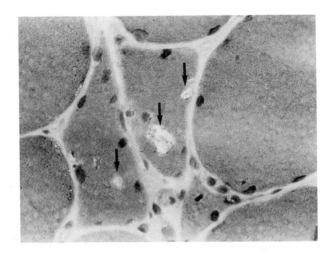

Figure 5 Oculopharyngeal muscular dystrophy. There is variation in muscle fiber size. Smaller, angulated fibers contain vacuoles (arrows). Hematoxylin and eosin, original magnification ×600.

small angulated fibers, rimmed vacuoles, moth-eaten fibers, rare fiber degeneration, and intranuclear filamentous inclusions on electron microscopy (131). Occasionally, ragged-red fibers are present (75).

   c. Pathogenesis and treatment.   The cause is unknown. It has been debated whether OPD is a myopathic or neurogenic disorder. The weight of the evidence in classical OPD favors a myopathic proceess, but there are variants (132) that seem to have a predominant neurogenic component. However, they may represent other disorders. It is likely that future genetic studies will settle the issue.

   The course is slowly progressive with the major funtional impairment being the dysphagia. Treatment is conservative, but may include ptosis surgery (or eyelid crutches) and cricomyotomy for dysphagia. Some patients require a gastrostomy for enteral feeding. Aspiration may become a concern.

2. *Distal myopathy* (*dystrophy*) (*of Welander*)

   a. Clinical features. Distal dystrophy (of Welander), which occurs primarily in Swedes, may also present late in life. Inheritance is primarily autosomal dominant. Onset usually occurs between ages 40 and 60 (range 20–77, mean 47) with slowly progressive hand intrinsic muscle and later tibialis anterior weakness. Patients may have clumsy, imprecise hand and finger movements as their chief complaint. Proximal weakness occurs rarely. There may be calf pseudohypertrophy (133). Affected males outnumber affected females (1.5:1).

   b. Laboratory features. The CK is normal or slightly elevated, and the EMG usually reveals myopathic MUP changes, occasionally with increased spontaneous activity. Muscle biopsy often reveals chronic myopathic changes with vacuolation (133).

   c. Pathogenesis and treatment. The disoder is inherited, but the underlying genetic abnormality is unknown. Treatment is supportive with physical and occupational activity, orthotics, and ambulatory assistive devices.

D. Other Inherited Myopathies Affecting the Elderly

Occasionally, patients with *myotonic dystrophy* (66) and metabolic myopathies involving disturbances in *mitochondrial* function (76) or glycogen metabolism (such as *McArdle's disease* [134] and *acid maltase deficiency* [73]) may first develop symptoms later in life. These disorders have been discussed earlier in the chapter. Other dystrophies (such as those with abnormalities in dystrophin) do not present late in life. Congenital myopathies do not generally present in the elderly either, but as an exception, a case of *centronuclear myopathy* has been reported in a 67-year-old woman who had longstanding leg weakness and calf pseudohypertrophy (135). This disorder is also unique among congenital myopathies because it is associated with increased insertional activity on EMG, simulating an inflammatory myopathy.

E. Acquired Myopathies

Endocrine and *toxic myopathies* may present at any age. The epidemiology of the endocrine myopathies reflects the age of onset and sex predilection of the endocrinopathy itself. Therefore, one might expect hypothyroid myopathy, for example, to be more common later in life since the mean age of onset of myxedema in females—who are more commonly affected than males—is 57 years. Infectious myopathies (viral, such as HIV; trichinosis; pyomyositis; etc.) may also occur at any age. These disorders have also been discussed earlier in the chapter.

1. Idiopathic inflammatory myopathies common in the elderly

In our experience, the idiopathic inflammatory myopathies make up the largest group of histologically proven muscle disease affecting the elderly (Table 4). As in younger adults, polymyositis is relatively common and dermatomyositis occurs as well; however, the major difference between these age groups is that inclusion-body myositis (IBM)—rare in younger patients—comprises at least a third of the inflammatory myopathies diagnosed after age 65 in our experience.

The features of PM an DM are discussed in the preceding sections. These features do not differ in the elderly. One caveat, however, is that the elderly tend to develop side effects from treatment with corticosteroids more frequently than do younger adults. Therefore, we tend to consider utilizing cytotoxic drugs, especially azathioprine in conjuction with corticosteroids, earlier and more frequently in the elderly as steroid-sparing agents that may be better tolerated than long-term high-dose prednisone. It is also helpful to obtain bone densitometry measurements before starting and during the course of corticosteroid administration in order to monitor for osteoporosis.

2. Inclusion-body myositis

a. Clinical features. Inclusion-body myositis is a relatively newly recognized entity first described in 1971 (136).

In part due to the more widespread examination of cryostat sections of muscle, the disorder has become increasingly recognized over the last 20 years (the characteristic rimmed vacuoles are not generally noted on paraffin sections).

The incidence is unknown. Approximately one-third of patients referred to the NIH with "treatment-resistant polymyositis" have been found to have IBM (79). Patients with IBM are usually over age 50 (137), and males are affected more frequently than females. Patients tend to develop very slowly progressive, usually painless weakness that may involve distal as well as proximal muscles. Finger flexors and quadriceps muscles may be especially affected. Dysphagia is a common accompaniment (138). Tendon reflexes, especially knee jerks, tend to be depressed. Systemic involvent is uncommon; a few patients with connective tissue diseases have been reported (138,139). Overall, the clinical diagnosis may often be delayed by as much as 3 years.

b. Laboratory features. Muscle enzymes may be normal or only mildly elevated. The EMG may reveal small, short-duration MUPs and fibrillation potential activity or mixed features of a myopathy with fibrillation potentials, as well as a reduced number of high-amplitude, long-duration MUPs that may be neurogenic in origin or more likely due to the longstanding myopathic process in which there is regeneration of myofibers (55). Approximately one-third of patients exhibit such mixed EMG features (140). Rarely, the EMG is solely neurogenic (140). However, none of these features clearly separate this entity from other inflammatory myopathies.

Muscle biopsy is necessary and diagnostic when the features include marked variation in fiber size with hypertrophic fibers (suggesting chronicity) as well as endomysial inflammation (mostly CD 8+ lymphocytes), grouped atrophic fibers, and fibers containing rimmed vacuoles (Figure 6A). The vacuoles contain amyloid (141) in addition to abnormal filamentous material—measuring 15–20 nm—that may be identified by electron microscopy (Figure 6B). Identification of these

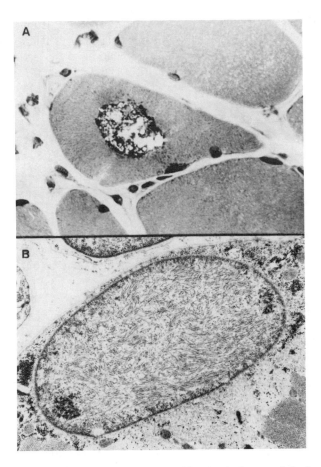

Figure 6 Inclusion-body myositis. A. A characteristic feature is the presence of vacuoles containing basophilic granules (rimmed vacuoles) within muscle fibers. Hematoxylin and eosin, original magnification ×1000. B. Intranuclear tubular inclusions 13–18 nm in diameter. Original magnification ×16,000. (From reference 139, with permission of American Medical Association.)

filaments by EM had been considered necessary for a definite diagnosis of IBM, but the presence of the classic light microscopic features alone is becoming acceptable for diagnosis.

c. **Pathogenesis and treatment.** The pathogenesis is unknown, although a viral etiology has been suspected (137). The immunopathology suggests an immune-mediated component. The presence of amyloid in vacuoles is of uncertain significance; it may be a secondary phenomenon. Recently, mitochondrial deletions have been identified in a small number of myofibers in patients with IBM (142). The significance of this finding requires further study. In rare instances, the disorder is inherited (143).

Unfortunately, IBM, unlike the other idiopathic inflammatory myopathies, does not usually respond to conventional immunosuppressive therapy, but we favor a trial of corticosteroids. Intravenous immunoglobulin, however, may be beneficial (144).

F.   Nonidiopathic Inflammatory Myopathies

1.   *Sarcoid myopathy*

a. **Clinical features.** Sarcoidosis, a multisystem disorder with a female predominance, usually presents in the 3rd to 4th decades, but it may occur much later, especially in postmenopausal women (145). Furthermore, patients who have sarcoid myopathy tend to become symptomatic later in life. Of the 51 patients included in Gardner-Thorpe's review of sarcoid myopathy, 20 developed muscle disease after age 59 (mean age of 58 for women and 39 for men) (146).

Overall, neurologic involvement occurs in about 5% of patients with sarcoidosis, and about 7–12% of these patients have a myopathy (147). Patients develop slowly progressive proximal weakness—or sometimes myalgia—with wasting that may be present for a mean of 4 years before patients seek medical attention (148). Acute myositis is rare (148) and may be associated with erythema nodosum (149). Involvement of facial, bulbar, and distal limb muscles has been occasionally noted. However, coexisting neuropathy could contribute to

distal weakness. More than half with myopathy have evidence
of sarcoidosis elsewhere, and the yield is likely to be higher
if the search is diligent.

   b. Laboratory features.   The CK may be normal or
increased (148), and needle EMG reveals myopathic MUPs
with or without fibrillation potentials. Muscle biopsy reveals
interstitial granulomas and lymphocytic inflammation (Figure
7). Muscle fiber degeneration as well as fibrosis may occur,
but often the myofibers surrounding the granulomas appear to
be undisturbed (149). Granulomas may also be detected in
muscle in between 50% and 80% of patients with sarcoidosis
who lack myopathic symptoms (149). Granulomatous myositis
is also associated with thymoma, inflammatory bowel disease,
and possibly Wegener's granulomatosis.

   c. Treatment.   The myopathy often, but not always,
responds favorably to corticosteroids.

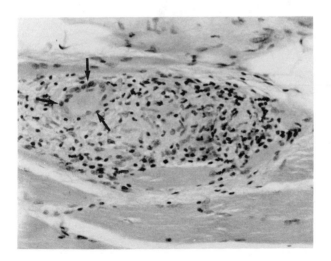

Figure 7   Sarcoid myopathy. A granuloma containing a Langhans'-
type giant cell (arrows) separates the muscle fibers. Hematoxylin and
eosin, original magnification ×370. (Reprinted with permission of
Continuing Professional Education Center, Inc.)

G. Miscellaneous Disorders

1. *Adult rod body myopathy*

a. Clinical features. Adult rod body myopathy is an example of a very rare myopathy that may affect the elderly patient (150–152). It is generally sporadic and affects patients in their 5th to 8th decades, causing progressive proximal more than distal weakness. Neck extensors may be preferentially affected.

b. Laboratory features. The CK is usually normal, and the EMG reveals myopathic or mixed features. Muscle histology reveals marked variation in fiber size with rod bodies (abnormalities of Z disk and alpha actinin) that seem to have a predilection for the atrophic fibers (Figure 8).

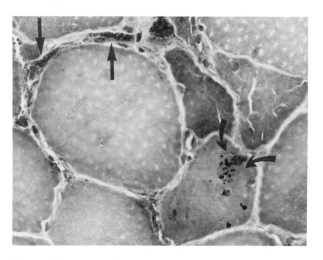

Figure 8 Adult rod body myopathy. There is marked variation in muscle fiber size. Rod bodies essentially fill the atrophic fiber (straight arrows), while fewer are present in normal-sized fibers (curved arrow). Hypertrophic fibers are devoid of rod bodies. Gomori trichrome, original magnification ×600. (Reprinted with permission, from reference 152.)

c. Pathogeneis and treatment. The origin of the rod bodies and the pathogenesis of the myopathy are unknown, although a seemingly related disorder, congenital nemaline myopathy, is of genetic origin (152). Rod bodies have been described in other disorders as well, and it has been argued that rod body myopathy is a pathologic phenomenon, not a distinct clinical entity.

The weakness is refractory to corticosteroids.

H. Amyloid Myopathy

Rarely, in systemic amyloidosis, amyloid infiltration of muscle may become symptomatic. Haleem reported (135) a 62-year-old woman with myalgia, stiffness, and muscle swelling with later heart, liver, and renal involvement. The EMG was "suggestive of a myopathic process," and amyloid was detected in muscle.

REFERENCES

1. Schulz R, Curnow C. Peak performance and age among superathletes: Track and field, swimming,baseball, tennis, and golf. J Gerontology 1988; 43:P113–120.
2. Stones MJ, Kozma A. Adult age trends in record running performances. Exp Aging Research 1980; 5:407–416.
3. Blumenthal HT. Biology of aging. In: Care of the Geriatric Patient, FU Steinberg, ed. St. Louis: Mosby, 1983;18–38.
4. Drachman DB. The role of acetylcholine as a neurotropic transmitter. Ann NY Acad Sci 1974; 228:160–175.
5. Drachman DB. The role of acetylcholine as a neurotrophic transmitter. Ann NY Acad Sci 1974; 228:160–176.
6. Giller EL, Neale JH, Bullock PN, Schrier BK, Nelson PG. Choline acetyltransferase activity of spinal cord cell cultures increased by co-culture with muscle and by muscle-conditioned medium. J Cell Biol 1977; 74:16–29.
7. Murphy R, Singer RH, Saide J, Pantagis NJ, et al. Synthesis and secretion of a high molecular weight form of nerve

growth factor by skeletal muscle cells in culture. Proc Natl Acad Sci 1977; 74:4496–4500.

8. DeGirolami U, Smith TW. Pathology of skeletal muscle. Am J Pathol 1982; 107:235–276.

9. Keynes RD, Aidley DJ. Nerve and muscle. New York: Cambridge University Press, 1991.

10. Pestronk A, Drachman DB, Griffin JW. Effects of aging on nerve sprouting and regeneration. Exp Neurol 1980; 70: 65–82.

11. Campbell MJ, McComas AJ, Petito F. Physiological changes in ageing muscles. J Neurol Neurosurg Psychiatry 1973; 36: 174–182.

12. Stålberg E, Thiele B. Motor unit fibre density in the extensor digitorum communis muscle. Single fibre electromyographic study in normal subjects at different ages. J Neurol Neurosurg Psychiatry 1975; 38:874–880.

13. Brown WF, Strong MJ, Snow R. Methods for estimating numbers of motor units in biceps-brachialis muscles and loss of motor units with aging. Muscle Nerve 1988; 11:423–432.

14. Tomlinson BE, Irving D. The numbers of limb motor neurons in the lumbosacral cord throughout life. J Neurol Sci 1977; 34:213–219.

15. Gardner E. Decrease in human neurons with age. Anat Rec 1940; 77:529–536.

16. Kawamura YI, Okazaki H, O'Brien PC, Dyck PJ. Lumbar motoneurons of man: (1) Number and diameter histogram of alpha and gamma axons of ventral root. J Neuropath Exp Neurol 1977; 36:853–860.

17. Gutman E, Hanzilikova V. Motor unit in old age. Nature 1966; 209:921–922.

18. Kanda K, Hashizume K. Changes in properties of the medial gastrocnemius motor units in aging rats. J Neurophysiol 1989; 61:737–746.

19. Buchthal F, Rosenfalck A. Evoked potentials and conduction velocities in human sensory nerves. Brain Res 1966; 3:1–122.

20. Dorfman LJ, Bosley TM. Age-related changes in peripheral and central nerve conduction in man. Neurology 1979; 29: 38–44.

21. Stevens JC, Lafgren EP, Dyck PJ. Histochemical evaluation of branches of peroneal nerve: Technique for combined bi-

opsy of muscle nerve and cutaneous nerve. Brain Res 1973; 52:37–59.

22. McMartin DN, O'Connor JA. Effect of age on axoplasmic transport of cholinesterase in rat sciatic nerves. Mech Ageing Dev 1979; 10:241–248.

23. Munsat TL. Aging of the neuromuscular system. In: Albert ML, ed., Clinical Neurology of Aging. New York: Oxford University Press, 1984:404–424.

24. Tomonaga M. Histochemical and ultrastructural changes in senile human skeletal muscle. J Am Ger Soc 1977; 25: 125–131.

25. Scelsi R, Marchetti C, Poggi P. Histochemical and ultrastructural aspects of m. vastus lateralis in sedentary old people (age 65–89 years). Acta Neuropath (Berl) 1980; 51:99–105.

26. Gimby G, Danneskiold-Samsoe B, Hvid K, Saltin B. Morphology and enzymatic capacity in arm and leg muscles in 78–82 year old men and women. Acta Phys Scand 1982; 115: 124–134.

27. Jennekens FGI, Tomlinson BE, Walton JN. Histochemical aspects of five limb muscles in old age. J Neurol Sci 1971; 14:259–276.

28. Engel AG, Banker BQ. Myology. New York: McGraw-Hill, 1986.

29. Florini JR. Minireview: Limitations of interpretation of age-related changes in hormone levels: Illustration by effects of thyroid hormones on cardiac and skeletal muscle. J Gerontol 1989; 44:B107–109.

30. Young A, Stokes M, Crowe M. Size and strength of the quadriceps muscle of old and young women. Eur J Clin Invest 1984; 14:82–87.

31. Larsson L, Karlsson J. Isometric and dynamic endurance as a function of age and skeletal muscle characteristics. Acta Physiol Scand 1978; 104:129–136.

32. Klitgaard H, Mantoni M, Schiaffino S, Ausoni S, Gorza L, et al. Function, morphology, and protein expression of ageing skeletal muscle: A cross-sectional study of elderly men with different training backgrounds. Acta Physiol Scand 1990; 140: 41–54.

33. Coggan AR, Spina RJ, King DS, Rogers MA, et al. Histochemical and enzymatic comparison of the gastrocnemius

muscle of young and healthy men and women. J Gerontol 1992; 47:B71–76.

34. Sadeh M. Effects of aging on skeletal muscle regeneration. J Neurol Sci 1988; 87:67–74.

35. Brooks SV, Faulkner JA. Cantraction-induced injury: Recovery of skeletal muscle in young and old mice. Am J Physiol 1990; 258:C436–442.

36. Zerba E, Komorowski TE, Faulkner JA. Free radical induced injury to skeletal muscle of young, adult, and old mice. Am J Physiol 1990; 258:C429–435.

37. Astrand I. Aerobic work capacity in men and women with special reference to age. Acta Physiol Scand 1960; 49(suppl 169):1–92.

38. Gersten JW. Effect of exercise on muscle function decline with aging. W J Med 1991; 154:579–582.

39. Tzankoff SP, Norris AH. Age-related differences in lactate distribution kinetics following maximal exercise. Eur J Appl Physiol 1979; 1:35–40.

40. Schlenska GK, Kleine TO. Disorganization of glycolytic and gluconeogenic pathways in skeletal muscle of aged persons studies by histometric and enzymatic methods. Mech Aging Dev 1980; 13;143–154.

41. Bass A, Gutmann E, Hanzlikova V. Biochemical and histochemical changes in energy supply–enzyme pattern of muscles in the rat during old age. Gerontologica 1975; 21: 31–45.

42. Farrar RP, Martin TP, Ardies CM. The interaction of aging and endurance exercises upon the mitochondrial function of skeletal muscle. J Gerontology 1981; 36:642–647.

43. Faulkner JA, Brooks SV, Zerba E. Skeletal muscle weakness and fatigue in old age: Underlying mechanisms. Ann Rev Gerontol and Geriatr 1990; 10:147–166.

44. Kallman DA, Plato CC, Tobin JD. The role of muscle loss in age-related decline of grip strength: Cross-sectional and longitudinal perspectives. J Gerontol 1990; 45:M82–88.

45. Grieg CA, Botella J, Young A. The quadriceps strength of healthy elderly people remeasured after 8 years. Muscle Nerve 1993; 16:6–10.

46. deVries H. Physiological effects of an exercise training regimen upon men aged 52–88. J Gerontol 1970; 25:325–336.

47. Suominen H, Heikkinen E, Liesen H, Michel D, Hollman W. Effects of 8 weeks endurance training on skeletal muscle metabolism in 56–70 year old sedentary men. Eur J Appl Physiol 1977; 37:173–180.

48. Frontera WR, Meredith CN, O'Reilly KP, Evans WJ. Strength training and determinants of VO2 max in older men. J Appl Physiol 1990; 68:329–333.

49. McCarter R, McGee J. Influence of nutrition and aging on the composition and function of rat skeletal muscle. J Gerontol 1987; 42:432–441.

50. Sharrard WJW. The distribution of the permanent paralysis in the lower limb in poliomyelitis. J Bone Joint Surg 1955; 37B:540–558.

51. Sobue G, Sahashi K, Takahashi A, Mitsuoka Y, Muroga T, Sobue I. Degenerating compartment and functioning compartment of motor neurons in ALS: Possible process of motor neuron loss. Neurology 1983; 33:654–657.

52. Wohlfart G. Collateral regeneration from residual motor nerve fibers in amyotrophic lateral sclerosis. Neurology 1957; 7:124–134.

53. Munsat TL, Hollander D, Andres P, Finison L. Clinical trials in ALS: Measurement and natural history. Adv Neurol 1991; 56:515–519.

54. Trainer PJ, Grossman A: The diagnosis and differential diagnosis of Cushing's syndrome. Clin Endocrinol 1991; 34: 317–330.

55. Kimura J. Electrodiagnosis in Diseases of Nerve and Muscle: Principles and Practice, 2nd ed. Philadelphia: FA Davis Co., 1989.

56. Uncini A, Lange DJ, Lovelace RE, Solomon M, Hays AP. Long-duration polyphasic motor unit potentials in myopathies: A quantitative study with pathologic correlation. Muscle Nerve 1990; 13:263–267.

57. Rowland LP. Clinical concepts of Duchenne muscular dystrophy. Brain 1988; 111:479–495.

58. Specht LA, Kunkel LM. Duchenne and Becker muscular dystrophies. In: The Molecular and Genetic Basis of Neurological Disease, Rosenberg RN, Pruisner SB, DiMauro S, Barchi RL, Kunkel LM, eds. Boston: Butterworth-Heinemann, 1993; 613–631.

59.   Hoffman EP, Fischbeck KH, Brown RH, Johnson M, et al. Characterization of dystrophin in muscle biopsy specimens from patients with Duchenne's or Becker's muscular dystrophy. N Engl J Med 1988; 38:1363–1368.

60.   Griggs RC, Moxley RT, Mendell JR, Fenichel GM, Brooke MH, et al. Duchenne dystrophy: Randomized, controlled trial of prednisone (18 months) and azathioprine (12 months). Neurology 1993; 43:520–527.

61.   Becker PE. Two new families with benign sex-linked recessive muscular dystrophy. Rev Can Biol 1962; 21:551–566.

62.   Emery AEH, Dreifuss FE. Unusual type of benign X-linked muscular dystrophy. J Neurol Neurosurg Psychiatry 1966; 29:338–342.

63.   Consalez GG, Thomas NST, Stayton CL, et al. Assignment of Emery-Dreifuss muscular dystrophy to the distal region of Xq28: The results of a collaborative study. Am J Hum Genet 1991; 48:468–480.

64.   Wimenga C, Padberg GW, Moerer P, Wiegant J, Liem L, Brower OF, et al. Mapping of facioscapulohumeral muscular dystrophy to chromosome 4q35-qter by multipoint linkage analysis and *in situ* hybridization. Genomics 1991; 5:570–575.

65.   Bradley WG. The limb girdle syndromes. In: Vinken PJ, Bruyn GW, eds., Handbook of Clinical Neurology: Diseases of Muscle. Amsterdam: North-Holland, 1975; 22:177–202.

66.   Harper PS. Myotonic Dystrophy, 2nd ed. Philadelphia: W.B. Saunders Co., 1989.

67.   Hawley RJ, Milner MR, Gottdiener JS, Cohen A. Myotonic heart disease: A clinical follow-up. Neurology 1991; 41: 259–262.

68.   Ptacek LJ, Johnson KJ, Griggs RC. Genetics and physiology of the myotonic muscle disorders. N Engl J Med 1993; 328: 482–489.

69.   O'Hoy KL, Tsilfidis C, Mani S, et al. Reduction in size of the myotonic dystrophy trinucleotide repeat mutation during transmission. Science 1993; 259:809–812.

70.   Streib EW. Differential diagnosis of the myotonic syndromes. Muscle Nerve 1987; 10:603–615.

71.   Bodensteiner J. Congenital myopathies. Neurologic Clinics 1988; 6:499–518.

72.   Servidei S, DiMauro S. Disorders of glycogen metabolism of muscle. Neurologic Clinics 1989; 7:159–178.

73. Engel AG, Gomez M, Seybold ME, Lambert EH. The spectrum and diagnosis of acid maltase deficiency. Neurology 1973; 23:95–106.

74. Carroll JE. Myopathies caused by disorders of lipid metabolism. Neurologic Clinics 1988; 6:563–574.

75. Chad DA, Drachman DA. Progressive external ophthalmoplegia. In: Vinken PJ, Bruyn GW, Klawans HL, DeJong JMB, eds., Handbook of Clinical Neurology 1991; 60:47–59.

76. Petty RKH, Harding AE, Morgan-Hughes JA. The clinical features of mitochondrial myopathy. Brain 1986; 109: 915–938.

77. Banker BQ, Engel AG. The polymyositis and dermatomyositis syndromes. In: Engel SG, Banker BQ, eds., Myology. New York: McGraw Hill, 1986;1396–1397.

78. Mastaglia FL. Ojeda VJ. Inflammatory myopathies. Ann Neurol 1985; 17:215–217, 317–323.

79. Dalakas MC. Polymyositis, dermatomyositis, and inclusion-body mysoitis. N Engl J Med 1991; 325:1487–1498.

80. Bohan A, Peter JB, Bowman RL, Pearson CM. A computer assisted analysis of 153 patients with polymyositis and dermatomyositis. Medicine (Baltimore) 1977; 56:255–286.

81. DeVere R, Bradley WG. Polymyositis. Its presentation, morbidity and mortality. Brain 1975; 98:637–666.

82. Sigurgeirsson B, Lindel_f B, Edhag O, Allander E. Risk of cancer in patients with dermatomyositis or polymyositis. N Engl J Med 1992; 326:363–367.

83. Sambrook P, Birmingham J, Kelly P, Kempler S, Nguyen T, et al. Prevention of corticosteroid osteoporosis. A comparison of calcium, calcitriol, and calcitonin. N Engl J Med 1993; 328:1747–1752.

84. Meunier PJ. Is steroid-induced osteoporosis preventable? [editorial]. N Engl J Med 1993; 328:1781–1782.

85. Carpenter JR, Bunch TW, Engel AG, O'Brien PC. Survival in polymyositis: Corticosteroids and risk factors. J Rheumatol 1977; 4:207–214.

86. Oddis C, Medsger TA, Hill P. Follow-up of a national cohort of 322 polymyositis-dermatomyositis (PM-DM) patients [abstract]. Arth Rheum 1991; 34(suppl):S148.

87. Bunch TW. Polymyositis: A case history approach to the differential diagnosis and treatment. Mayo Clin Proc 1990; 65: 1480–1497.

88. Dalakas MC, Illa I, Dambrosia JM, et al. A controlled trial of high-dose intravenous immune globulin infusions as treatment for dermatomyositis. N Engl J Med 1993; 329:1993-2000.

89. Miller FJ, Leitman SF, Cronin ME, Hick JE. Controlled trial of plasma exchange and leukapharesis in polymyositis and dermatomyositis. N Engl J Med 1992; 326:1380-1384.

90. Simpson DM, Citak KA, Godfrey E, Godbold J, Wolfe DE. Myopathies associated with human immunodeficiency virus and zidovudine: Can their effects be distinguished? Neurology 1993; 43:971-976.

91. Felice K, DeGirolami U, Chad DA. Pyomyositis presenting as rapidly progressive generalized weakness. Neurology 1991; 41:944-945.

92. Urbanic RC, George JM. Cushing's disease—18 years experience. Medicine 1981; 60:14-24.

93. Dropcho EJ, Soong SJ. Steroid-induced weakness in patients with primary brain tumors. Neurology 1991; 41:1235-1239.

94. Bowyer SL, LaMothe MP, Hollister JR. Steroid myopathy: Incidence and detection in a population with asthma. J Allergy Clin Immunol 1985; 76:234-242.

95. Afifi A, Bergman RA, Harvey JC. Steroid myopathy. Johns Hopkins Med J 1968; 123:158-173.

96. Lacomis D, Samuels MA. Adverse neurologic effects of glucocorticosteroids. J Gen Intern Med 1991; 6:367-377.

97. Chad DA, Lacomis D. Critically ill patients with newly acquired weakness: The clinicopathologic spectrum. Ann Neurol 1994; 35:257-259.

98. Lacomis D, Chad DA, Smith T, Aronin N. Myopathy of Cushing's syndrome. Muscle Nerve 1993; 16:880

99. Ruff RL. Endocrine myopathies. In: Engel AG, Banker BQ, eds., Myology. New York: McGraw Hill, 1986; 1871-1906.

100. Nickel SN, Frame B, Bebin J, Tourtellotte WW, Parker JA, Hughes BR. Myxedema myopathy and neuropathy. A clinical and pathologic study. Neurology 1961; 11:125-137.

101. Engel AG. Metabolic and endocrine myopathies. In: Walton, J, ed., Disorders of Voluntary Muscle, 5th ed. Edinburgh: Churchill Livingstone, 1988; 811-868.

102. Laroche CM, Cairns T, Moxham J, Green M. Hypothyroidism presenting with respiratory muscle weakness. Am Rev Respir Dis 1988; 138:472-474.

103. Halverson PB, Kozin F, Ryan LM, Sulaiman AR. Rhab-domyolysis and renal failure in hypothyroidism. Ann Intern Med 1979; 91:57–58.

104. Mastaglia FL, Ojeda VJ, Sarnat HB, Kakulas BA. Myo-pathies associated with hypothyroidism: A review based upon 13 cases. Aust NZ J Med 1988; 18:799–806.

105. Torres CF, Moxley RT. Hypothyroid neuropathy and myo-pathy: Clinical and electrodiagnostic longitudinal findings. J Neurol 1990; 237:271–274.

106. McKeran RO, Slavin G, Ward P, Paul E, Mair WGP. Hypo-thyroid myopathy. A clinical and pathological study. J Pathol 1980; 132:35–54.

107. Samuels HH, Forman BM, Horowitz ZD, Ye Z. Regulation of gene expression by thyroid hormone. Ann Rev Physiol 1989; 51:623–639.

108. Moore DM, Brent GA. Thyroid hormone: Half-sites and in-sights. New Biologist 1991; 3:835–844.

109. Ianuzzo D, Patel P, Chen V, O'Brien P, Williams C. Thy-roidal trophic influences on skeletal muscle myosin. Nature 1977; 270:74–76.

110. Havard CWH, Campbell EDR, Ross HB, Spence AW. Elec-tromyographic and histological findings in the muscle of pa-tients with thyrotoxicosis. Q J Med 1963; 32:145–163.

111. Ramsay ID. Muscle dysfunction in hyperthyroidism. Lancet 1966; 2:931–933.

112. Puvanendran E, Cheah JS, Naganathan N, Wong PK. Thy-rotoxic myopathy. A clinical and quantitiative analytic elec-tromyographic study. J Neurol Sci 1979; 42:441–451.

113. Patten BM, Bilezikian JP, Mallette LE, Prince A, Engel WK, Aurbach GD. Neuromuscular disease in primary hyper-parathyroidism. Ann Intern Med 1974; 80:182–193.

114. Frame B, Heinze EG, Block MA, Manson GA. Myopathy in primary hyperparathyroidism. Observations in 3 patients. Ann Intern Med 1968; 68:1022–1027.

115. Mastaglia FL, Barwick DD, Hall R. Myopathy in acro-megaly. Lancet 1970; 2:907–909.

116. Stern LZ, Payne CM, Hannapel LK. Acromegaly: Histo-chemical and electron microscopic changes in deltoid and in-tercostal muscles. Neurology 1974; 24:589–593.

117. Smith R, Stern G. Myopathy, osteomalacia, and hyperparathyroidism. Brain 1967; 40:593–602.

118. Kuncle RW, Wiggins WW. Toxic myopathies. Neurol Clin 1988; 6:593–619.

119. Estes ML, Ewing-Wilson D, Chou SM, Mitsumoto H, Hanson M, et al. Chloroquine neuromyotoxicity. Clinical and pathologic perspective. Am J Med 1987; 82:447–455.

120. Kuncl RW, Duncan G, Watson D, Alderson K, Rogawski MA, Peper M. Colchicine myopathy and neuropathy. N Engl J Med 1987; 316:1562–1568.

121. London SF, Gross KF, Ringel SP. Cholesterol-lowering agent myopathy (CLAM). Neurology 1991; 41:1159–1160.

122. Dalakas MC, Illa I, Pezeshkpour GH, Laukaitis JP, et al. Mitochondrial myopathy caused by long-term zidovudine therapy. N Engl J Med 1990; 322:1098–1105.

123. Goodwin JS. Progress in gerontology: Polymyalgia rheumatica and temporal arteritis. J Am Ger Soc 1992; 40: 515–525.

124. Engel AG. Myasthenia gravis and myasthenic syndromes. Ann Neurol 1984; 16:519–534.

125. O'Neill JH, Murray NMF, Newsom-Davis J. The Lambert-Eaton myasthenic syndrome. Brain 1988; 111:577–596.

126. Black JT, Bhatt GP, Dejesus PV, Schotland DL, Rowland LP. Dignositic accuracy of clinical data, quantitative electromyography, and histochemistry in neuromuscular disease. J Neurol Sci 1974; 21:59–70.

127. Buchthal F, Kamieniecka Z. The diagnostic yield of quantified muscle biopsy in neuromuscular disorders. Muscle Nerve 1982; 5:265–280.

128. Daube JR. AAEM mini-monograph #11. Needle examination in clinical electromyography. Muscle Nerve 1991; 14: 685–700.

129. Lacomis D, Chad DA, Smith TW. Myopathy in the elderly: Evaluation of the histopathological spectrum and the accuracy of clinical diagnosis. Neurology 1993; 43:825–828.

130. Victor M, Hayes R, Adams RD. Oculopharyngeal muscular dystrophy. A familial disease of late life characterized by dysphagia and progressive ptosis of the eyelids. N Engl J Med 1962; 267:1267–1272.

131. Tom FMS, Fardeau M. Nuclear inclusions in OPD. Acta Neuropath (Berl) 1980; 49:85–87.

132. Hardiman O, Halperin JJ, Farrell MA, Shapiro BE, Wray SH, Brown RH. Neuropathic findings in oculopharyngeal muscular dystrophy. Arch Neurol 1993; 50:481–488.

133. Welander L. Myopathia distalis tarda heredetaria. 249 examined cases in 72 pedigrees. Acta Med Scand 1951; 264(suppl):1–124.

134. Felice KJ, Sneebaum AB, Jones HR. McArdle's disease with late-onset symptoms: Case report and review of the literature. J Neurol Neurosurg Psychiatry 1992; 40:407–408.

135. Haleem MA. Myopathies in the elderly. Gerontol Clin 1972; 14:361–377.

136. Yunis EJ, Samaha FJ. Inclusion body myositis. Lab Invest 1971; 25:240–248.

137. Carpenter S, Karpati G, Heller I, Eisen A. Inclusion body myositis: A distinct variety of idiopathic inflammatory myopathy. Neurology 1978; 28:8–17.

138. Lotz BP, Engel AG, Nishino H, Stevens JC, Litchy WJ. Inclusion body myositis. Observations in 40 patients. Brain 1989; 112:727–747.

139. Chad DA, Good P, Adelman L, Bradley WG, Mills J. Inclusion body myositis associated with Sjogren's syndrome. Arch Neurol 1982; 39:186–188.

140. Joy JL, Oh SJ, Baysal AI. Electrophysiological spectrum of inclusion body myositis. Muscle Nerve 1990; 13:949–951.

141. Mendell JR, Sahenk Z, Gales T, Paul L. Amyloid filaments in inclusion body myositis. Novel findings provide insight into nature of filaments. Arch Neurol 1991; 48:1229–1234.

142. Oldfors A, Larsson N, Lindberg C, Holme E. Mitochondrial DNA deletions in inclusion body myositis. Brain 1993; 116:325–336.

143. Neville HE, Baumbach LL, Ringel SP, Russo LS, Sujansky, Garcia CA. Familial inclusion body myositis: Evidence for autosomal dominant inheritance. Neurology 1992; 42:897–902.

144. Soueidan SA, Dalakas MC. Treatment of inclusion-body myositis with high-dose intravenous immunoglobulin. Neurology 1993; 43:876–879.

145. Rudberg-Roos I. The course and prognosis of sarcoidosis as observed in 296 cases. Acta Tuberc Scand 1962; 52(suppl):1–42.

146. Gardner-Thorpe C. Muscle weakness due to sarcoid myopathy. Six case reports and an evaluation of steroid therapy. Neurology 1972; 22:917–928.

147. Stern BJ, Krumholz A, Johns C, Scott P, Nissim J. Sarcoidosis and its neurological manifestations. Arch Neurol 1985; 42:909–917.

148. Wolfe SM, Pinals RS, Aelion JA, Goodman RE. Myopathy in sarcoidosis: Clinical and pathologic study of four cases and review of the literature. Sem Arthritis Rheum 1987; 16: 300–306.

149. Silverstein A, Siltzbach LE. Muscle involvement in sarcoidosis. Asymptomatic, myositis, and myopathy. Arch Neurol 1969; 21:235–241.

150. Engel AG. Late-onset rod myopathy (a new syndrome?): Light and electron microscopic observations in 2 cases. Mayo Clin Proc 1966; 41:713–741.

151. Paulus W, Peiffer J, Becker I, Roggendorf W, Schumm F. Adult-onset rod disease with abundant intranuclear rods. J Neurol 1988; 235:343–347.

152. Lacomis D, Chad DA, Smith TW. Adult rod body myopathy: Case report and approach to the diagnosis of myopathy in the elderly. Neurology Chronicle 1992; 2:11–15.

7

Neuropathic Disorders

Anthony A. Amato
Wilford Hall Medical Center and
University of Texas Health Science Center at San Antonio
San Antonio, Texas

Richard J. Barohn
University of Texas Southwestern Medical Center at Dallas
Dallas, Texas

Neuropathic disorders are an important group of neurologic disorders in the elderly population. A discussion of neuropathic disorders encompasses those diseases that affect the neuron's cell body, or neuronopathies, and those affecting the peripheral process, or peripheral neuropathies (Table 1). Neuronopathies can be further subdivided into those that affect only the anterior horn cells, or motor neuron disease, and those involving only the sensory neurons, also called sensory neuronopathies or ganglionopathies. Peripheral neuropathies can be broadly subdivided into those that affect myelin, or myelinopathies, and those that affect the axon, or axonopathies. This is primarily a pathologic approach to neuropathic disorders in which the first question asked by the clinician is "Where is the lesion?" Each of these categories has distinct clinical and electrophysiologic features that allow the clinician to place a patient's disease into one of these broad groups. Subsequently, the clinician attempts to determine the etiology of the disorder (Table 2). For example, is the disor-

The views expressed herein are those of the authors and do not necessarily reflect the views of the U.S. Air Force or the Department of Defense.

Table 1 Pathologic Classification of Neuropathic Disorders

Neuronopathies (pure sensory or pure motor):
  Sensory neuronopathies (ganglionopathies)
  Motor neuronopathies (motor neuron disease)
Peripheral neuropathies (usually sensorimotor):
  Myelinopathies
  Axonopathies

Table 2 Etiology of Neuropathic Disorders

I. Acquired
  Dysmetabolic states
    Diabetes mellitus[a]
    Neuropathy related to renal disease[a]
    Vitamin deficiency states (e.g., vitamin B_{12} deficiency[a])
    Primary amyloidosis[a]
  Immune mediated
    Guillain-Barré syndrome[a]
    Chronic inflammatory demyelinating polyneuropathy (CIDP)[a]
    Vasculitis[a]
    Neuropathy associated with a monoclonal antibody[a]
    Plexitis—cervical and lumbosacral[a]
    Multifocal motor neuropathy
  Infectious
    Herpes zoster[a]
    Leprosy, Lyme, HIV, and sarcoid related
  Cancer related
    Lymphoma,[a] myeloma,[a] and carcinoma[a] related
    Paraneoplastic subacute sensory neuronopathy[a]
  Drugs or toxins
    Chemotherapy induced[a]
    Other drugs
    Heavy metals and industrial toxins
  Mechanical/compressive
    Radiculopathy[a]
    Mononeuropathy
  Unknown etiology
    Idiopathic sensory and sensorimotor neuropathy[a]
    Amyotrophic lateral sclerosis[a]

Table 2   Continued

II. Hereditary
    Hereditary motor sensory neuropathy (Charcot-Marie-Tooth
      disease)
    Hereditary neuropathy with predisposition to pressure palsies
    Familial brachial plexopathy
    Familial amyloidosis
    Porphyria
    Other rare peripheral neuropathies
      (Fabry's, metachromatic leukodystrophy, adrenoleukody-
        strophy, Refsum's disease, etc.)
    Motor neuron disease
      Spinal muscular atrophy
      Familial amyotrophic lateral sclerosis
      X-linked bulbospinal muscular atrophy

---

[a]These disorders need to be considered more often in the elderly.

der hereditary or acquired? If it is acquired, is the neuropathic disorder due to a systemic dysmetabolic state? Is it drug or toxin induced? Is it mediated by an immune or infectious process, or is the cause unknown? The final step in approaching the patient with a neuropathic disorder is to determine whether or not therapy is possible, and if so, what the course of therapy should be. These final two steps are often frustrating as it is not always possible to determine the cause or alter the natural history of neuropathic disorders.

What is the chance of correctly determining the pathologic type and etiology of a neuropathic disorder? If one considers only peripheral neuropathies, some information is available. Of 205 patients referred to the Mayo Clinic with an undiagnosed peripheral neuropathy, a diagnosis was made in 76% of cases (1). A hereditary neuropathy was found in 42%, an inflammatory demyelinating disorder (chronic inflammatory demyelinating polyneuropathy or CIDP) was diagnosed in

21%, and 13% were diagnosed as having a peripheral neuropathy associated with other diseases (diabetes and other metabolic disorders, nutritional deficiency, toxins, and cancer). In our experience, these figures may be somewhat overly optimistic with regard to identifying hereditary neuropathy and CIDP, which we would place at 20% and 10%, respectively. In addition, approximately 50% of patients in our clinic are ultimately found to have no identifiable cause for their peripheral neuropathy, which is a figure compatible with at least one published series (2). No good data are available regarding these percentages if one includes all neuropathic disorders (motor neuron disease along with peripheral neuropathy).

While neuropathic disorders can occur at any age, some diseases are more likely to develop in the elderly. On the other hand, there are relatively few differences in the clinical manifestations of neuropathic disorders between old and young patients. Therefore, the format for this chapter will differ somewhat from most of the others in this book. In the first part of this chapter, we will present a simplified clinical approach to the patient with a neuropathic disorder. As we go through this clinical approach, we will highlight diseases that need to be considered more often in the elderly. In the next section, we will address the various morphologic, clinical, and electrophysiologic aspects of motor neurons and peripheral nerves that are affected by age. Finally, we will discuss in detail a number of the neuropathic disorders that need to considered in the elderly patient.

I. APPROACH TO THE PATIENT WITH A NEUROPATHIC DISORDER

A. Important Information from the History and Physical

Our initial approach is to determine if the patient's symptoms and signs are pure motor, pure sensory, or both. If the patient has only weakness without any evidence of sensory loss, a motor neuronopathy, or motor neuron disease, is the most likely diagnosis (Table 3). In motor neuron disease, the initial weakness is nearly always asymmetric, beginning in either arm, leg, or bulbar muscles. Cramps and fasciculations are also frequent associated features. The majority of patients with adult-onset motor neuron disease have evidence of both upper and lower motor neuron dysfunction on examination (i.e., amyotrophic lateral sclerosis), which is the primary diagnostic hallmark of this disorder (3). On the other hand, nearly one-third of adult patients with motor neuron disease may present initially without upper motor neuron findings (3).

While some peripheral neuropathies may present with only motor symptoms, evidence of sensory involvement on neurologic examination is generally found in these cases. The clinician should be aware of those neuropathic disorders that may present with pure motor symptoms (Table 3). Of the disorders listed in Table 3, motor neuron disease and the acquired demyelinating polyneuropathies need to considered strongly in the elderly.

The distribution of the patient's weakness is crucial for an accurate diagnosis and in this regard two questions should be asked: (1) Does the weakness only involve the distal extremity or is it both proximal and distal? (2) Is the weakness focal and asymmetric or is it symmetric? The finding of weak-

Table 3 Neuropathic Disorders that May Be Purely Motor at Presentation

---
Motor neuron disease[a]
Guillain-Barré syndrome[a]
CIDP[a]
Lead intoxication
Acute porphyria
Multifocal motor neuropathy
Hereditary motor sensory neuropathy (Charcot-Marie-Tooth disease)

---
[a]These disorders need to be considered more often in the elderly.

ness in both proximal and distal muscle groups in a symmetric fashion is the hallmark for acquired immune demyelinating polyneuropathies, both the acute form (Guillain-Barré syndrome) and the chronic form (CIDP). Patients with proximal muscle weakness will complain of difficulty raising their arms to brush their teeth or comb their hair as well as problems climbing stairs or rising from a chair. On the neurologic examination, the clinician needs to pay particular attention for the presence of facial, neck, shoulder, and hip weakness in addition to the more distal muscle groups in the hands and feet. The importance of finding symmetric proximal and distal weakness in a patient who presents with both motor and sensory symptoms cannot be overemphasized because this identifies the important subset of patients who may have a treatable acquired demyelinating neuropathic disorder. On the other hand, if a patient with both symmetric sensory and motor findings has weakness involving only the distal lower and upper extremities, the disorder generally reflects a primarily axonal peripheral neuropathy and is much less likely to represent a treatable entity. A rare exception is the uncommon and still incompletely understood entity of multifocal motor neuropathy, presumably an acquired primarily motor demyelinating disorder, but which presents with distal, and often asymmetric, extremity weakness (see below).

Asymmetry or focality of the weakness is also a feature that can narrow the diagnostic possibilities (Table 4). Some neuropathic disorders may present with unilateral leg weakness. If sensory symptoms and signs are absent, and an elderly patient presents with painless foot drop evolving over weeks or months, motor neuron disease is the leading and most worrisome diagnostic possibility. On the other hand, if a patient presents with subacute or acute sensory and motor symptoms of one leg, lumbosacral radiculopathies, plexopathies, vasculitis, and compressive mononeuropathy need to be carefully considered. Similarly, if the clinical manifestations are pure motor weakness in one arm or hand, motor neuron disease is probably the leading consideration. If sen-

Table 4 Neuropathic Disorders that Produce Asymmetric/ Focal Weakness

---

Motor neuron disease
  Amyotrophic lateral sclerosis
Radiculopathy—cervical or lumbosacral
  Root compression from osteoarthritis[a]
  Root compression from herniated disk
  Herpes zoster focal paresis (with rash)[a]
  Meningeal carcinomatosis and lymphomatosis[a]
Plexopathy—brachial or lumbosacral
  Immune mediated/idiopathic (primarily brachial)[a]
  Neoplastic infiltration[a]
  Diabetic radiculoplexopathy (primarily lumbosacral)[a]
  Familial brachial plexopathy
Mononeuropathy multiplex due to:
  Vasculitis[a]
  Multifocal motor neuropathy
  Lyme disease
  Sarcoid
  Leprosy
  HIV infection
  Hereditary neuropathy with predisposition to pressure palsy
Compressive/entrapment mononeuropathies
  Median neuropathy (carpal tunnel syndrome)
  Ulnar neuropathy (cubital tunnel syndrome, Guyon's canal)
  Peroneal neuropathy at the fibular head

---

[a]These disorders need to be considered more often in the elderly.

sory symptoms are also present, cervical radiculopathy, brachial plexopathy, or a mononeuropathy are likely possibilities. All of these disorders are reasonable diagnostic considerations in an elderly patient. On the other hand, hereditary neuropathy with predisposition to pressure palsies (HNPP) or familial brachial plexus neuropathies are conditions that can present with focal, asymmetric leg or arm weakness, but would be unlikely to present initially in an elderly patient.

Complaints of numbness or tingling, while implicating sensory involvement, are in general not very helpful in suggesting a specific diagnosis as these symptoms can accompany many peripheral neuropathies. Two sensory features may be helpful to the clinician in arriving at a diagnosis. If severe pain is one of the patient's symptoms, certain peripheral neuropathies should be considered (Table 5). The idiopathic distal sensory neuropathy and neuropathy due to diabetes mellitus are the most common neuropathies in elderly patients that are associated with severe pain. In addition, painful peripheral neuropathies due to peripheral nerve vasculitis or Guillain-Barré syndrome (GBS) are important to recognize because these disorders are treatable. The pain in vasculitic neuropathy is generally distal in the most severely involved extremity. Some patients with GBS have severe back pain associated with symmetric numbness and paresthesia in the extremities. The pain associated with idiopathic and diabetic distal sensory neuropathy is symmetric (usually worse in the feet). Another painful form of diabetic neuropathy is lumbosacral radiculoplexopathy (also known as diabetic amyotrophy), in which patients may present with the abrupt onset of hip or thigh pain that may precede weakness by hours to days. In contrast, the quality or other descriptive characteristics of the pain (i.e., burning, aching, sharp, lancinating, needle-like, etc.) are rather nonspecific.

Table 5 Peripheral Neuropathies that May Be Associated with Pain

---

Idiopathic distal sensory or sensorimotor neuropathy[a]
Diabetes mellitus[a]
Vasculitis[a]
Guillain-Barré syndrome[a]
Amyloidosis (familial and acquired)[a]
Toxic (arsenic, thallium)
HIV-related distal symmetrical polyneuropathy
Fabry's disease

---

[a]These disorders need to be considered more often in the elderly.

Another important sensory abnormality that significantly narrows the differential diagnosis is severe proprioceptive loss. This is sometimes difficult to discern from the history but complaints of loss of balance, especially in the dark, or symptoms suggesting disequilibrium may be helpful. If the neurologic examination reveals a dramatic loss of proprioception (usually accompanied by a significant vibration sensation deficit), the clinician should immediately consider a sensory neuronopathy (i.e., ganglionopathy) (Table 6). A subacute sensory neuronopathy associated with malignancy is the most important of these disorders to consider in the elderly population.

Of obvious importance is the onset, duration, and evolution of symptoms. Does the disease have an acute (days to 4 weeks), subacute (4–8 weeks), or chronic (greater than 8 weeks) course? Is the course monophasic, progressive, or relapsing? Neuropathies with acute and subacute presentations include GBS, vasculitis, and diabetic lumbosacral radiculoplexopathy. A relapsing course can be present in CIDP and porphyria. It is also important to inquire about preceding or concurrent infections, associated medical conditions, drug use including over-the-counter vitamin preparations (B_6), alcohol, and dietary habits.

Some peripheral neuropathies are associated with significant autonomic nervous system dysfunction (Table 7). Inquire

Table 6 Causes of Sensory Neuronopathy (Ganglionopathy)

Cancer[a]
Cisplatin and other analogues[a]
Idiopathic sensory neuronopathy
Sjögren's syndrome
Vitamin B_6 toxicity
HIV-related sensory neuronopathy

[a]These disorders need to be considered more often in the elderly.

Table 7 Peripheral Neuropathies with Autonomic Nervous System Involvement

Diabetes mellitus[a]
Amyloidosis (familial and acquired)[a]
Guillain-Barré syndrome[a]
Vincristine induced[a]
Porphyria
HIV-related autonomic neuropathy
Idiopathic pandysautonomia

[a]These disorders need to be considered more often in the elderly.

if the patient has had fainting spells or orthostatic lightheadedness, heat intolerance, or any bowel, bladder, or sexual dysfunction. If these symptoms are present, check for an orthostatic fall in blood pressure without an appropriate increase in heart rate. Autonomic dysfunction in the absence of diabetes should alert the clinician to the possibility of amyloid polyneuropathy. Rarely, an idiopathic pandysautonomic syndrome can be the only manifestation of a peripheral neuropathy without other motor or sensory findings.

Finally, a hereditary cause for a peripheral neuropathy in an elderly patient will not be as likely as in a younger population but should not be overlooked. In patients with a chronic, very slowly progressive distal weakness over many years, with very little in the way of sensory symptoms, the clinicians should pay particular attention to the family history and inquire about foot deformities in immediate relatives. On examining the patient, the clinician must look carefully at the feet for arch and toe abnormalities (high or flat arches, hammer toes), and look at the spine for scoliosis.

B. Important Information from the Electrophysiologic Study

The electrophysiologic evaluation of patients with a suspected peripheral neuropathy consists of nerve conduction studies

(NCS) and needle electromyography (EMG). The electrophysiologic data provide information about the nature of the neuropathy. Thus, whether the neuropathic disorder is a mononeuropathy, multiple mononeuropathy (mononeuropathy multiplex), radiculopathy, plexopathy, or generalized polyneuropathy can be confirmed. Similarly, it can be ascertained whether the process involves only sensory nerves, only motor nerves, or both. Finally, the electrophysiologic data can help distinguish axonopathies from myelinopathies.

It is beyond the scope of this chapter to provide an extensive discussion about how the electrophysiologic data lead the clinician to make the conclusions noted above; the reader is referred to standard sources on the subject (4,5,6). However, the basic electrophysiologic paradigm by which one classifies a neuropathy as being due to axonal degeneration or segmental demyelination is outlined in Table 8. In general, low-amplitude potentials with relatively preserved distal latencies, conduction velocities, and late potentials, along with fibrillations on needle EMG, constitute the findings of an axonal neuropathy. On the other hand, slow-conduction velocity, prolonged distal latencies and late potentials, relatively preserved amplitudes (unless there is conduction block), temporal dispersion, and the absence of fibrillations on needle EMG characterize a pure demyelinating neuropathy.

Unfortunately, many neuropathic disorders cannot always be neatly categorized into one of two groups. For example, in motor neuropathies or neuronopathies in which the compound motor action potential (CMAP) amplitude is significantly reduced due to axonal degeneration, the conduction velocity may be mildly slow. Motor conduction velocity can be slowed to as much as 80% of the lower limit of normal (LLN) (i.e., reduced by 20% below the LLN) due to axonal degeneration. Thus, a peroneal or tibial conduction velocity (in which the LLN is 42 meters/sec) can be reduced to 33 meters/second in an axonal neuropathy or neuronopathy in which the CMAP is very small. In addition, it is not uncommon to find indications of some degree of secondary axonal

Table 8 Axonal Degeneration vs. Segmental Demyelination: Electrophysiologic Features

	Axonal degeneration	Segmental demyelination
Motor nerve conduction studies		
CMAP amplitude	Decreased	Normal (except with CB)
Distal latency	Normal	Prolonged
Conduction velocity	Normal	Slow
Conduction block	Absent	Present
Temporal dispersion	Absent	Present
F wave	Normal	Prolonged or absent
H reflex	Normal	Prolonged or absent
Sensory nerve conduction studies		
SNAP amplitude	Decreased	Normal
Distal latency	Normal	Prolonged
Conduction velocity	Normal	Slow
Needle EMG		
Spontaneous activity		
Fibrillations	Present	Absent
Fasciculations	Present	Absent
Voluntary motor unit potentials		
Recruitment	Decreased	Decreased
Morphology	Long duration/normal	Polyphasic

CMAP = compound motor action potential
SNAP = sensory nerve action potential
CB = conduction block

degeneration in neuropathies that are predominantly demyelinating. Thus, fibrillation potentials on needle EMG can be seen in over 70% of patients with CIDP (7).

Recently, a committee appointed through the American Academy of Neurology (AAN) attempted to define the nerve conduction studies constituting an acquired demyelinating polyneuropathy (Table 9) (8). While these criteria provide

Table 9　AAN Electrophysiologic Criteria for Chronic Inflammatory Demyelinating Polyneuropathy (CIDP)

A.　Mandatory
　　Must have three of four:
　　1.　Reduction in conduction velocity (CV) in two or more motor nerves
　　　　a.　<80% of lower limit of normal (LLN) if amplitude >80% of LLN
　　　　b.　<70% of LLN if amplitude <80% of LLN
　　2.　Partial conduction block or abnormal temporal dispersion in one or more motor nerves: either peroneal nerve between ankle and below fibular head, or median nerve between wrist and below elbow

　　　　Criteria suggestive of partial conduction block: <15% change in duration between proximal and distal sites and >20% drop in negative-peak (–p) area or peak-to-peak (p-p) amplitude between proximal and distal sites

　　　　Criteria for abnormal temporal dispersion and possible conduction block: >15% change in duration between proximal and distal sites and >20% drop in –p area or p-p amplitude between proximal and distal sites. These criteria are only suggestive of partial conduction block as they are derived from studies of normal individuals. Additional studies, such as stimulation across short segments or recording of individual motor unit potentials, are required for confirmation.
　　3.　Prolonged distal latencies in two or more:
　　　　a.　>125% of upper limit of normal (ULN) if amplitude >80% of LLN
　　　　b.　>150% of ULN if amplitude <80% of LLN
　　4.　Absent F waves or prolonged minimum F-wave latencies (10–15 trials) in two or more motor nerves:
　　　　a.　>120% of ULN if amplitude >80% of LLN
　　　　b.　> 150% of ULN if amplitude <80% of LLN
B.　Supportive
　　1.　Reduction in sensory CV <80% of LLN
　　2.　Absent H reflexes

Source: Neurology 1991; 47:617.

reasonable guidelines, they are meant primarily for research purposes. For example, many patients who clinically have CIDP and respond to treatment do not fulfill these strict criteria. In a recent study (9), only approximately two-thirds of patients with CIDP fulfilled the AAN criteria for demyelinating neuropathy. Despite these limitations, nerve conduction studies and needle EMG can provide extremely useful information and should be performed on most patients being evaluated for a neuropathic disorder.

C.   Important Information from the Nerve Biopsy

There are relatively few diseases that require a nerve biopsy for diagnosis. Peripheral nerve vasculitis and amyloidosis are the two most likely neuropathies in the elderly in which a nerve biopsy may be necessary. The sural nerve is the most common nerve biopsied, but the superficial peroneal nerve can also be used for this purpose. Nerve biopsy is useful but probably not mandatory in supporting the clinical diagnosis of CIDP. Finding thinly myelinating axons with Schwann cell proliferation (so-called "onion bulbs") and mild perivascular inflammation can be quite helpful in this regard. Unfortunately, the sensory nerve biopsy in patients with clinical and electrophysiologic evidence of a demyelinating neuropathy may not always show these classic pathologic features. In addition, the normal aging process can produce some degree of pathologic abnormalities irrespective of clinical evidence for a neuropathy (see below). In our opinion, in a patient who fulfills clinical and electrophysiologic criteria for CIDP, and who has an elevated spinal fluid protein, a nerve biopsy is probably not mandatory.

D.   Other Important Laboratory Information

There are relatively few blood tests that should be routinely done in the evaluation of all (or nearly all) patients who present with a neuropathic disorder (Table 10). Additional studies can be ordered in selective cases in which there is a

Table 10 Useful and Nonuseful Blood Studies in Evaluating Patients with Neuropathic Disorders

Useful tests in all or some cases:

  CBC[a]

  SMA 20[a]

  Serum protein electrophoresis and immunofixation electrophoresis[a]

  Thyroid function tests[a]

  B_{12} level[a]

  VDRL and FTA-ABS[a]

  Methylmalonic acid and homocysteine[b]

  Parathyroid hormone[b]

  Hemoglobin A1C[b]

  Erythrocyte sedimentation rate[b]

  Antinuclear antibodies (including SS-A and SS-B)[b]

  Rheumatoid factor[b]

  Antineuronal nuclear antibody type I (ANNA-1 or anti-Hu)[b]

  Lyme antibody[b]

  HIV antibody[b]

  Myelin-associated glycoprotein (MAG) antibody[b]

  Molecular genetic analysis for CMT-1A[b], hereditary neuropathy with liability for pressure palsy (HNPP)[b], and the familial amyloid polyneuropathies[b]

Not proven to be useful:

  GM1 antibody

  Asialo-GM1 antibody

  GD1b antibody

  Sulfatide antibody

  CY ratio

[a]Obtained in the evaluation of most neuropathic disorders.
[b]Obtained in selective cases.

strong clinical index of suspicion for a particular disorder. For example, an elderly patient with known small-cell lung cancer who develops a subacute sensory neuronopathy should have a serologic determination for antineuronal antibodies. There are a number of antibodies to various glycolipids in myelin (Table 10) that are now commercially available. However, the significance and utility of these antibodies has not been proven in controlled prospective clinical studies.

The cerebrospinal fluid protein determination is important in the evaluation of possible demyelinating neuropathies. The CSF protein is elevated in over 90% of patients with acute and chronic inflammatory demyelinating polyneuropathy, although the cell count is seldom abnormal (7).

II. NEUROPATHIC DISORDERS AND AGING

A. Morphologic and Physiologic Effects of Aging on the Peripheral Nervous System

Morphologic changes in nerve fibers of the peripheral neuron system (PNS) occur with normal aging. One of the most obvious changes is the accumulation of lipofuscin in aging cell bodies of motor and sensory neurons as well as in autonomic ganglia (10). Melanin pigment also accumulates in sensory and autonomic ganglion cells but not in motor neurons. Neurofibrillary tangles similar to those observed in Alzheimer's disease have been reported in spinal ganglia cells of old Wistar rats (11) and in the upper cervical ganglia of a 76-year-old man (12). In addition, a decrease in the number of anterior horn cells within the spinal cord occurs with age (13). Similar observations with loss of cell bodies within the cervical sympathetic chain (10) and intermediolateral cell column of the autonomic nervous system (14) have been noted. Data regarding sensory ganglia are conflicting, with some reporting loss of sensory neurons (15,16) whereas others report no change in cell numbers with aging (17).

A loss of myelinated nerve fibers has been documented with the spinal roots and peripheral nerves in the elderly (18–22). Axonal degeneration and regeneration as well as segmental demyelination and remyelination occur with advancing age (22). There is shortening of internodal segments that can be variable between successive internodal segments along individual nerves and between different nerve fibers (22,23). In addition, loss of axons with empty Schwann cell bands occurs among unmyelinated nerve fibers with age (24).

Electrophysiologic techniques that estimate the number of motor units supplying a muscle have consistently documented a 30–50% loss of motor units in patients over 60 years old (25–27). For example, in the study by Sica et al., the thenar muscle was supplied by 340 ($\pm$79) motor units in young adults, compared to 83 ($\pm$46) motor units in patients over 60 years of age (25–27). The remaining motor units are larger (i.e., they innervate more muscle fibers presumably due to re-innervation) (28–30) and have increased twitch tension (31, 32). It is unknown to what extent motor unit losses with age and the adaptive changes of surviving motor units are due to biologic aging or to repeated trauma and injury.

Nerve conduction studies reflect the morphologic changes in nerves observed as people age. Distal latencies of compound muscle and sensory nerve action potentials become mildly prolonged with age (33–35). The latencies of F waves and somatosensory evoked potentials also increase with age. Motor, sensory, and mixed nerve conduction velocities decrease with age (36–39) but significant changes do not occur until after the 60th (40,41) year of life. Robinson et al. estimate that ulnar motor nerve conduction velocity decreases by about 0.2 meters/second/year, although they found no change in the ulnar motor latency with age (39). On the other hand, the ulnar sensory distal latency increased by 0.01 milliseconds/year (39). In interpreting nerve conduction velocities in general, Oh (42) allows for a 1 meter/second/decade decline in motor nerves and 2 meters/second/decade decline in sensory nerves per decade over the age of 60 years. Temporal dispersion and reduction in amplitude of sensory nerve and to a lesser extent compound muscle action potentials occur with advancing age (34,38,39,43–45).

With needle EMG, motor unit durations increase with age. In the biceps brachii, there is an increase in motor unit potential durations by 0.05 milliseconds/year (46). With regard to spontaneous potentials, we are unaware of any reliable studies that would indicate that fibrillation or fasciculation potentials are more often seen in "normal" elderly patients. One situation in which this issue occasionally arises is during the needle EMG examination of a foot muscle such as the abductor hallucis in an elderly patient. Anecdotal experience leads one to believe that occasional fibrillation may occur in these muscles in older individuals, presumably as a result of recurrent trauma over the years, and thus their presence may not necessarily imply a more diffuse neurogenic disorder. However, this observation needs confirmation in a prospective clinical study. On the other hand, a number of neuropathic disorders are more likely to occur in the elderly (see below) that can produce denervation potentials.

Quantitative sensory testing of vibratory sensation by various methods has shown a definite increase in vibratory perception thresholds with age (47–51). While this phenomenon can be seen as early as the third decade, the most significant changes occur after age 50 (47). Thermal discrimination thresholds also increase with age (48,51).

While many clinicians do not have access to sophisticated quantitative sensory equipment, the bedside use of a 120 Hz tuning fork can reveal decreased vibration sensation in older patients. Our examination technique consists of striking the tuning to obtain a maximal vibratory stimulus and immediately applying the tip of the handle to the interphalangeal joint of the great toe. Using a clock, one determines how long the patient can perceive the vibratory stimulus. In children and young adults, this maximal vibratory stimulus is appreciated for at least 15 seconds over the great toe. As patients age, this time decreases even in the absence of overt peripheral neuropathy. As a basic rule of thumb, we allow 1 second of vibration perception loss per decade (authors' unpublished observations). Thus, it is not uncommon for a 70-year-old patient to have only 9 or 10 seconds of maximal vibration perception over the great toe. Other bedside measurements of sensation (pin prick, touch, proprioception, temperature) are not as easily quantified with age.

B. Specific Neuropathic Disorders that Can Affect the Elderly

1. *Motor neuron disease*

Motor neuron disease (MND) comprises a heterogeneous group of disorders involving degeneration of the upper motor neurons (UMN) of the brain and the lower motor neurons (LMN) of the brainstem and spinal cord. The most common subset of MND is amyotrophic lateral sclerosis (ALS). In ALS there is involvement of both upper and lower motor neurons. Progressive bulbar palsy, progressive muscular atrophy, and spinal muscular atrophy are characterized by pure LMN abnormalities while primary lateral sclerosis (PLS) is characterized by pure UMN dysfunction. However, pathologic findings on autopsies may reveal evidence of UMN involvement in what was clinically felt to be a lower motor neuron syndrome (progressive bulbar palsy or muscular atrophy) while evidence of LMN degeneration may be seen on EMG or muscle biopsy in what appeared to be PLS.

a. Amyotrophic lateral sclerosis.   ALS is a fatal disorder characterized by progressive degenerative UMNs and LMNs. The annual incidence is about 2 per 100,000 with a peak age of onset in the sixth decade (52,53). The male-to-female ratio is 2:1. LMN involvement manifests with atrophy, weakness, and fasciculation. UMN degeneration results in spasticity and frequently a pseudobulbar affect.

Onset of weakness may begin in the extremities, usually distal, or in the musculature. When onset occurs in an extremity, spread to the contralateral myotomes generally ensues before other extremity or bulbar muscle involvement. Cramps are common. Sensory symptoms may be reported in 25% of patients, but objective sensory loss is not observed (53). Ocular muscles are generally spared, but may rarely be affected late in the course of the disease when life is prolonged by mechanical ventilation (53). Bowel, bladder, and autonomic functions are preserved. Deep tendon reflexes are hyperreflexic given the degree of muscle atrophy. Plantar responses eventually are extensor. Needle EMG reveals fibrillation and fasciculation potentials, large polyphasic MUPs, and decreased recruitment. Sensory nerve conduction studies are normal. Decreased amplitudes of CMAPs and "pseudo" conduction block may be observed over atrophic muscles (3). However, true conduction block demonstrated over a discrete segment of nerve (as is seen in some cases of multifocal motor neuropathy) is not seen in ALS.

In general, the course is relentlessly progressive with death in 2 years in 50% of patients. In some patients the course of the disease is unusually prolonged with stabilization or rarely reversal of deficits (52). The age of onset is the most significant predictor determining duration. Shorter survival times correlate with later age of onset (54,55). One study found a mean illness duration of 2.6 years for patients ages 61–70 compared to 8.2 years for patients <40 years old (54). Dementia has been reported in up to 5% of sporadic and familial ALS (52).

There is no known treatment for ALS. There are ongoing drug trials with antioxidants as well as various neurotrophic growth factors. Studies involving steroids, immunosuppressants, thyroid-releasing hormone, L-threonine, branch-chain amino acids, and various glutamate receptor inhibitors have been unrewarding (3). Recently, a preliminary report suggested that riluzole, a glutamate antagonist, can prolong survival for a short time in ALS patients (56,57). A subsequent riluzole study has apparently confirmed these preliminary findings, but at this time the data from this follow-up study have not been published. Nevertheless, if the new riluzole data stands up to Federal Drug Administration scrutiny, many ALS patients will probably be placed on this drug within a year or two. Orthotic devices may help with activities of daily living. Many patients have problems handling secretions and anticholinergic drugs may be beneficial. In patients with situational depression, a tricyclic antidepressant is useful and may also aid in drying secretions. Computer-assisted language devices can be used late in the course of the illness to prolong communication. Baclofen and benzodiazepines can be helpful in patients with significant spasticity; however, some degree of spasticity may be necessary in weak leg muscles in order to ambulate.

There are a number of conditions that can mimic ALS and are treatable. Multifocal motor neuropathy, characterized by slowly progressive asymmetric weakness, conduction block on motor NCS, and perhaps elevated anti-GM1 ganglioside titers, can resemble ALS but is treatable with intravenous immunoglobulin or cyclophosphamide (3,58,59). Therefore, nerve conduction studies of proximal and distal segments of motor nerves should be assessed in all motor neuron disorders to evaluate for the presence of localized conduction block. This disorder is possibly a pure motor variant of chronic inflammatory demyelinating polyneuropathy (CIDP). It occurs primarily in young and middle-aged adults (males more often than females). However, several males in their 60s have been reported with this disease (59). Since it is potentially treatable, conduction block needs to be excluded in all patients with motor neuron disease.

Thyrotoxicosis and hyperparathyroidism can result in muscle weakness, fasciculations, and hyperreflexia. Therefore, serum calcium, parathyroid hormone levels, and thyroid function tests should be obtained in all patients with a motor neuron syndrome. Occasionally a motor neuronopathy occurs in patients with lymphoma and can be the presenting feature (60). Thus, serum immunoelectrophoresis or immunofixation should also be obtained. The presence of a monoclonal gammopathy, markedly elevated cerebral spinal fluid protein, or pleocytosis should lead to an aggressive work-up for lymphoma. In addition, exposure to inorganic or organic mercury (61) and lead intoxication (62) may mimic ALS.

b. Hereditary ALS.   Five to ten percent of ALS may be inherited in an autosomal-dominant pattern. Some, but not all, familial ALS (FALS) pedigrees are linked to chromosome 21q. Tight genetic linkage between FALS and the gene that encodes for a copper-zinc binding superoxide dismutase

(SOD1) enzyme has been reported (63). Missense mutations in the SOD1 gene have been discovered and are the putative cause of the disorder in some FALS families. There may be an earlier onset in the familial compared with the sporadic type of ALS (52). DNA analysis may potentially be useful for confirmation and genetic counseling, but it is not commercially available at this time.

c. **Hereditary spinal muscular atrophy.** The spinal muscular atrophies (SMAs) comprise a group of hereditary disorders characterized by degeneration of lower motor neurons without upper motor neuron or sensory abnormalities. Currently, the SMAs are classified according to age of onset, distribution of weakness, mode of inherence, and prognosis. In general, SMA presents in children or young adults. Some cases, however, develop and go undiagnosed until late in life. Onset symptoms of adult-onset autosomal-recessive SMA range from 15 to 60 years (64,65). Muscle weakness is slowly progressive and predominantly involves the proximal arms and legs. Eventually distal weakness occurs, but bulbar involvement is unusual. Life expectancy is not significantly reduced (64). Some forms of autosomal-recessive SMA have been mapped to chromosome 5q (66). Rare adult-onset autosomal-dominant (AD) SMA with onset beginning as late as 65 years of age has been reported (64). An additional type of AD-SMA with a scapuloperoneal distribution has been described with onset at age 70 (64).

X-linked bulbar and spinal muscular atrophy or bulbospinal neuronopathy is caused by a mutation in the androgen receptor gene (67–69). Onset of the weakness begins in the third to seventh decade of life. The presence of an X-linked inheritance of androgen insufficiency (gynecomastia, impotence, infertility) in combination with LMN abnormalities should lead to the correct diagnosis. In addition, despite the lack of sensory symptoms, sensory SNAPs are frequently of low amplitude or absent. This electrophysiologic feature distinguishes the disorder from other motor neuron diseases.

2. *Idiopathic Sensory or Sensorimotor Polyneuropathy*

This is the most common neuropathy the clinician faces in clinical practice, and specifically in the elderly patient. Surprisingly few good clinical studies have been done to clarify the clinical presentation, course, and management of this common disorder. The age of onset is usually between ages 45 and 65 (2). Patients complain of distal numbness, tingling, and often burning pain that invariably begins in the feet, and may eventually involve the fingers and hands. Patients exhibit a stocking or stocking-and-glove loss to pain, temperature, touch, and vibration, with proprioception being significantly involved in a minority of cases. Neither subjective nor objective evidence of weakness is a prominent feature. The ankle muscle stretch reflex is frequently absent, but in cases with predominantly small-fiber loss, this may be preserved.

The electrophysiologic findings in this common disorder range from isolated sensory nerve action potential abnormalities (usually with loss of amplitude), to evidence for an axonal sensorimotor neuropathy, to a completely normal study (if primarily small fibers are involved). It is not uncommon to find abnormalities on peroneal and tibial nerve conduction studies (low amplitudes, mild slowing) and denervation potentials on needle EMG in distal leg and feet muscles without evidence for motor involvement on the neurologic examination.

The work-up of these patients consists of the blood tests outlined in the section on "Other Important Laboratory Information." An extensive screen for serum glycolipid antibodies is not indicated. In addition, a screen for cancer does not go beyond a good history and physical examination in most cases. Neither a CSF examination nor a sural nerve biopsy are necessary in these cases, because they will seldom yield information that will change management.

Therapy primarily involves the control of neuropathic pain, if this is one of the patient's symptoms. If the patient has only numbness, or numbness and tingling without sharp or burning pain, placing the patient on the medications outlined below is of no benefit. The most frequently used medications for neuropathic pain are the tricyclic antidepressants (70–72) (Table 11). Unfortunately, these medications often are accompanied by intolerable anticholinergic and sedating side effects, especially in elderly patients. The pharmacokinetics of the tricyclic antidepressants is altered with age so that the elimination half-life increases (73,74). Some authors suggest beginning tricyclic antidepressants with smaller doses in elderly patients, such as 10 mg at bedtime, and increasing by 10 mg increments every 5–7 days as tolerated (75). Extreme caution is required to ensure an elderly male patient has not had symptoms of prostatic hypertrophy, as tricyclic antidepressants can significantly exacerbate urinary hesitancy. Other oral medications that can be used include anticonvulsants (76) and, more recently, the antiarrhythmic drug, mexiletine (77) (Table 11). All can cause some degree of sedation or mental confusion, especially in older patients.

Topical capsaicin ointment is effective in no more than half of the patients with painful neuropathy, but is usually worth a trial before using oral medication (78,79). Some patients can not tolerate the caustic sensation of the ointment itself, and caution needs to be used in applying the ointment so that none is rubbed inadvertently on the face or eyes. Capsaicin ointment needs to be applied three or four times a day to be effective and a reasonable trial consists of at least 4 weeks of therapy. We usually begin with the 0.025% ointment and will proceed to the 0.075% preparation if necessary. Another "topical" therapy is transcutaneous nerve stimulation (TENS), but it also is effective in only a minority of patients (80,81). Immunotherapy with corticosteroids, other immunosuppressive agents, intravenous immune globulin, or plasmapheresis is not indicated in these patients.

We are aware of only one prospective study of idiopathic sensory and sensorimotor polyneuropathy and this involved a cohort of 75 elderly patients, mean age 56.5 years (82). On

Table 11 Symptomatic Therapy for Peripheral Neuropathy

Therapy	Route	Dose	Monitor
Amitriptyline/ Nortriptyline	po	10–100 mg at bedtime	mental status blood pressure (orthostasis) heart rate difficulty urinating (males)
Carbamazepine	po	200–300 mg tid to qid	mental status blood count serum drug level
Phenytoin	po	300–400 mg at bedtime	mental status gingival hyperplasia serum drug level
Mexiletine	po	200–300 mg tid	heart rate, blood pressure, blood count, liver enzymes serum drug level
Capsaicin	cutaneous	0.025% or 0.075% tid to qid	skin irritation; avoid eye contact (wear gloves when applying)
Transcutaneous nerve stimulation (TENS)	cutaneous	daily (frequency variable)	—

clinical grounds, 39% had a pure sensory neuropathy, 57% had a sensorimotor neuropathy, and 4% (2 patients) had a pure motor neuropathy. Sixty-four patients (85%) had electrophysiologic evidence for an axonal sensorimotor neuropathy, which therefore included most of the patients who had only evidence for sensory involvement on the history and physical examination. An important finding in this study is that patients had either a very slowly progressive (56%) or a nonprogressive (44%) course over the years. In addition, 71% of the patients remained independent, 28% needed the use of a cane or ankle brace, and only one patient was wheelchair dependent. As there is no treatment available that can reverse an idiopathic distal peripheral neuropathy, a significant amount of time needs to be spent by the clinician in explaining to the patient the relatively benign course of this disorder.

3. *Diabetic neuropathy*

In industrialized nations, diabetes mellitus represents the most common cause of peripheral neuropathy, and this is especially true for the elderly population. It has been observed that while only 8% of diabetics have a neuropathy when their disease is first diagnosed, after 25 years, 50% will have developed a neuropathy (83). Therefore, neuropathy is a particular concern for the elderly patient with diabetes mellitus.

The pathologic basis for diabetic neuropathy remains controversial. There is evidence that both vascular and metabolic derangements may be responsible for peripheral nerve pathology in diabetes (84,85). A detailed discussion of this data is beyond the scope of this chapter and readers are referred to more detailed reviews (84–86). However, from a purely clinical view, diabetic neuropathies can be broadly divided into those that are focal or multifocal, and those that are symmetrical polyneuropathies (Table 12). A simplified pathophysiologic scheme would account for the focal and multifocal neuropathies on a primarily vascular basis, and the symmetrical polyneuropathies on a primarily metabolic basis. In general, patients with strict control of blood glucose have fewer dia-

Table 12   Clinical Classification of Diabetic Neuropathies

I. Symmetric Polyneuropathies
    Distal sensory neuropathy
    Autonomic neuropathy
    Diabetic neuropathic cachexia
    Hyperglycemic neuropathy
    Treatment-induced diabetic neuropathy
II. Asymmetric/Focal and Multifocal Diabetic Neuropathies
    Cranial neuropathies
    Limb mononeuropathies
    Truncal neuropathies (thoracic polyradiculopathy)
    Lumbosacral polyradiculoneuropathy (Bruns-Garland syndrome;
        diabetic amyotrophy)

---

betic neuropathy complications (87,88), although there are often exceptions to this rule (89).

   a.   Symmetric neuropathies.   Distal symmetric polyneuropathy is the most common form of diabetic neuropathy. Clinically, this is primarily a sensory neuropathy, and significant distal weakness is uncommon. However, as in idiopathic distal sensory neuropathy, there is usually electrophysiologic evidence for subclinical motor involvement. Indeed, the clinical and electrophysiologic findings in both idiopathic and diabetic distal sensory and sensorimotor neuropathy are virtually indistinguishable. Dysesthesia, usually burning pain, may be present, although the majority of diabetic patients with a distal sensory neuropathy do not complain of significant discomfort. If severe foot ulcers and neurogenic arthropathies develop, this is often labeled pseudosyringomyelic diabetic neuropathy. Severe proprioceptive loss is uncommon, but occasionally it can occur, and it has been called the pseudotabetic form of diabetic neuropathy. Finally, significant autonomic insufficiency symptoms can accompany the distal sensory loss. Autonomic manifestations can affect cardiovascular, genitourinary, or gastrointestinal organ systems so that patients develop orthostasis, gastroparesis, impotence, or bladder atony. Other autonomic manifestations include profuse nocturnal or post-prandial sweating and abnormal pupillary light responses. Rarely, an acute severe painful diabetic neuropathy can be associated with excessive weight loss (so-called diabetic neuropathic cachexia) (90,91), initiation of insulin treatment, or new-onset hyperglycemia.

b. Asymmetric/focal neuropathies. Focal diabetic neuropathies may involve isolated limb (carpal tunnel syndrome, peroneal neuropathies) or cranial nerve (oculomotor, abducens, facial) mononeuropathies (92). The most common, and often misdiagnosed, multifocal diabetic neuropathy is lumbosacral radiculoplexopathy syndrome. This disorder has been referred to by many names including proximal diabetic neuropathy, ischemic mononeuropathy multiplex, femoral or femoral-sciatic neuropathy, and most often, diabetic amyotrophy. Diabetic amyotrophy is perhaps the most misleading term as it implies a disorder of muscle, when in fact this is a neuropathic process affecting the roots and lumbosacral plexus. An older eponym that we have recently reintroduced, Bruns-Garland syndrome, gives recognition to the physicians who were responsible for defining this clinical entity (89).

Bruns-Garland syndrome affects an older group of diabetics, usually over age 50. Most patients have noninsulin-dependent diabetes mellitus and the development of this neuropathy is often unrelated to glucose control or the duration of glucose intolerance. The neuropathy begins with severe pain in the back, hip, or thigh, and patients are frequently misdiagnosed as having a compressive lumbosacral radiculopathy. Within several days or weeks after the onset of pain, patients develop weakness in both proximal and distal leg muscles. On examination there is weakness of hip flexors and extensors, knee flexors and extensors, and ankle dorsiflexors and plantar flexors of varying degree. It is the exception rather than the rule for the weakness to be isolated to proximal hip and thigh muscles. There is usually distal sensory loss, but this is often indistinguishable from the sensory abnormalities of a distal sensory neuropathy, which often was present prior to the development of the radiculoplexopathy. Loss of knee and ankle reflexes is common. While the condition usually begins in one leg, spread to the other leg within weeks or months is rather frequent. The disorder worsens in a gradually progressive or stepwise manner. Cases have been documented in which there is worsening for 18 months. Eventually, the process stabilizes and gradually improves, although the recovery may take many months. In many cases, some degree of permanent weakness may persist.

Electrophysiologically, the nerve conduction study findings may not be able to be differentiated from a distal sensorimotor polyneuropathy. The needle EMG, however, reveals abundant fibrillation potentials in weak proximal and distal leg muscles as well as in the lumbosacral paraspinous muscles (93). The CSF protein is often strikingly elevated.

Another common focal form of diabetic radiculopathy involves isolated thoracic roots (94,95). Cervical root or brachial plexus involvement is extremely rare. The presumed pathophysiologic basis for radiculoplexopathy in diabetics is ischemic infarction.

The management of diabetic neuropathy involves the control of glucose (if this is found to be abnormal) and pain relief. For the most part, the therapies for pain management are similar to those outlined in the section on idiopathic painful distal sensory neuropathies (78,79,96,97). However, patients with focal or multifocal diabetic neuropathies may have such severe discomfort that the temporary use of narcotics may be indicated. At times, in lumbosacral radiculoplexopathy syndrome, more aggressive pain relief therapies through an anesthesia pain clinic are required. Once the pain is controlled, an aggressive physical therapy program is required. Motor rehabilitation cannot, however, be accomplished until significant pain relief has been achieved.

4. *Uremic neuropathy*

The evidence of peripheral neuropathies in patients with renal failure is quite variable, but at least 60% of dialysis patients have signs of neuropathy (98–100). The etiology of the neuropathy is felt to be secondary to the accumulation of toxins normally excreted by the kidneys. In addition, systemic conditions responsible for the renal failure (i.e., diabetes mellitus, amyloid, systemic lupus erythematosus, polyarteritis nodosa, etc.) can also cause peripheral neuropathy. As patients with chronic renal insufficiency live longer, this group of neuropathies is of particular concern for clinicians caring for elderly patients.

Uremic neuropathy is generally considered to be distal symmetric, axonal, sensorimotor neuropathy. Initial symptoms consist of numbness and paresthesia affecting the legs more than the arms (98). Painful burning sensation of the feet can occur. The earliest manifestation of motor involvement is usually ankle dorsiflexor weakness. Autonomic dysfunction can occur in severe cases (101). Muscle cramps and restless leg syndrome may herald symptoms of peripheral nerve involvement (98). Onset of the neuropathies is usually gradual and slowly progressive. However, the severity and tempo of uremic neuropathy can be quite variable (98). Abrupt or gradual onset of severe weakness resembling that seen in GBS or CIDP has been reported (102).

Electrophysiologic studies reveal decreased amplitudes, prolonged distal latencies, and slow conduction velocities (103,104). Electromyography may demonstrate distal denervation changes. Cerebrospinal fluid is acellular, but protein may be markedly elevated (98). The predominant features on nerve biopsies are axonal atrophy and degeneration with secondary demyelination (105).

The prognosis of untreated uremic neuropathy is poor. Successful renal transplantation can result in resolution of the neuropathy, but in advanced cases the recovery may be prolonged and incomplete (106–108). Chronic hemodialysis may stabilize or improve symptoms but is generally felt to be less effective than renal transplantation (108,109).

5. *Vitamin B_{12} deficiency neuropathy*

Vitamin B_{12} deficiency is an important treatable cause of peripheral neuropathy in the elderly. It is estimated that 3–10%

of patients >65 years old have low serum vitamin B_{12} levels (110–114). In addition, the mean age of onset of pernicious anemia, the most common cause of vitamin B_{12} deficiency, is 60 years. Deficiency of vitamin B_{12} leads to axonal degeneration and myelin loss of both central and peripheral nerve fibers. In the spinal cord, this results in the classic *combined systems degeneration* of the posterior sensory columns and the lateral corticospinal tracts. In biopsied peripheral sensory nerves, the pathology reflects a primary axonal degeneration (114).

The mechanism of vitamin B_{12} deficiency is usually due to malabsorption (115). Inadequate dietary intake of this vitamin is unusual in developed countries, where it occurs predominantly in patients on strict vegetarian diets. In classic pernicious anemia, the lack of vitamin B_{12} absorption is due to the absence of intrinsic factor, which in turn results from the autoimmune destruction of gastric parietal cells. Other causes include gastric and small bowel disease and surgery, overgrowth of intestinal bacteria, chronic pancreatitis, and interference of absorption by certain drugs (ethanol, cholestyramine, colchicine, neomycin, cimetidine, oral contraceptives).

There are clues from the history and neurologic exam that should alert the clinician to possible vitamin B_{12} deficiency. Numbness and paresthesia can begin in the hands or feet. In a patient complaining of numb hands and gait unsteadiness, one should suspect vitamin B_{12} deficiency. Additionally, the coexistence of ataxia, hyperreflexia in the arms and knees, hyporeflexia at the ankles, and vibration loss at the toes should raise a red flag for this disorder. Such findings reflect simultaneous pathology in both the central and peripheral nervous system. Lhermitte's sign may be present in some cases.

The electrophysiologic evaluation also may reflect the involvement of central or peripheral nerves, or both. Motor and sensory NCS may be entirely normal if most of the pathology is central. When NCS is abnormal, this usually consists of amplitude loss out of proportion with latency and conduction velocity abnormalities, although mild slowing can occur. Evidence of central nervous pathology can be reflected by abnormal latencies on somatosensory-evoked potentials and visual-evoked potentials (116). Patients with the isolated "numb hands syndrome" may have normal NCS but abnormal somatosensory-evoked potential latencies, indicating that the site of lesions in this syndrome is central rather than peripheral (117).

The diagnosis can be confirmed by demonstrating a very low serum vitamin B_{12} level (115). Only 60–70% of patients with pernicious anemia, however, have levels below 100 ng/L. In addition, anemia and macrocytosis may be not be present in 30–40% of cases. Thus, even if these studies are normal, in the appropriate clinical setting further tests for vitamin B_{12} deficiency should be obtained. Serum or urine methylmalonic acid and homocysteine are frequently elevated, even if the serum vitamin B_{12} is normal (118). Finally, the Schilling test is extremely useful both in finding evidence of vitamin B_{12} deficiency in cases with normal serum levels and in determining if the lesion is due to intrinsic factor deficiency.

Vitamin B_{12} should be replaced parenterally with intramuscular injections, usually for the rest of the patient's life. A typical recommended version is 1000 µg daily for the first week, then weekly for 1 month, then monthly (115). However, all of the symptoms and signs of vitamin B_{12} deficiency may not be corrected even with vigorous therapy (117). More often, there will be a partial improvement, but this may not occur for 6–12 months. In severe cases, vitamin B_{12} replacement may simply stop further progression of the disease.

6. *Inflammatory demyelinating polyneuropathy*

a. **Guillain-Barré syndrome.** Guillain-Barré syndrome (GBS) or acute inflammatory demyelinating polyneuropathy (AIDP) is associated with rapidly evolving weakness, sensory loss, and areflexia. GBS is the most common cause of acute generalized weakness and has an incidence of 1–2 cases per 100,000 people (119). GBS can occur at any age. The incidence is several times higher in the age group over 60 (3.2 per 100,000) as compared to individuals under 18 years of age (0.8 per 100,000) (119). In addition, in a large multicenter study, 22% of patients (53 of 245) were over the age of 60 (120). In many patients, there is an antecedent infection that is usually viral. Campylobacter jejuni enteritis precedes GBS in 15–38% of patients and is the most common antecedent bacterial infection (121). In addition, recent surgery is a recognized premonitory event (122).

Initial symptoms are usually numbness and tingling of the extremities. Aching pain in the extremities and back is common. Subsequent weakness involving proximal and distal muscles ensues. Usually the lower-extremity muscles are initially affected. Patients become hypo- or areflexic. Over 50% of patients reach their nadir by 2 weeks, 80% by 3 weeks, and 90% by 4 weeks (123). Tempo of progression is variable and some can become flaccid and ventilator dependent in a few days.

In addition to the classic presentation of GBS, variants have been described. Fisher syndrome (124) with ophthalmoplegia, ataxia, and areflexia is well recognized. In addition, other variants including areflexic paraparesis with bilateral lower-extremity numbness and weakness sparing the arms; pharyngeal-cervical-brachial weakness with ptosis sparing the arms; bifacial paresis, paresthesia, and reduced deep-tendon reflexes; lateral rectus paresis, paresthesia, and diminished deep-tendon reflexes have been well described (125, 126). Also, rare cases of pure sensory, pure motor, or dysautonomia occur. An axonal variant manifested by rapidly progressive weakness with prolonged paralysis and respiratory failure has been reported (127). This axonal variant may be associated with antecedent *Campylobacter jejuni* enteritis and has a poor prognosis (121).

Cerebrospinal fluid (CSF) is remarkable for elevated protein with minimal, if any, lymphocytic pleocytosis (albuminocytologic disassociation) after the first week. Early electrophysiologic features include low-amplitude or prolonged CMAPs and prolonged or absent F waves, indicating a predilection for the nerve roots and terminals (128,129). Later, slowed conduction velocities with temporal dispersion and conduction block can be demonstrated. The disorder is felt to be autoimmune, involving both the cellular and humoral mechanisms. Autopsy studies and nerve biopsies demonstrate lymphocyte and macrophage infiltration of nerves with demyelination (130). The axonal variant has been associated with low-amplitude CMAPs, prominent denervation on EMG, and axonal degeneration without significant demyelination on nerve biopsies (127).

The most important component of treatment is supportive care. Patients need to be monitored closely for respiratory and autonomic instability. Forced vital capacities (FVCs) need to be followed, and FVCs below 15–20 ml/kg require endotracheal tube intubation. Progressive neck, flexor, and extensor weakness closely correlates with respiratory compromise and can also be used to monitor for impending respiratory failure. Leg stockings and subcutaneous heparin, 5000 units twice daily, are indicated for prevention of deep venous thrombosis and pulmonary emboli. Aggressive physical therapy is useful for prevention of muscle contractures in a severely weak patient.

Most patients with GBS recover spontaneously; however, 10–23% require mechanical ventilation, 7–22% have residual defects, 3–10% relapse, and 2–5% die (120). Age over 60 years and low-amplitude CMAPs are poor prognostic indicators (131). In the study by McKhann et al (131), older patients took a significantly larger time to walk or improve a grade on a standardized disability scale. Plasma exchange, involving 200–250 ml of plasma per kg body weight over 7–10 days, has been shown to be an effective therapy (120) (Table 13). Recently, one study reported intravenous immunoglobulin (IVIG) to be at least as effective as plasma exchange (132). Anecdotal reports suggest IVIG may be associated with higher incidence of relapse compared to plasma exchange (133,134). However, in elderly patients with hemodynamic instability or poor venous access, IVIG may represent the treatment of choice. Unlike in CIDP, corticosteroids are not of benefit in the treatment of GBS (see below).

b.   Chronic inflammatory demyelinating polyneuropathy.   Chronic inflammatory demyelinating polyneuropathy (CIDP) represents a significant number of all initially undiagnosed acquired neuropathies (7,135). Diagnosis is important because CIDP is treatable with various immunomodulating therapies. CIDP occurs at any age, but the peak age of onset is 40–60 years. In order to fulfill diagnostic criteria for CIDP (7,136), weakness must be present for at least 2 months. Weakness can vary in severity, but is symmetric and involves proximal and distal muscles of the upper and lower extremities. Facial and neck flexor weakness can occur. Rarely, extraocular and respiratory muscles are involved. Sensory complaints usually consist of numbness and tingling. Painful paresthesia is less common. Many patients describe a loss of balance. Deep tendon reflexes are usually absent or depressed.

A diagnosis of CIDP is supported by CSF showing typical albuminocytologic disassociation. Nerve conduction studies are suggestive of demyelination with prolonged distal latencies, slowed conduction velocities, and prolonged or absent F waves in the presence of conduction block or temporal dispersion (7,135,136). Nerve biopsy may be helpful in excluding other etiologies such as amyloidosis, vasculitis, and various hereditary or toxic neuropathies. However, no feature on nerve biopsy is pathognomonic for CIDP. In fact, in one large series of CIDP cases (7), demyelination was seen in only 48% while 21% had axonopathy, 13% had mixed demyelinating and axonal features, and 18% were normal. In addition, only 11% had evidence of inflammatory infiltrate.

Based on clinical, electrophysiologic, and pathologic features, diagnostic categories have been introduced: definite, probable, and possible CIDP (7,136). In addition to idiopathic

Table 13 Immunosuppressive Therapy for Immune-Mediated Neuropathies

Therapy	Route	Dose	Monitor
Prednisone	po	100 mg/day for 2–4 weeks, then 100 mg every other day; single a.m. dose	Weight, blood pressure, serum glucose/potassium, cataract formation
Methylprednisone	IV	1 g in 100 m/normal saline over 1–2 hours, 3–6 doses, daily or every other day	Heart rate, blood pressure, serum glucose/potassium
Azathioprine	po	2–3 mg/kg/daily; single a.m. dose	Monthly blood count and liver enzymes
Cyclophosphamide	po	1.5–2 mg/kg/day; single a.m. dose	Monthly blood count and urinalysis

Cyclosporine	p.o.	3–6 mg/kg/day; single a.m. or b.i.d. dose	Blood pressure, cyclosporine level, creatinine/BUN, liver enzymes
Plasmapheresis	IV	Remove total of 200–250 cc/kg plasma over 7–14 days; may require periodic exchanges	Heart rate, blood pressure, blood count, electrolytes, PT/PTT, volume removed and replaced
Immune globulin	IV	0.4 g/kg/day over 5 days, or 1 g/kg/day over 2 days; then 0.4 to 1.0 g/kg single doses every 4–8 weeks as needed	Heart rate, blood pressure, creatinine/BUN, blood count

CIDP, there is a category of concurrent diseases with CIDP, which include systemic lupus erythematosus, HIV infection, monoclonal or biclonal gammopathies, and concomitant central nervous system demyelination.

Randomized control trials have confirmed that steroids (137) and plasma exchange (138) are beneficial in CIDP. Plasma exchange generally needs to be repeated every few months; otherwise patients relapse. We generally prefer treating with high-dose prednisone and initiate treatment with 100 mg a day as a one-time dose in the morning (Table 13) (7). Once improvement begins, usually within 2–4 weeks, we switch to alternate-day prednisone with a dose of 100 mg every other day (Table 13). When the strength has returned to normal or improvement has plateaued (usually within 3–6 months), we slowly taper the prednisone by 5 mg every 2–3 weeks. A few patients can eventually be tapered completely off the prednisone; however, many patients relapse. It is important for both the patients and physician to realize CIDP is a chronic disorder and may require immunosuppressant therapy for many years. Although 95% of patients with CIDP show initial improvement, the relapse rate is very high. In one series, 50% of patients relapsed after a mean follow-up of 49 months (7). Only 51% of patients made a complete recovery. In a retrospective study, age did not appear to be a poor prognostic variable (7) as it is in GBS (131). However, this needs to be confirmed in a prospective study. In patients who relapse during prednisone taper, we add azathioprine as a second-line immunosuppressive drug. There are important risks of long-term steroids including glucose intolerance, hypertension, weight gain, cataracts, glaucoma, osteoporosis, and infection, and these are often more significant problems in elderly patients. The use of alternate-day prednisone as a one-time dose in the morning, in combination with a low-carbohydrate, low-salt diet, and vitamin D and calcium supplements, reduces the side effects of prednisone. Recently, IVIG has been shown to be useful in the treatment of CIDP (139,140), although a double-blind, placebo-controlled trial did not demonstrate benefit (141).

7. Vasculitic neuropathy

Vasculitis is characterized by inflammation and necrosis of blood vessel walls resulting in ischemia in the distribution of damaged vessels. Average age of onset is in the sixth decade (142) and thus this disease constitutes another important treatable neuropathy in the elderly. The vasculitides have been classified according to the type and size of the blood vessel involved and by the emphasis on primary (i.e., polyarteritis nodosa, Wegener's granulomatosis) versus secondary (i.e., associations with connective tissue disease, infection, drugs, or malignancy) (143) (Table 14). Peripheral neuropathy may complicate systemic vasculitis and can be the presenting manifestation (143). In addition, nonsystemic or isolated peripheral nerve vasculitis can occur (144).

Table 14 Vasculitic Diseases that Can Produce Peripheral Neuropathy

Systemic necrotizing vasculitis
    Polyarteritis nodosa
    Wegener's granulomatosis
    Churg-Straus disease
    Vasculitis associated with other connective tissue disease
        (systemic lupus erythematosus, rheumatoid arthritis, Sjögren's
        syndrome)
Hypersensitivity vasculitis
    Henoch-Schönlein purpura
    Serum sickness
    Drug reactions
    Vasculitis associated with infection or malignancy
Giant-cell arteritis
    Temporal arteritis
    Takayasu's arteritis
Isolated peripheral nervous system vasculitis (nonsystemic)

Systemic necrotizing vasculitis refers to a potentially life-threatening group of disorders affecting multiple organ systems. These vasculitides classically involve small- and medium-size arteries. Polyarteritis nodosa (PAN) is the most common of the necrotizing vasculitides (145). It involves the kidneys, bowels, liver, skin, and muscle. Importantly, the pulmonary circulation is spared. Peripheral nerve involvement occurs in up to 50% of patients (145). Hepatitis B antigenemia and immune complexes are found in about 30% of cases (143). Abdominal angiography can demonstrate vasculitis involvement of renal, hepatic, and visceral blood vessels. Churg-Strauss syndrome, or allergic angiitis and granulomatosis, is a rare condition with prominent involvement of the pulmonary system (143,145). Prominent eosinophilic infiltration of blood vessels is seen. The frequency of peripheral nerve involvement is similar to that observed in PAN. Wegener's granulomatosis affects the upper and lower respiratory track accompanied by glomerulonephritis (143,145). Peripheral nervous system involvement is evident in about 20% of cases (143). The lack of an asthma history and peripheral eosinophilia can distinguish Wegener's granulomatosis from Churg-Strauss syndrome. Peripheral nerve vasculitis may complicate connective tissue diseases, most commonly with rheumatoid arthritis, but also with systemic lupus erythematosus and Sjögren's syndrome (143,146).

Hypersensitivity vasculitis involves small vessels and implies exposure to an antigen that may be exogenous or endogenous (143). It can occur in Henoch-Schönlein purpura, serum sickness, infections, drug reactions, and neoplasms. The association between neoplasm and vasculitis usually occurs in the setting of myelo- or lymphoproliferative disorder and not solid tumors (143). In contrast to systemic necrotizing vasculitis, hypersensitivity vasculitis rarely causes irreversible damage to the vital organs and is usually a self-limited disorder.

The large and medium arteries are affected in the giant cell arteritis with particular involvement of the branches of the carotid artery, temporal artery, and retinal vessels (143). The inflammatory infiltrate consists of mononuclear and giant cells. Peripheral nerve involvement is rare in Takayasu's arteritis but can complicate temporal arteritis in about 14% of cases (143,147).

Isolated peripheral vasculitis or nonsystemic vasculitic neuropathy involves small- and medium-sized arteries of the epineurium and perineurium (143,144). The clinical presentation histologic features are similar to the systemic vasculitis with exception of sparing of other organs. However, constitutional symptoms of fever, malaise, weight loss, and nonspecific arthralgias can occur in both isolated and systemic vasculitis (148). Patients with clinical manifestations restricted to peripheral nerve have better prognosis than patients with systemic vasculitis (143).

The pattern of neuropathic involvement depends on the duration and extent of the ischemic-induced damage (143). Burning pain and dysesthesias in the distribution of involved nerves occur in 70–80% of patients (148). Usually both motor and sensory nerves are affected, although rarely some patients have only sensory loss. True multiple mononeuropathy with deficits restricted to the multiple individual peripheral nerves occurs in only 10–15% of cases (148). An overlapping multiple mononeuropathy obscuring individual nerve involvement occurs much more commonly in about 50–60% of patients (148). Because of the multiple and overlapping nerve involvement, it may be difficult to distinguish individual neuropathies, although examination may reveal asymmetries between the limbs. Approximately 20–30% of patients with a diffuse overlapping neuropathy may present with a distal, symmetric "stocking-glove" sensory motor neuropathy (148).

All patients suspected of vasculitis should be evaluated for an underlying systemic vasculitis. Laboratory evaluations should include erythrocyte sedimentation rate, antinuclear antibody titer, rheumatoid factor, serum protein or immunoelectrophoresis, complement levels, quantitative immunoglobulins, hepatitis B serology, and eosinophil count. In addition, routine CBC, urinalysis, renal, and liver functions should be obtained for underlying systemic involvement. Electrophysiology studies may demonstrate an asymmetric axonopathy. Nerve conduction studies can also be useful to determine appropriate nerves to biopsy. The sural nerve is most commonly biopsied. However, the yield of biopsy can be increased by biopsying the superficial peroneal nerve and the underlying peroneus brevis muscle (149). Even in so-called isolated peripheral nervous system vasculitis, involvement of blood vessels supplying muscle can be demonstrated. Characteristic findings on nerve and muscle biopsy include both perivascular and transmural inflammatory cell infiltration with necrosis of the blood vessel wall. The inflammatory cells are predominantly T cells and macrophages with most of the T cells being CD8 positive cytotoxic/suppressor cells (150). Immunoglobulin, complement, and membrane attack complex deposition can be seen accompanying cellular infiltrates in 80% of nerve specimens (150).

There are no prospective, randomized, controlled trials of therapy in vasculitis involving the peripheral nervous system. However, most patients respond to the combination of cyclophosphamide and corticosteroids (143). We generally initiate treatment with oral cyclophosphamide at a dose of 2 mg/kg/ day in combination with prednisone 1.5 mg/kg/day (Table 13). Prednisone is given as a single morning daily dose for 2–4 weeks. Once improvement is evident, we switch to an alternate-day regimen. When the condition stabilizes, prednisone is slowly tapered by 5 mg every 2–3 weeks. Cyclophosphamide is generally maintained for a least 1 year. It is important to monitor for side effects of prednisone (i.e., glucose intolerance, hypertension, weight gain, cataracts, glaucoma, osteoporosis, increased risk of infection) and risks of cyclophosphamide (pancytopenia with risk of infection and bleeding, hemorrhagic cystitis, and secondary malignancy). Frequent CBCs, electrolytes, glucose, and urinalysis should be obtained. Patients should be encouraged to follow a low-carbohydrate, low-salt diet and to adequately hydrate themselves for prophylaxis against hemorrhagic cystitis. Vitamin D and calcium supplements are helpful for prevention of osteoporosis. Because isolated peripheral nervous system vasculitis may be more benign than systemic vasculitis (142–144), a trial of steroids alone or a shorter course of cyclophosphamide may be indicated in these cases (143).

8. Neuropathies associated with monoclonal gammopathies

Peripheral neuropathies associated with paraproteins or monoclonal gammopathies are an important category of late-onset peripheral neuropathy (151). Monoclonal gammopathies are present in 0.1% of the general population in the third decade. However, the frequency increases to 3% by age 70 (152,153). An increased incidence of monoclonal gammopathies has been observed in patients with peripheral neuropathy. About 10% of patients with idiopathic peripheral neuropathies have monoclonal gammopathies compared to 2.5% of patients with peripheral neuropathies secondary to other diseases (154). In addition, peripheral neuropathies may be more frequent in patients with monoclonal gammopathies than in the general population (155,156). A causal relationship between monoclonal gammopathies and peripheral neuropathies has been suggested by studies demonstrating binding of monoclonal IgM to myelin sheaths (157,158). Antibodies directed against myelin-associated glycoprotein (anti-MAG) are present in 50% of patients with IgM monoclonal gammopathies and peripheral neuropathies (159). However, what connection, if any, these antibodies have to the pathogenesis of the peripheral neuropathies is unknown. In IgA and IgG monoclonal gammopathies, immunoglobulin deposition is generally not seen on nerve sheaths, and a causal link is not strongly established.

All patients with peripheral neuropathies of unknown etiology should be tested for the presence of monoclonal gammopathies. The serum protein electrophoresis (SPEP) is a useful screening test, but it is not as sensitive as immuno-electrophoresis (IEP) or immunofixation (IFE). Serum IEP or IFE should be performed to identify the nature of monoclonal proteins, and in patients suspected of having a myelo-proliferative disorder even with a normal SPEP, because a small monoclonal protein may not be apparent. The presence of monoclonal gammopathies should lead to an aggressive work-up for amyloidosis, multiple myeloma, osteosclerotic myeloma, Waldenström's macroglobulinemia, cryoglobul-inemia, leukemia, and lymphoma. If a monoclonal gammo-pathy is detected, urine protein electrophoresis and immuno-electrophoresis should be performed along with hematologic studies, bone marrow biopsy and aspirate, and a radiographic skeletal survey (159). In the majority of patients with mono-clonal gammopathies, no underlying disease is found in pa-tients, and these patients are designated as having monoclonal gammopathies of undetermined significance (MGUS). MGUS has replaced the term *benign monoclonal gammopathy* because 20% of patients initially classified as having MGUS eventu-ally develop malignant disorders with long-term follow-up (160,161).

a. **Neuropathies associated with a monoclonal gammopathy of uncertain significance.** Some investigators separate the IgM-MGUS group from IgG- and IgA-MGUS groups because of possible differences in clinical, electro-physiologic features, pathogenesis, and response to treatment (151,162,163). The relationship of IgG and IgA monoclonal gammopathies and peripheral neuropathy is not as well docu-mented as the relationship of IgM monoclonals and peripheral neuropathy as previously described. Clinically, IgM-MGUS neuropathies are similar to IgG- and IgA-MGUS peripheral neuropathies. Some authorities have noted a higher frequency of sensory loss, tremor, and ataxia in the IgM-MGUS group (162,164), while others have not (163). In both groups, dis-tal, symmetric, sensory greater than motor, polyneuropathy develops. Distal pain, parathesia, and sensory loss are the ini-tial complaints. If weakness develops, it is usually distal (162).

Nerve conduction studies reveal prolonged distal latencies and slowed conduction velocities in both the IgM- and non-IgM-MGUS groups (162). However, a higher frequency of nerve conduction abnormalities may be present in the IgM-MGUS group (162). The IgG- and IgA-MGUS groups are more heterogeneous with nerve conduction features suggesting primary axonopathy in some cases (151,165,166). Studies have shown that the IgG- and IgA-MGUS groups are more responsive to plasma exchange than the IgM group (151,163). Some authorities suggest that MGUS peripheral neuropathies, especially the IgG and IgA groups, may be a variant of CIDP given the similar clinical, electrophysiologic features and response to treatment (7). Others suggest that paraprotein-related neuropathies should be separated from CIDP until the pathogenesis of both the paraprotein and idiopathic CIDP neuropathies is resolved (151,162,163).

Rarely patients with an IgM-related neuropathy will be found to have Waldenström's macroglobulinemia. These patients have a serum IgM monoclonal protein greater than 3 grams/liter, anemia, and increased numbers of lymphocytes, plasma cells, or both in the bone marrow (154). These patients may respond to chemotherapy and plasmapheresis (167).

b. Neuropathies associated with multiple myeloma. Peripheral neuropathies associated with multiple myeloma are uncommon, occurring in 5–13% of cases (168, 169). Electrophysiologic abnormalities, however, may be detected in 40% of cases, indicating possible subclinical peripheral neuropathy (169). The majority of patients have a distal, axonal, sensory, or sensorimotor neuropathy (168,169). Epidural cranial and spinal root compression by expanding plasmacytomas is common and may be superimposed upon and overshadow the peripheral neuropathy. Less frequently, a sensory neuronopathy or a demyelinating polyradiculoneuropathy may develop (168). Amyloid deposition may be responsible for up to two-thirds of neuropathy in multiple myeloma patients (168). Peripheral involvement of small fibers with painful paresthesia, loss of pinprick and temperature discrimination, autonomic dysfunction, as well as superimposed carpal tunnel syndrome are suggestive of amyloid neuropathy (159). Abdominal fat pad, rectal, or sural nerve biopsy should be performed to look for amyloid deposition. Unfortunately, the treatment of the underlying multiple myeloma does not usually affect the course of the neuropathy.

    c.   **Neuropathies associated with osteosclerotic myeloma.** Osteosclerotic myeloma occurs in less than 3% of patients with myeloma. However, unlike multiple myeloma, polyneuropathy is present in almost one-half of cases of osteosclerotic myeloma (170). The neuropathy is slowly progressive and symmetric with both distal and proximal weakness (similar to CIDP). CSF protein levels are often elevated, suggesting that the disorder is a polyradiculoneuropathy. Nerve conduction studies may reveal prolonged distal latencies, slowed conduction velocities, temporal dispersion along with low amplitudes, suggesting prominent demyelination in addition to axonal degeneration (170). Sural nerve biopsies demonstrate axonal atrophy with or without degeneration and secondary demyelination (171). Systemic manifestations are common and include hepatosplenomegaly, cutaneous pigmentation, hypertrichosis, edema, leukonychia, finger clubbing, gynecomastia, and testicular atrophy (172). This complex constitutes the Crow-Fukase or POEMS syndrome (P = polyneuropathy, O = organomegaly, E = endocrinopathy, M = monoclonal gammopathy, S = skin changes) (172,173). Patients may display all or none of these features. The neuropathy may respond to a radiation or surgical excision of the isolated plasmacytoma or to chemotherapy.

    d.   **Neuropathies associated with primary amyloidosis.** Primary amyloidosis is a systemic disorder that typically affects men past the sixth decade of life (174,175). Primary amyloidosis occurs in association with multiple myeloma, Waldenström's macroglobulinemia, or as a primary plasma cell dyscrasia without any underlying disease. The amyloid is composed of the complete or variable portion of the monoclonal light chain (176). Lambda is more common than kappa light chain (2:1) in primary amyloidosis (176).

Peripheral neuropathy occurs in 15–30% of patients with primary amyloidosis and may be the presenting manifestation in one-sixth of cases (174,176,177). Initially small-fiber modalities are affected, resulting in painful dysesthesia along with diminished pain and temperature sensation. The neuropathy is slowly progressive and eventually symmetric weakness develops, beginning in the distal lower extremities along with large-fiber, discriminatory sensory loss. Most patients develop autonomic involvement with postural hypertension, syncope, impotence, gastrointestinal disturbance, impaired sweating, and loss of bladder control (159). Carpal tunnel syndrome occurs in 25% of patients and may be the presenting manifestation (176).

Electrophysiologic studies are suggestive of a primary axonopathy with low-amplitude compound motor and sensory nerve action potentials with normal or only mildly prolonged distal latencies and mildly slow conduction velocities. Nerve biopsies may reveal amyloid deposition in either the globular or diffuse pattern infiltrating the epineural and endoneural connected tissue and in blood vessel walls. Active axonal degeneration and severe loss of small myelinated and unmyelinated fibers are observed.

The prognosis of patients with primary amyloidosis is poor with a median survival of 2 years (176). Death is generally secondary to progressive congestive heart failure or renal failure. Chemotherapy with melphalan, prednisone, and colchicine have generally been unsatisfactory (159,176).

9. *Neuropathy associated with malignancy*

It is difficult to estimate the frequency of peripheral neuropathies accompanying malignancies since it is dependent on a number of factors, including the type, stage, and location of the cancer, duration of disease, degree of malnutrition, and neurotoxic effects of chemotherapy. In an elderly patient with a neuropathic disorder, an underlying malignancy must be considered.

Clinically evident peripheral neuropathy has been reported in 1.7–5.5% (178,179) of patients with malignancy. Quantitative sensory testing reveals peripheral neuropathy in 12% (180) while nerve conduction studies demonstrate peripheral neuropathy in 30–40% (178).

Peripheral neuropathy is most common in carcinoma of the lung, but also accompanies carcinoma of the stomach, colon, rectum, and other organs including the lymphoproliferative system (178,181–183). Most any tumor type can potentially compress or invade roots, plexi, or individual nerves. This section will deal predominantly with paraneoplastic, or remote, effects of cancer, and peripheral neuropathy. Toxic neuropathies due to chemotherapy are dealt with in the next section.

Subacute sensory neuronopathy was the first neuropathy described that is a complication of carcinoma (184). The site of the lesion is at the level of the sensory cell body and, therefore, the disorder is also referred to as ganglionopathy. In the vast majority of cases, the underlying tumor is small-cell carcinoma of the lung, but cases of carcinoma of the esophagus, breast, ovary, kidney, and lymphoma have also been reported (178). The disorder is rare and most commonly affects females in late–middle life with a mean age of onset of 59 years (185). The predominant symptoms are the subacute onset of numbness, dysesthesia, and paresthesia, beginning distally then spreading proximally. Occasionally, the onset can be quite acute. Diminished touch, pin and temperature sensation, prominent loss of vibratory and position sense occurs, resulting in sensory ataxia and pseudoathetosis (186,187). Deep tendon reflexes are diminished or absent. Autonomic dysfunction and cranial nerve abnormalities may occur. Alterations in mental status may occur in patients with superimposed paraneoplastic encephalomyelitis (187).

While most cases of sensory neuronopathy have only sensory abnormalities, mild weakness may occasionally be evident (188). This may reflect an associated sensorimotor neuropathy or a superimposed myasthenic (Lambert-Eaton) syndrome.

The neuropathy generally evolves over a few months, then stabilizes. The symptoms of the neuropathy may precede those of the cancer by several months or years (185,187,188). Discovery of a sensory neuronopathy should lead to an aggressive workup for an underlying malignancy. Treatment of the underlying cancer may prolong survival but generally does not affect the course of the underlying neuronopathy (186, 187). However, rare cases of remission following treatment of the tumor have been reported (189).

Nerve conduction studies in pure sensory neuronopathy reveal low-amplitude or absent SNAPs with normal CMAPs (186–188). CSF may be normal or may demonstrate mild lymphocytic pleocytosis and elevated protein (187,188). Type 1 antineuronal nuclear antibodies (ANNA-1), also known as anti-Hu, can be demonstrated in serum and CSF in patients with small-cell carcinoma of the lung complicated by paraneoplastic sensory or sensorimotor polyneuropathy, encephalitis, and cerebellar degeneration (188,190,191). The antibodies are directed against a 35–40 kD nuclear protein and are highly specific for small-cell lung carcinoma (192). Patients with a positive ANNA-1, a sensory neuronopathy, but no identifiable cancer should have periodic chest imaging; some advise chest x-ray every 3 months and chest CT or MRI every 6 months (192).

Pathologic features of the disease include inflammation and degeneration of the dorsal root ganglia, and secondary degeneration of sensory neurons and the posterior columns. Occasionally, degeneration and inflammation involve neurons in the brainstem and limbic system (178,184). The etiology of the neuropathy is unclear. Perhaps there is antigenic similarity between proteins in the tumor cells and the neuron cells, leading to an immune response against both tumor and neuronal cells (190).

Mixed sensorimotor polyneuropathy complicating cancer is much more common than pure sensory neuronopathy (178, 193,194). It is more frequent in individuals with small-cell cancer of the lung, but can also complicate carcinoma of the breast, ovary, uterus, testis, kidney, and gastrointestinal tract (178). The neuropathy is a distal symmetric axonopathy. Nerve biopsies and postmortem tissue most commonly reveal axonal degeneration and regeneration, but segmental demyelination and remyelination have been reported (184,188). Lymphocytic infiltration and vasculitic changes within peripheral nerves have been described (195,196). The neuropathy manifests clinically with distal symmetric numbness and weakness beginning in the feet and gradually progressing to involve the proximal lower extremities and distal upper extremities. All sensory modalities can be affected, but the prominent sensory ataxia that is seen in sensory neuronopathies is generally not observed.

The etiology of sensorimotor neuropathy in malignancy is unknown. Chemotherapies can be toxic to peripheral nerves (see below), but neuropathy can occur in untreated individuals with cancer. Although weight loss frequently accompanies malignancies, patients often are neither cachectic nor manifest other signs of malnutritional deficiency when neuropathy initially manifests (178,179,181,194). Vitamin supplementation is of no benefit (178). Toxic factors released by the tumor may result in axonal degeneration (178). Metabolic disturbance such as an alteration in protein and fat metabolism and enzyme activity occurs with malignancy and may result in neuropathy (188).

Peripheral neuropathy can occur in the setting of lymphoma (183). The majority of non-Hodgkin's lymphoma occurs after age 60, whereas less than 10% of Hodgkin's disease occurs after age 60. Peripheral neuropathy can complicate both Hodgkin's and non-Hodgkin's lymphoma (183). The incidence of neuropathy in lymphoma patients is generally felt to be less than that observed in small-cell carcinoma the lung (183). However, a prospective study reported clinically evident neuropathy in 8% and electrophysiologic evidence of neuropathy in 35% of patients with lymphoma (197). The presentation is variable. The neuropathy may be purely sensory (187,198) or motor (199), but is most commonly sensorimotor (197), and can be symmetric, asymmetric, or multifocal (183,200). Autonomic dysfunction may occur. The course may be acute (201,202), subacute (203–205), chronic progressive (194,197,203), or relapsing and remitting (185,202,205,206). Nerve conduction studies may reveal axonal changes (197) or features of prominent demyelination (183,202,205), as observed in acute and chronic inflammatory demyelinating polyneuropathies. CSF may reveal lymphocytic pleocytosis and elevated protein (183,200,204,205). The etiology may be secondary to direct endoneurial infiltration or direct compression of nerves by lymphoma cells (183,200, 204,206), but more commonly is a remote effect of the cancer (183,197,202,204). From a clinical and electrophysiologic standpoint it may be impossible to distinguish neuropathy caused by direct tumor infiltration from the paraneoplastic variant. Nerve biopsy may reveal axonal degeneration along with segmental demyelination (183,194,197). Inflammatory cells within the endoneurium may be demonstrated in both the infiltrative and presumed paraneoplastic neuropathies complicating lymphoma. The presence of a monoclonal population of inflammatory cells within the nerve fascicles would suggest infiltration of tumor cells rather than an immunologic paraneoplastic etiology. The neuropathy may respond to treatment of the underlying lymphoma (198,200,205).

An unusual complication of lymphoma is subacute motor neuropathy or neuronopathy (199). Its recognition is important because it may clinically resemble amyotrophic lateral sclerosis. The motor neuropathy may begin at any stage and can precede the diagnosis of lymphoma. Subacute onset of painless asymmetric weakness usually initially involving the lower extremities is associated with widespread fasciculations and diminished or absent reflexes. There is an absence of sensory or corticospinal tract abnormalities. CSF studies may reveal lymphocytic pleocytosis and an elevated protein. A monoclonal gammopathy may be demonstrated in the serum in lymphomas of B-cell lineage. Nerve conduction studies reveal a decrease in CMAP amplitude and mild conduction velocity slowing. Needle EMG reveals evidence of active denervation. Pathologic features include marked anterior horn cell degeneration with axonal loss and demyelination of the ventral motor roots (199). Interestingly, the course of the neuropathy appears independent of the activity of the underlying lymphoma and there is a high incidence of spontaneous remission (199).

Peripheral neuropathy is an uncommon complication of acute leukemia, but has been reported in up to 5.5% of cases (183,206–209). Mononeuropathy or mononeuropathy multiplex may develop secondary to hemorrhage or leukemic infiltration into cranial or peripheral nerves and spinal roots (207,209–213). Symmetric peripheral neuropathy is unusual but has been described (183). Acute, subacute, and chronic sensorimotor polyneuropathies complicating chronic leukemia, especially chronic lymphocytic leukemia, are well documented (183,197,203,205). Leukemic infiltration of the nerve, axonal degeneration, and segmental demyelination have been reported (205,212). The neuropathy may respond to corticosteroids and treatment of the underlying leukemia (205,213).

10. *Neuropathy produced by chemotherapeutic agents and other drugs*

Peripheral neuropathies due to chemotherapeutic drugs are important considerations in elderly patients with malignancies. The commonly used anticancer drugs that can cause neuropathy fall into three groups: platinum agents (cisplatin); vinca alkaloids (vincristine); and most recently, Taxol and its derivative, Taxotere (Table 15) (214–219). In addition, etoposide (VP-16), a derivative of podophyllin, is associated with an axonal sensory or sensorimotor neuropathy. The pathologic process in chemotherapy-induced neuropathies is either a distal axonopathy due to axonal degeneration or a ganglionopathy

Table 15 Chemotherapeutic Drugs that Can Produce Peripheral Neuropathy

Platinum agents
Cisplatin
Vinca alkaloid agents (microtubule formation inhibitors)
Vincristine
Vinblastine
Taxol alkaloid agents (microtubule assembly promoters)
Taxol
Taxotere[a]
Etoposide (VP-16)

[a]Investigational drug.

(219). These agents generally produce neuropathy in a dose-dependent relationship, so that the higher the dose and the longer the time of exposure, the more likely a neuropathy will occur.

The mechanism by which the axonal degeneration occurs is probably different for these drugs. Cisplatinum given to rats produces changes in the dorsal root ganglion and axonal degeneration on both central and peripheral nerve processes (216). Vinca alkaloids inhibit microtubule formation by binding to tubulin and by this mechanism the drugs interfere with axoplasmic transport (214,215). Taxol, on the other hand, stimulates microtubule aggregation in experimental models, and there is an accumulation of abnormal bundles of microtubules in dorsal root ganglia, axons, and Schwann cells (217, 218). It is hypothesized that axoplasmic transport is disrupted by the mechanical obstruction of the abnormal collections of microtubules.

The clinical manifestations of neuropathy are somewhat different for these various agents. Cisplatin, used widely for the treatment of ovarian, testicular, and bladder cancer, produces a predominantly sensory neuronopathy (ganglionopathy) at cumulative doses of 225–500 mg/m^2 (216,219). The degree of sensory loss can be dramatic, so that there is not only distal sensory loss, but also gait ataxia and even pseudoathetoid finger movements. Weakness rarely occurs. Vincristine, the most commonly used Vinca alkaloid, produces a sensorimotor and autonomic neuropathy (214,215,219). The earliest symptoms are paresthesia and numbness, which can at times occur in the fingers before the toes. These symptoms have been reported as early as 2 weeks after a single 2 mg/m^2 dose. With further dose accumulation, distal weakness of the hands and feet can occur. Proximal weakness, on the other hand, is not a feature of this neuropathy. Constipation, gastrointestinal ileus, and bladder atony are thought to be due to autonomic nerve involvement. Taxol is a new chemotherapy agent that has recently been approved as a second-line treatment for ovarian cancer (217,218). Taxol produces predominantly sensory symptoms with doses above 200 mg/m^2. Paresthesia and dysesthesia in the hands and feet can occur within days after the first course, but can improve before the next dose. However, with further therapy, the sensory symptoms persist. Distal motor weakness is uncommon, even with large cumulative doses, but there may be electrophysiologic evidence of subclinical motor involvement.

When sensory symptoms first begin, nerve conduction studies are often normal. With further doses, abnormalities eventually occur, but again these may differ among the chemotherapeutic drugs. Electrophysiologic studies of cisplatin neuropathy show sensory nerve action potentials that are either low amplitude or absent (216). Motor nerve conduction studies and needle EMG are usually normal. Vincristine and Taxol produce both sensory and motor nerve conduction abnormalities and denervation potentials in distal muscles, reflecting an axonal neuropathy (214,215). However, in the case of Taxol, the electrophysiologic motor involvement is more likely to be subclinical and to occur later (217,218).

Neurotoxicity is more common and severe if there is a preexisting neuropathy (for example, diabetic neuropathy) or if patients take other potentially neurotoxic drugs (for example, nitrofurantoin, isoniazid, disulfiram, gold, phenytoin, pyridoxine) (Table 16).

It is often a difficult decision whether or not to stop one of these drugs in the setting of neuropathy, if the tumor is responding the therapy. Occasionally, a dose reduction can ameliorate some of the neuropathy symptoms or halt them from progressing. In general, withdrawal of these drugs will lead to some improvement of the neuropathy. However, complete resolution of symptoms and signs is more likely to happen if the drug is stopped at the early stages of the peripheral neuropathy. After significant cumulative doses, some

Table 16 Other Drugs that Can Produce a Peripheral Neuropathy

Amiodarone
Chloramphenicol
Colchicine
Cyclosporine A
ddC, ddI
Disulfiram
Ethambutol
Glutethimide
Gold
Hydralazine
Isoniazid
Metronidazole
Nitrofurantoin
Nitrous oxide
Phenytoin
Pyridoxine
Sodium cyanate
Suramin
Tacrolimus (FK506)
Thalidomide
Tryptophan

symptoms and signs may persist, especially mild distal sensory loss and hypo- or areflexia.

Table 16 lists the drugs other than the chemotherapeutic agents discussed above that can produce a peripheral neuropathy. Age alone is probably not a major factor that predisposes a patient to develop a neuropathy from these drugs. Therefore, a discussion of all of these drugs will not be covered here and the reader is referred to detailed reviews (219–221).

11. *Infectious neuropathy*

a. Herpes zoster radiculitis and cranial neuritis. The neuropathic disorder of infectious etiology (Table 2) that is sufficiently common enough in the elderly population to warrant discussion is the radiculitis produced by the varicella zoster virus, or shingles. Shingles presumably results from a reactivation of varicella zoster virus infection. Over 90% of adults are seropositive for antibodies against the varicella zoster virus and the virus presumably becomes latent in many sensory ganglia after the primary infection (222,223).

There are generally no identifiable factors that precipitate reactivation of the infection. The reactivation produces a vesicular rash in a dermatomal distribution. The thoracic dermatomes are involved in over half of the cases, but the eruption can also occur in cranial nerve distributions (trigeminal and facial) and in cervical and lumbosacral roots. The vesicular rash may be preceded by pain and paresthesia in the dermatome region by a week or more. Systemic signs such as fever, malaise, and headache can occur. In the majority of patients who are not immunocompromised, the vesicles dry up and resolve within 2–3 weeks and there are no sequelae. A persistent pain syndrome lasting beyond 4 weeks, or post-herpetic neuralgia, occurs in 10–20% of patients. In addition, a small number of patients, approximately 5%, develop segmental motor paresis after the rash has resolved (224). Segmental paresis is manifested by muscle weakness and atrophy in the root or cranial nerve distribution in which there had been shingles. This is observed more often in cervical and lumbosacral zoster compared to thoracic zoster, probably because weakness of thoracic muscles is overlooked (225).

Herpes zoster radiculitis is a disease of the elderly and there is a direct correlation between increasing age and the incidence of shingles (222,226–229). Overall, two-thirds of the patients are over 45 years old. The annual incidence rate for 50-year-olds is 2–4 cases per 1000, and this figure doubles for individuals over 80 (222). Why there is an increased risk of zoster reactivation with age is unclear, but it is believed to reflect the gradual senescence of the immune containment of the virus in the ganglia (227,230,231).

In addition, the complication rate for postherpetic neuralgia is significantly higher for the elderly (222,226–229). Postherpetic neuralgia is actually quite uncommon before age 50 (229). Persistent pain beyond 4 weeks occurs in nearly 50% of patients over age 60 (222). While postherpetic neuralgia resolves by 3 months in most patients, prolonged periods of pain for up to several years can occur, and this is particularly a potential problem in patients over age 70. In one series, patients with shingles who developed postherpetic neuralgia had a mean age of 67, whereas those with uncomplicated herpes zoster had a mean age of 46 (226).

The treatment of an acute eruption of shingles consists of oral acyclovir, 800 mg five times daily for 10 days. It has been shown in several studies that this regimen significantly reduces the duration of the rash and the severity of the pain during the acute illness (232). On the other hand, there is no convincing evidence that acyclovir can reduce the frequency of postherpetic neuralgia. Thus, some authors advocate acyclovir therapy only in immunocompromised patients. Corticosteroids have been employed in the treatment of acute shingles. However, the efficacy of either oral prednisone or subcutaneous triamcinolone has not been clearly demonstrated; thus their use in shingles is still controversial.

Several options are available for the treatment of postherpetic neuralgia, although none are uniformly successful.

Topical capsaicin ointment applied three or four times daily for 2–4 weeks is of benefit to some patients (233,234). A number of placebo-controlled studies have demonstrated that tricyclic antidepressants reduce the pain in many postherpetic neuralgia patients (235). However, as mentioned previously, elderly patients are particularly prone to side effects with these agents (73–75), and therefore it may be prudent to begin with smaller doses in elderly patients (75). Carbamazepine can be helpful in some cases that have intermittent lancinating, as opposed to constant, burning pain (228). Transcutaneous electrical nerve stimulation has been useful at times (236). Finally, if these therapies are not effective, short courses of narcotics may be necessary (237).

12. *Other focal neuropathic disorders*

Focal neuropathic disorders can involve the cervical and lumbosacral roots and plexi and individual nerves (238). Most of these conditions, especially those involving the roots and nerves, are due to mechanical compression or entrapment. A detailed discussion of these conditions is beyond the scope of this chapter. However, a number of pertinent points related to aging deserve mention.

   a. Radiculopathy.   Cervical and lumbosacral roots can be compressed by soft (disk) or hard (bone) structures (239, 240). However, patients over 50 years of age who present with a radiculopathy are much more likely to have bone pathology and excessive calcification as the source of the root injury (239). Osteoarthritis can produce posterior osteophyte formation, facet subluxation, and hypertrophy. Calcification and bulging of the ligamentum flavum is also another potential factor. In the older age group, compressive radiculopathy may also be associated with a myelopathy due to cervical stenosis. These patients will have a combination of upper and lower motor neuron signs (241,242).

   Nonmechanical medical disorders can also produce focal radicular disease. Diabetes mellitus, herpes zoster, and malignancy are the most common of these conditions that occur in the elderly and have been previously discussed.

b. Plexopathy. Idiopathic brachial plexitis, or so-called Parsonage-Turner syndrome, is a frequently overlooked diagnosis in all age groups, but especially in the elderly (243–245). The disorder is characterized by the rapid onset of shoulder and arm pain, which is followed in 1–2 weeks by arm weakness. Sensory loss is variable and may be confined to sensory disturbance in the distribution of the axillary nerve over the lateral arm. Muscles supplied by the upper trunk of the plexus are most commonly involved. The syndrome may be preceded by a viral illness, vaccination, or surgery. Pain usually lasts for days to weeks, whereas the weakness may last for many months. One-third of patients may develop bilateral arm involvement. The recovery process may be slow and take up to 1–3 years. While 80–90% of patients reach a satisfactory recovery, a small number of patients fail to regain useful function of the arm. Although prednisone therapy early in the course of a brachial plexitis may reduce the pain, there is no evidence that it alters the ultimate prognosis.

Idiopathic brachial plexitis can occur at any age. However, in the large series of 146 patients from the Mayo Clinic, the majority of patients were over 50 years old and many were in their eighth decade of life (243). We have diagnosed this disorder in a number of patients over 80 years old. We are unaware of any good data on prognosis and the age of onset.

The most frequent misdiagnosis in elderly patients with an idiopathic brachial plexitis is cervical root compression. Patients are often referred after neuroimaging fails to find a mechanical etiology. The electrophysiologic study may help to differentiate patients with plexitis from those with root disease. Sensory nerve potentials often are abnormal and needle EMG of paraspinous muscles is normal in plexitis, whereas the opposite is true for radiculopathies (245,246).

Although rare, an idiopathic inflammatory process can also affect the lumbosacral plexus (247–250). Considerably less is known about the epidemiology and natural history of this disorder compared to the more common brachial plexitis.

In one series of six cases, all patients were in their seventh to eighth decade at the time of diagnosis (250). In addition, the patients in this series improved only after aggressive immunosuppressive therapy (250). Recently, intravenous immune globulin was reported to improve the course of two patients (one who was 76 years of age) with a progressive lumbosacral plexitis (251). Thus, it appears that idiopathic lumbosacral plexitis may not be nearly so benign as the brachial plexus counterpart in that spontaneous recovery does not always occur. Some patients with painful idiopathic lumbosacral plexitis may have extremely high erythrocyte sedimentation rates (250). Of course, the most common medical cause for a lumbosacral plexopathy in the elderly is diabetes mellitus (see above), and in some patients diabetes is not discovered until the patient presents with this focal radiculoplexopathy (89).

Both brachial and lumbosacral plexopathy can be caused by infiltration of tumor (245,248,252,253). This diagnosis needs to be considered in any patient with a known malignancy and a plexopathy and in a patient whose course is atypical for an idiopathic plexitis. Radiographic imaging of the plexus by CT or MRI is useful in this regard. In addition, cancer patients who have received radiation therapy in the region of the brachial or lumbosacral plexus can develop a radiation plexopathy. Radiation plexopathy can be distinguished from tumor infiltration plexopathy by the absence of pain and myokymic discharges on needle EMG (245,246); however, the definitive diagnosis depends on the absence of an infiltrating mass on imaging studies.

c. **Mononeuropathies**. The most common mononeuropathies involve the median nerve at the wrist (carpal tunnel syndrome) (254–256), the ulnar nerve at the elbow (cubital tunnel syndrome) (254,255,257), and the peroneal nerve at the fibular head (254,258). These conditions are due to compression or entrapment at these sites. Entrapment neuropathies can occur in adults of any age and the clinical presentation of these disorders, as well as their management, is not significantly different in elderly patients. An exception to this rule might be diabetic patients who have an increased incidence of compressive neuropathies correlating with the duration of the disease (83). In addition, patients who undergo prolonged hospitalizations or extensive weight loss are more predisposed to develop a peroneal neuropathy (258). Readers are referred to standard treatises on mononeuropathies for detailed discussions (238,254–259). While these particular risk factors can occur at any age, the elderly patient may be particularly susceptible.

13. *Hereditary neuropathies*

a. **Hereditary motor sensory neuropathy (HMSN).** The majority of peripheral neuropathies presenting in the elderly population are acquired; however, some forms of hereditary neuropathies may manifest late in life. Most cases of HMSN type I, the so-called demyelinating form of Charcot-Marie-Tooth disease, present in the first decades of life. HMSN type II, or the "neuronal" form of Charcot-Marie-Tooth disease, generally presents in the second decade, but cases presenting as late as the seventh decade of life have been reported (260–262). HMSN-II is generally autosomal dominant, but autosomal recessive and sporadic cases have been described (260–262). Patients initially develop weakness and atrophy of the distal lower extremities. Pes cavus and hammer toe deformities of the feet are frequently present. Subjective sensory loss is not a common complaint. Unlike acquired neuropathies, paresthesia and dysesthesia are infrequently present, although some patients do develop distal cramps. Despite the lack of subjective sensory complaints, sensory loss, in particular vibratory sensation, can be demonstrated on examination. Nerve conduction studies reveal normal or only mildly slow conduction velocities and absent or reduced amplitude of SNAPs and CMAPs (260–262). Needle EMG reveals denervation potentials in distal muscles. The treatment for HMSN involves prophylactic meticulous foot care in order to prevent ulcers and infection. In addition, ankle-foot orthotics are beneficial in patients with significant ankle dorsiflexion weakness. The genetic defect for HMSN-II is unknown at the present time.

b. Hereditary neuropathy with predisposition to pressure palsies. Hereditary neuropathy with predisposition to pressure palsies (HNPP), or tomaculous neuropathy, is an autosomal-dominant disorder that appears to be the result of a large deletion on chromosome 17 p11.2-12, (263,264). Interestingly, this is a reciprocal mutation to the duplication mutation present in the majority of HMSN-IA cases (264, 265). Patients often present in the second to fifth decade of life with recurrent pressure palsies. However, some patients remain asymptomatic or develop symptoms later in life. In addition to recurrent pressure palsies, some patients are found to have a generalized sensorimotor polyneuropathy (263,266). Nerve conduction studies reveal conduction slowing that is accentuated across common pressure sites and prolonged distal latencies (263,266). Nerve biopsies demonstrate the "tomacula" or sausage-shaped myelin thickening characteristic of the disorder. There is no specific treatment other than avoidance of activities or positions causing compression on nerves.

c. Familial amyloidotic polyneuropathy. Familial amyloidotic polyneuropathy (FAP) is a group of autosomal-dominant inherited disorders characterized by amyloid deposition in the peripheral nerves and in various system organs (267–269). Unlike the primary and secondary amyloid neuropathies (see above), there is no associated monoclonal gammopathy. The most common forms of FAP are associated with point mutations in the transthyretin (TTR) or prealbumin gene on chromosome 18. FAP associated with TTR mutations usually presents as (1) a symmetric polyneuropathy beginning in the distal lower extremities; (2) carpal tunnel syndrome followed by a slowly progressive generalized axonal polyneuropathy; and (3) an amyloid cardiomyopathy with which the polyneuropathy is not prominent (268,269). While familial amyloid polyneuropathy usually presents in the third to fifth decade, late onset in the seventh decade can occur (267–269).

The initial symptom is distal sensory loss. Autonomic dysfunction characterized by orthostatic hypotension, impotence, hypohidrosis, and bowel and bladder dysfunction are frequently present (269). Mild to moderate weakness of distal muscle groups can develop. Involvement of systemic organs usually leads to death within 10 years (268); however, survival may be longer in some allelic variants. No treatment is currently available. The diagnosis is confirmed by skin, rectal, abdominal fat pad, or nerve biopsy, and more recently by DNA analysis for TTR mutations.

REFERENCES

1. Dyck PJ, Oviatt KF, Lambert EH. Intensive evaluation of referred unclassified neuropathies yields improved diagnosis. Ann Neurol 1981; 10:222–226.

2. Grahmann F, Winterholler M, Neundorfer B. Cryptogenetic polyneuropathies: An out-patient follow-up study. Acta Neurol Scand 1991; 84:221–225.

3. Tan E, Lynn DJ, Amato AA, Kissel JT, Rammohan KW, Sahenk Z, Warmolts JR, Jackson CE, Barohn RJ, Mendell JR. Immunosuppressive treatment of motor neuron syndromes: Attempts to distinguish a treatable disorder. Arch Neurol 1994; 51:194–200.

4. Kimura J. Electrodiagnosis in diseases of nerve and muscle. Principles and practice, 2nd ed. Philadelphia: FA Davis, 1989.

5. Oh SJ. Clinical electromyography: Nerve conduction studies, 2nd ed. Baltimore: Williams and Wilkins, 1993.

6. Brown WF, Bolton CF. Clinical electromyography, 2nd ed. Boston: Butterworth-Heinemann, 1993.

7. Barohn RJ, Kissel JT, Warmolts JR, Mendell JR. Chronic inflammatory demyelinating polyradiculoneuropathy: Clinical characteristics, course, and recommendations for diagnostic criteria. Arch Neurol 1989; 46:878–884.

8. Ad Hoc Subcommittee of the American Academy of Neurology AIDS Task Force. Research criteria for diagnosis of chronic inflammatory demyelinating polyneuropathy (CIDP). Neurology 1991; 41:617–618.

9.   Bromberg MB. Comparison of electrodiagnostic criteria for primary demyelination in chronic polyneuropathy. Muscle Nerve 1991; 14:968–976.

10. Thomas PK, Scaravilli F, Belai A. Pathologic alterations in cell bodies of peripheral neurons in neuropathy. In: Dyck PJ, Thomas PK, Griffin JW, Low PA, Paduslo JF, eds. Peripheral Neuropathies, 3rd ed. Philadelphia: WB Saunders, 1993; 488–492.

11. Wisniewski HM, Narang HK, Terry RD. Neurofibrillary tangles of paired helical filaments. J Neurol Sci 1976; 27:173–181.

12. Kawasaki H, Murayama S, Tomonaga M, Izumiyama N, Shimada H. Neurofibrillary tangles in human upper cervical ganglia. Morphological study with immunohistochemistry and electron microscopy. Acta Neuropathol 1987; 75:156–159.

13. Kawamura Y, O'Brien P, Okazaki H, Dyck PJ. Lumbar motoneurons of man II: The number and diameter distribution of large- and intermediate-diameter cytons in "motoneuron columns" of spinal cord of man. J Neuropathol Exp Neurol 1977; 36:861–870.

14. Dyck PJ, Jedrzejowska H, Karnes J, Kawamura Y, Low PA, O'Brien PC, Offord K, Ohnishi A, Ohta M, Pollock M, Stevens JC. Reconstruction of motor, sensory, and autonomic neurons based on morphometric study of sampled levels. Muscle Nerve 1979; 2:399–405.

15. Gardner ED. Decrease in human neurons with age. Anat Rec 1940; 77:529–536.

16. Nagashima K, Oota K. A histopathological study of the human spinal ganglia. 1. Normal variations in aging. Acta Pathol Jpn 1974; 24:333–344.

17. Ota M, Offord K, Dyck PJ. Morphometric evaluations of first sacral ganglion of man. J Neurol Sci 1974; 22:73–82.

18. Corbin KB, Gardner ED. Decrease in number of myelinated nerve fibers in human spinal roots with age. Anat Rec 1937; 68:63–74.

19. Cottrell JL. Histologic variations with age in apparently normal nerve trunks. Arch Neurol Psychiatry 1940; 43:1138–1150.

20. Tohgi H, Tsukagoshi H, Toyokura Y. Quantitative changes with age in normal sural nerves. Acta Neuropathol 1977; 38:213–220.

21. Ochoa J, Mair WGP. The normal sural nerve in man II. Changes in axons and Schwann cells due to aging. Acta Neuropathol 1969; 13:217–239.

22. Jacobs JM, Love S. Qualitative and quantitative morphology of human sural nerve at different ages. Brain 1985; 108:897–924.

23. Lascelles RG, Thomas PK. Changes due to age in internodal length in the sural nerve in man. J Neurol Neurosurg Psychiatry 1966; 29:40–44.

24. Ochoa J. Recognition of unmyelinated fiber disease: Morphology criteria. Muscle Nerve 1978; 1:375–387.

25. Brown WF. A method for estimating the number of motor units in thenar muscles and the change in motor unit count with aging. J Neurol Neurosurg Psychiatry 1972; 35:845–852.

26. Brown WF, Strong MJ, Snow RS. Methods for estimating numbers of motor units in biceps-brachialis muscles and losses of motor units with aging. Muscle Nerve 1988; 11:423–432.

27. Sica REP, McComas AJ, Upton ARM. Motor unit estimations in small muscles of the hand. J Neurol Neurosurg Psychiatry 1974; 37:55–67.

28. Doherty TJ, Vandervoort AA, Brown WF. Effects of ageing on the motor unit: A brief review. Can J Appl Physiol 1993; 18(4):331–358.

29. Doherty TJ, Vandervoort AA, Taylor AW, Brown WF. Effects of motor unit losses on strength in older men and women. J Appl Physiol 1993; 74:868–874.

30. Stalberg E, Fawcett PRW. Macro EMG in healthy subjects of different ages. J Neurol Neurosurg Psychiatry 1982; 45:870–878.

31. Campbell MJ, McComas AJ, Petito F. Physiological changes in aging muscles. J Neurol Neurosurg Psychiatry 1973; 36:174–182.

32. Galganski M, Fuglevand AJ, Enoka RM. Reduced control of motor output in a human hand muscle of elderly subjects during submaximal contractions. J Neurophysiol 1993; 69:2108–2115.

33. Rigshospitalet Laboratory of Clinical Neurophysiology. EMG-Sensory and Motor Conduction Findings in Normal Subjects. Copenhagen, Denmark: RLCN, 1975;27–29.

34. Dorfman LJ, Bosley TM. Age-related changes in peripheral and central nerve conduction in man. Neurology 1979; 29:38–44.
35. Kimura J. Nerve conduction studies and electromyography. In: Dyck PJ, Thomas PK, Griffin JW, Low PA, Paduslo JF, eds. Peripheral Neuropathies, 3rd ed. Philadelphia: WB Saunders, 1993;605.
36. Rivner MH, Swift TR, Crout BO, Rhodes KP. Toward more rational nerve conduction interpretations: The effect of height. Muscle Nerve 1990; 13:232–239.
37. Falco FJ, Hennessey WJ, Braddom RL, Goldberg G. Standardized nerve conduction studies in the upper limb of the healthy elderly. Am J Phys Med Rehabil 1992; 71:263–271.
38. Falco FJE, Hennessey WJ, Goldberg G, Braddom RL. Standardized nerve conduction studies in the lower limb of the healthy elderly. Am J Phys Med Rehabil 1994; 73:168–174.
39. Robinson LR, Rubner DE, Wahl PW, Fujimoto WY, Stolov WC. Influences of height and gender on normal nerve conduction studies. Arch Phys Med Rehabil 1993; 74:1134–1138.
40. Taylor PK. Non-linear effects of age on nerve conduction in adults. J Neurol Sci 1984; 66:223–234.
41. Norris AH, Schock NW, Wagman IH. Age changes in maximum conduction velocity of motor fibers of human ulnar nerves. J Appl Physiol 1953; 5:589–593.
42. Oh, SJ. Physiologic factors affecting nerve conduction. Clinical electromyography. In: Nerve Conduction Studies, 2nd ed. Baltimore: Williams and Wilkins, 1993;307.
43. LaFratta CW, Canestrari R. A comparison of sensory and motor nerve conduction velocity as related to age. Arch Phys Med Rehab 1966; 47:286–290.
44. LaFratta CW. Relation of age to amplitude of evoked antidromic sensory nerve potentials: A supplemental report. Arch Phys Med Rehab 1972; 53:388–389.
45. Buchthal F, Rosenfalck A. Evoked action potentials and conduction velocities in human sensory nerves. Brain Res 1966; 3:1–122.
46. Rosenfalck P. Electromyography in normal subjects of different age. Methods Clin Neurol Physiol 1991; 2:47–52.
47. Goldberg JM, Lindblom U. Standardized method of determining vibratory perception thresholds for diagnosis and screen-

ing in neurological investigation. J Neurol Neurosurg Psychiatry 1979; 42:793–803.

48. de Neeling JND, Beks PJ, Bertelsmann FW, Heine RJ, Bouter LM. Sensory thresholds in older adults: Reproducibility and reference values. Muscle Nerve 1994; 17:454–461.

49. Armstrong FM, Bradbury JE, Ellis SH, Owens DR, Rosen I, Sonksen P, Sundkvist G. A study of peripheral diabetic neuropathy. The application of age-related reference values. Diabetic Med 1991; 8:S94–99.

50. Wiles PG, Pearce SM, Rice PJS, Mitchell JMO. Vibration perception threshold: Influence of age, height, sex, and smoking, and calculation of accurate centile values. Diabetic Med 1991; 8:157–161.

51. De Neeling JND, Beks PJ, Bertelsmann FW, Heine RJ, Bouter LM. Sensory thresholds in older adults: Reproducibility and reference values. Muscle Nerve 1994; 17:454–461.

52. Tandan R, Bradley WG. Amyotrophic lateral sclerosis: Part 1. Clinical features, pathology, and ethical issues in management. Ann Neurol 1985; 18:271–280.

53. Williams DB, Windebank AJ. Motor neuron disease (amyotrophic lateral sclerosis). Mayo Clin Proc 1991; 66:54–82.

54. Eisen A, Schulzer M, MacNeil M, Pant B, Mak E. Duration of amyotrophic lateral sclerosis is age dependent. Muscle Nerve 1993; 16:27–32.

55. Jablecki CK, Berry C, Leach J. Survival prediction in amyotrophic lateral sclerosis. Muscle Nerve 1989; 12:833–841.

56. Bensimon G, Lacomblez L, Meininger V, and the ALS/Riluzole Study Group. A controlled trial of riluzole in amyotrophic lateral sclerosis. N Engl J Med 1994; 330:585–591.

57. Rowland LP. Riluzole for the treatment of amyotrophic lateral sclerosis—too soon to tell? N Eng J Med 1994; 330:636–637.

58. Pestronk A, Cornblath DR, Ilyas AA, Baba H, Quarles RH, Griffin JW, Alderson K, Adams RN. A treatable multifocal motor neuropathy with antibodies to GM1 ganglioside. Ann Neurol 1988; 24:73–78.

59. Feldman EL, Bromberg MB, Albers JW, Pestronk A. Immunosuppressive treatment in multifocal motor neuropathy. Ann Neurol 1991; 30:397–401.

60. Younger DS, Rowland LP, Latov N, Hays AP, Lange DJ,

Sherman W, Inghirami G, Pesce MA, Knowles DM, Powers J, et al. Lymphoma, motor neuron disease, and amyotrophic lateral sclerosis. Ann Neurol 1991; 29:78–86.

61. Adams CK, Gegler DK, Linn JT. Mercury intoxication simulating amyotrophic lateral sclerosis. JAMA 1983; 250:642–643.

62. Boothby JA, DeJesus PV, Rowland LP. Reversible forms of motor neuron disease. Lead "neuritis." Arch Neurol 1974; 31:18–23.

63. Rosen DR, Siddique T, Patterson D, Figlewicz DA, Sapp P, Hentati A, Donaldson D, Goto J, O'Regan JP, Deng HX, et al. Mutations in Cu/Zn superoxide dismutase gene are associated with familial amyotrophic lateral sclerosis. Nature 1993; 362:59–62.

64. Harding AE. Inherited neuronal atrophy and degeneration predominately of lower motor neurons. In: Dyck PJ, Thomas PK, Griffin JW, Low PA, Poduslo JF, eds., Peripheral Neuropathy, 3rd ed. Philadelphia: WB Saunders, 1993; 1051–1093.

65. Pearn JH, Hudgson P, Walton JN. A clinical and genetic study of spinal muscular atrophy of adult onset: The autosomal recessive form as a discrete disease entity. Brain 1978; 101:591–606.

66. Munsat TL, Skerry L, Korf B, Pober B, Schapira Y, Gascon GG, al-Rajeh SM, Dubowitz V, Davies K, Brzustowicz LM, Penchaszadeh GK, Gilliam TC. Phenotypic heterogeneity of spinal muscular atrophy mapping to chromosome 5q 11.2-13.3 (SMA 5q). Neurology 1990; 40:1831–1836.

67. Kennedy WR, Alter M, Sung JH. Progressive proximal spinal and bulbar muscular atrophy of late onset. A sex-linked recessive trait. Neurology 1968; 18:671–680.

68. Amato AA, Prior TW, Barohn RJ, Synder P, Papp A, Mendell JR. Kennedy's disease: A clinicopathologic correlation with mutations in the androgen receptor gene. Neurology 1993; 43:791–794.

69. La Spada AR, Wilson EM, Lubahn DB, Harding AE, Fishbeck KH. Androgen receptor gene mutations in X-linked spinal and bulbar muscular atrophy. Nature 1991; 352:77–79.

70. Dalessio DJ. Chronic pain syndromes and disordered cortical inhibition: Effects of tricyclic compounds. Dis Nerv System 1967; 28:325–328.

71. Atkinson JH Jr, Kremer EF, Garfin SR. Psychopharmacological agents in the treatment of pain. J Bone Joint Surg-Amer Vol 1985; 67:337–342.

72. Walsh TD. Antidepressants in chronic pain. Clin Neuropharmacol 1983; 6:271–295.

73. Nies A, Robinson DS, Friedman MJ, Green R, Cooper TB, Ravaris CL, Ives JO. Relationship between age and tricyclic antidepressant plasma levels. Amer J Psychiatry 1977; 134:790–793.

74. Schulz P, Turner-Tamiyasu K, Smith G, Giacomini KM, Blaschke TF. Amitriptyline deposition in young and elderly normal men. Clin Pharmacol Ther 1983; 33:360–366.

75. Watson CP. Therapeutic window effect for amitriptyline analgesia. Can Med Assoc J 1984; 130:105–106.

76. Swerdlow M. Anticonvulsant drugs and chronic pain. Clin Neuropharmacol 1984; 7:51–82.

77. Rumsfield JA, West DP. Topical capsaicin in dermatologic and peripheral pain disorders. DICP Ann Pharmacother 1991; 25:381–387.

78. Dejgard A, Petersen P, Kastrup J. Mexiletine for treatment of chronic painful diabetic neuropathy. Lancet 1988; 1:9–11.

79. Ross DR, Varipapa RJ. Treatment of painful diabetic neuropathy with topical capsaicin. N Engl J Med 1989; 321:474–475.

80. Bates JA, Nathan PW. Transcutaneous electrical nerve stimulation for chronic pain. Anesthesia 1980; 35:817–822.

81. Gersh MR, Wolf SC, Rao VR. Evaluation of transcutaneous electrical nerve stimulation for pain relief in peripheral neuropathy. Phys Ther 1980; 60:48–52.

82. Notermans NC, Wokke JHJ, Franssen H, van der Graaf Y, Vermeulen M, van den Berg LH, Bar PR, Jennekens FGI. Chronic idiopathic polyneuropathy presenting in middle or old age: A clinical and electrophysiological study of 75 patients. J Neurol Neurosurg Psychiatry 1993; 56:1066–1071.

83. Melton LJ, Dyck PJ. Clinical features of the diabetic neuropathies: Epidemiology. In: Dyck PJ, Thomas PK, Asbury AK, Winegrad AI, Porte DJ, eds., Diabetic Neuropathy. Philadelphia: WB Saunders, 1987;27–35.

84. Brown MJ, Asbury AK. Diabetic neuropathy. Ann Neurol 1984; 15:2–12.

85. Low PA, Recent advances in the pathogenesis of diabetic neuropathy. Muscle Nerve 1987; 10:121–128.

86. Dyck PJ, Thomas PK, Asbury AK, Winegrad AI, Porte D Jr. Diabetic Neuropathy. Philadelphia: WB Saunders, 1987.

87. Service FJ, Rizza RA, Daube JR, O'Brien PC, Dyck PJ. Near normoglycaemia improved nerve conduction and vibration sensation in diabetic neuropathy. Diabetologia 1985; 28:722–727.

88. The Diabetes Control and Complication Trial Research Group. The effect of intensive treatment of diabetes on the development and progression of long-term complications in insulin-dependent diabetes mellitus. N Engl J Med 1993; 329:977–986.

89. Barohn RJ, Sahenk Z, Warmolts JR, Mendell JR. The Bruns-Garland syndrome (diabetic amyotrophy): Revisited 100 years later. Arch Neurol 1991; 48:1130–1135.

90. Ellenberg M. Diabetic neuropathic cachexia. Diabetes 1974; 23:418–423.

91. Archer AG, Watkins PJ, Thomas PK, Sharma AK, Payan J. The natural history of acute painful neuropathy in diabetes mellitus. J Neurol Neurosurg Psychiatry 1983; 46:491–499.

92. Asbury AK, Aldredge H, Hershberg R, Fisher CM. Oculo-motor palsy in diabetes mellitus: A clinico-pathological study. Brain 1970; 93:555–566.

93. Bastron JA, Thomas JE. Diabetic polyradiculopathy: Clinical and electromyographic findings in 105 patients. Mayo Clin Proc 1981; 56:725–732.

94. Sun SF, Streib EW. Diabetic thoracoabdominal neuropathy: Clinical and electrodiagnostic features. Ann Neurol 1981; 9:75–79.

95. Waxman SG, Sabin TD. Diabetic truncal polyneuropathy. Arch Neurol 1981; 38:46–47.

96. Max MB, Lynch SA, Muir J, Shoaf SE, Smoller B, Dubner R. Effects of desipramine, amitriptyline, and fluoxetine on pain in diabetic neuropathy. N Engl J Med 1992; 326:1250–1256.

97. Ross DR, Varipara RJ. Treatment of painful diabetic neuropathy with topical capsaicin. N Engl J Med 1989; 321:474–475.

98. Asbury AK. Neuropathies with renal failure, hepatic disorders, chronic respiratory insufficiency and critical illness. In:

Dyck PJ, Thomas PK, Griffin JW, Low PA, Poduslo JF, eds., Peripheral Neuropathy, 3rd ed. Philadelphia: WB Saunders, 1993;1251–1265.

99. Bolton CF. Peripheral neuropathies associated with chronic renal failure. Can J Neurol Sci 1980; 7:89–96.

100. Bolton CF, Young GB. Neurologic Complications of Renal Disease. Stoneham: Butterworth, 1990.

101. Solders G. Autonomic function tests in healthy controls and in terminal uremia. Acta Neurol Scand 1986; 73:638–639.

102. Ropper AH. Accelerated neuropathy of renal failure. Arch Neurol 1993; 50:536–539.

103. Bolton CF. Electrophysiologic changes in uremic neuropathy after successful renal transplantation. Neurology 1976; 26:152–161.

104. Ackil AA, Shahani BT, Young RR, Rubin NE. Late response and sural conduction studies. Usefulness in patients with chronic renal failure. Arch Neurol 1981; 38:482–485.

105. Dyck PJ, Johnson WJ, Lambert EH, O'Brien PC. Segmental demyelination secondary to axonal degeneration in uremic neuropathy. Mayo Clin Proc 1971; 46:400–431.

106. Bolton CF, Baltzan MA, Baltzan RB. Effects of renal transplantation on uremic neuropathy. A clinical and electrophysiologic study. N Engl J Med 1971; 284:1170–1175.

107. Nielsen VK. The peripheral nerve function in chronic renal failure. IX. Recovery after renal transplantation. Electrophysiological aspects (sensory and motor nerve conduction). Acta Med Scand 1974; 195:171–180.

108. Fraser CL, Arieff A. Nervous system complications in uremia. Ann Int Med 1988; 109:143–153.

109. Tegner R, Lindholm B. Vibratory perception threshold compared with nerve conduction velocity in the evaluation of uremic neuropathy. Acta Neurol Scand 1985; 71:284–289.

110. Carethers M. Diagnosing vitamin B12 deficiency, a common geriatric disorder. Geriatrics 1988; 43:89–94, 105–107, 111–112.

111. Gross JS, Weintraub NT, Neufeld RR, Libow LS. Pernicious anemia in the demented patient without anemia or macrocytosis. A case for early recognition. J Amer Geriat Soc 1986; 34:612–614.

112. Marcus DL, Shadick N, Crantz J, Gray M, Hernandez F, Freedman ML. Low serum B12 levels in a hematologically

normal elderly subpopulation. J Amer Geriatr Soc 1987; 35:635–638.

113. Normal EJ. Vitamin B12 deficiency in the elderly [Letter]. J Amer Geriatr Soc 1985; 33:374.

114. McCombe PA, McLeod JG. The peripheral neuropathy of vitamin B12 deficiency. J Neurol Sci 1984; 66:117–126.

115. Pruthi RK, Tefferi A. Pernicious anemia revisited. Mayo Clin Proc 1994; 69:144–150.

116. Fine EJ, Soria E, Paroski MW, Petryk D, Thomasula L. The neurophysiological profile of vitamin B12 deficiency. Muscle Nerve 1990; 13:158–164.

117. Jackson CE, Barohn RJ. Lesion localization of the numb hand syndrome in B12 deficiency. Muscle Nerve 1993; 16:1111–1112.

118. Lindenbaum J, Healton EB, Savage DG, Brust JCM, Garrett TJ, Podell ER, Marcell PD, Stabler SP, Allen RH. Neuropsychiatric disorders caused by cobalamin deficiency in the absence of anemia or macrocytosis. N Engl J Med 1988; 318:1720–1728.

119. Alter M. The epidemiology of Guillain-Barré syndrome. Ann Neurol 1990; 27(suppl.):S7–12.

120. Guillain-Barré Syndrome Study Group. Plasmapheresis and acute Guillain-Barré syndrome. Neurology 1985; 35:1096–1104.

121. Griffin JW, Ho TW. The Guillain-Barré syndrome at 75: The Campylobacter connection. Ann Neurol 1993; 34:125–127.

122. Arnason BG, Asbury AK. Idiopathic polyneuritis after surgery. Arch Neurol 1968; 18:500–507.

123. Loffel NB, Rossi LN, Mumenthaler M, Lutschg J, Ludin HP. The Landry-Guillain-Barré syndrome. Complications, prognosis, and natural history in 123 cases. J Neurol Sci 1977; 33:71–79.

124. Fisher CM. An unusual variant of acute idiopathic poly-neuritis (syndrome of ophthalmoplegia, ataxia, and areflexia). N Engl J Med 1956; 255:57–65.

125. Ropper AH. Unusual clinical variants and signs in Guillain-Barré syndrome. Arch Neurol 1986; 43:1150–1152.

126. Ropper AH. Further regional variants of acute immune poly-neuropathy. Arch Neurol 1994; 51:671–675.

127. Feasby TE, Gilbert JJ, Brown WF, Bolton CF, Hahn AF,

Koopman WF, Zochodne DW. An acute axonal form of Guillain-Barré polyneuropathy. Brain 1986; 109:1115–1126.

128. Albers JW, Donofrio PD, McGonagle TK. Sequential electro-diagnostic abnormalities in acute inflammatory demyelinating polyradiculoneuropathy. Muscle Nerve 1985; 8:528–539.

129. Cornblath DR, Mellits ED, Griffin JW, McKhann GM, Albers JW, Miller RG, Feasby TE, Quaskey SA, and the Guillain-Barré Study Group. Motor conduction studies in Guillain-Barré syndrome: Description and prognostic value. Ann Neurol 1988; 23:354–359.

130. Asbury AK, Arnason BG, Adams RD. The inflammatory lesion in idiopathic polyneuritis. Its role in pathogenesis. Medicine 1969; 48:173–215.

131. McKhann GM, Griffin JW, Cornblath DR, Mellits ED, Fisher RS, Quaskey SA, and the Guillain-Barré Study Group. Plasmapheresis and Guillain-Barré syndrome: Analysis of prognostic factors and the effect of plasmapheresis. Ann Neurol 1988; 23:347–353.

132. van der Meche FGA, Schmitz PIM, and the Dutch Guillain-Barré Study Group. A randomized trial comparing intravenous immune globulin and plasma exchange in Guillain-Barré syndrome. N Engl J Med 1992; 326:1123–1129.

133. Irani DN, Cornblath DR, Chaudhry V, Borel C, Hanley DF. Relapse in Guillain-Barré syndrome after treatment with human immune globulin. Neurology 1993; 43:857–858.

134. Castro LHM, Ropper AH. Human immune globulin in Guillain-Barré syndrome: Worsening during and after treatment. Neurology 1993; 43:1034–1036.

135. Dyck PJ, Lais AC, Ohta M, Bastron JA, Okazaki H, Groover RV. Chronic inflammatory demyelinating polyradiculoneuropathy. Mayo Clin Proc 1975; 50:621–637.

136. Ad Hoc Subcommittee of the American Academy of Neurology AIDS Task Force. Research criteria for diagnosis of chronic inflammatory demyelinating polyneuropathy (CIDP). Neurology 1991; 41:617–618.

137. Dyck PJ, O'Brien PC, Oviatt KF, Dinapoli RP, Daube JR, Bartleson JD, Mokri B, Swift T, Low PA, Windebank RJ. Prednisone improves chronic inflammatory demyelinating polyradiculoneuropathy more than no treatment. Ann Neurol 1982; 11:136–141.

138. Dyck PJ, Daube J, O'Brien P, Pineda A, Low PA, Windebank AJ, Swanson C. Plasma exchange in chronic inflammatory demyelinating polyradiculoneuropathy. N Engl J Med 1986; 314:461–465.

139. Faed JM, Day B, Pollock M, Taylor PK, Nukada H, Hammond-Tooke GD. High- dose intravenous human immunoglobulin in chronic inflammatory demyelinating polyneuropathy. Neurology 1989; 39:422–425.

140. van Doorn PA, Vermeulen M, Brand A, Mulder PGH, Busch HFM. Intravenous immunoglobulin treatment in patients with chronic inflammatory demyelinating polyneuropathy. Clinical and laboratory characteristics associated with improvement. Arch Neurol 1991; 48:217–220.

141. Vermeulen M, van Doorn PA, Brand A, Strengers PFW, Jennekens FG, Busch HFM. Intravenous immunoglobulin treatment in patients with chronic inflammatory demyelinating polyneuropathy: A double-blind, placebo controlled study. J Neurol Neurosurg Psychiatry 1993; 56:36–39.

142. Gordon M, Luqumani RA, Adu D, Greaves I, Richards N, Michael J, Emery P, Howie AJ, Bacon PA. Relapses in patients with a systemic vasculitis. Quart J Med 1993; 86:779–789.

143. Kissel JT, Mendell JR. Vasculitic neuropathy. Neurol Clinics 1992; 10:761–781.

144. Dyck PJ, Benstead TJ, Conn DL, Stevens JC, Windebank AJ, Low PA. Nonsystemic vasculitic neuropathy. Brain 1987; 110:843–853.

145. Fauci AS. The vasculitis syndromes. In: Wilson JD, Braunwald E, Issellbacher KJ, et al, eds., Harrison's Principles of Internal Medicine, 12th ed. New York: McGraw Hill, 1991;1456–1463.

146. Olney RK. Neuropathies in connective tissue disease. Muscle Nerve 1992; 15:531–542.

147. Caselli RJ, Daube JR, Hunder GG, Whisnant JP. Peripheral neuropathic syndromes in giant cell (temporal) arteritis. Neurology 1988; 38:685–689.

148. Kissel JT, Slivka AP, Warmolts JR, Mendell JR. The clinical spectrum of necrotizing angiopathy of the peripheral nervous system. Ann Neurol 1985; 18:251–257.

149. Said G, Lacroix-Ciaudo C, Fujimura H, Blas C, Faux N. The

peripheral neuropathy of necrotizing arteritis: A clinicopathological study. Ann Neurol 1988; 23:461–465.

150. Kissel JT, Riethman JL, Omerza J, Rammohan KW, Mendell JR. Peripheral nerve vasculitis: Immune characterization of the vascular lesions. Ann Neurol 1989; 25:291–297.

151. Yeung KB, Thomas PK, King RHM, Waddy H, Will RG, Hughes RA, Gregson NA, Leibowitz S. The clinical spectrum of peripheral neuropathies associated with benign monoclonal IgM, IgG and IgA paraproteinemia. Comparative clinical, immunological and nerve biopsy findings. J Neurol 1991; 238:383–391.

152. Kyle RA, Finkelstein S, Elveback LR, Kurland LT. Incidence of monoclonal proteins in a Minnesota community with a cluster of multiple myeloma. Blood 1972; 40:719–724.

153. Axelsson U, Bachman R, Hallen J. Frequency of pathological proteins (M components) in 6,995 sera from an adult population. Acta Medica Scand 1966; 179:235–247.

154. Kelly JJ Jr, Kyle RA, O'Brien PC, Dyck PJ. Prevalence of monoclonal protein in peripheral neuropathy. Neurology 1981; 31:1480–1483.

155. Osby E, Noring L, Hast R, Kjellin KG, Knutsson E, Siden A. Benign monoclonal gammopathy and peripheral neuropathy. Brit J Haematol 1982; 51:531–539.

156. Vrethem M, Cruz M, Wen-Xin H, Malm C, Holmgren H, Ernerudh J. Clinical, neurophysiological and immunological evidence of polyneuropathy in patients with monoclonal gammopathies. J Neurol Sci 1993; 114:193–199.

157. Latov N, Sherman WH, Nemni R, Galassi G, Shyong JS, Penn AS. Plasma cell dyscrasia and peripheral neuropathy with a monoclonal antibody to peripheral nerve myelin. N Engl J Med 1980; 303:618–621.

158. Mendell JR, Sahenk Z, Whitaker JN, Trapp BD, Yates AJ, Griggs RC, Quarles RH. Polyneuropathy and IgM monoclonal gammopathy: Studies on the pathogenic role of anti-myelin-associated glycoprotein antibody. Ann Neurol 1985; 17:243–254.

159. Bosch EP, Smith BE. Peripheral neuropathies associated with monoclonal proteins. Med Clin N Amer 1993; 77:125–139.

160. Kyle RA. "Benign" monoclonal gammopathy. A misnomer? JAMA 1984; 251:1849–1854.

161. Kyle RA, Garton JP. The spectrum of IgM monoclonal gammopathy in 430 cases. Mayo Clin Proc 1987; 62:719–731.

162. Gosselin S, Kyle RA, Dyck PJ. Neuropathy associated with monoclonal gammopathies of undetermined significance. Ann Neurol 1991; 30:54–61.

163. Dyck PJ, Low PA, Windebank AJ, Jaradeh SS, Gosselin S, Bourque P, Smith BE, Kratz KM, Karnes JL, Evans BA, et al. Plasma exchange in polyneuropathy associated with monoclonal gammopathy of undetermined significance. N Engl J Med 1991; 325:1482–1486.

164. Suarez GA, Kelly JJ Jr. Polyneuropathy associated with monoclonal gammopathy of undetermined significance: Further evidence that IgM-MGUS neuropathies are different than IgG-MGUS. Neurology 1993; 43:1304–1308.

165. Kelly JJ Jr. The electrodiagnostic findings in peripheral neuropathy associated with monoclonal gammopathy. Muscle Nerve 1983; 6:504–509.

166. Nemni R, Feltri ML, Fazio R, Quattrini A, Lorenzetti I, Corbo M, Canal N. Axonal neuropathy with monoclonal IgG kappa that binds to a neurofilament protein. Ann Neurol 1990; 28:361–364.

167. Dalakas MC, Flaum MA, Rick M, Engel WK, Gralnick HR. Treatment of polyneuropathy in Waldenstrom's macroglobulinemia: Role of paraproteinemia and immunologic studies. Neurology 1983; 33:1406–1410.

168. Kelly JJ Jr, Kyle RA, Miles JM, O'Brien PC, Dyck PJ. The spectrum of peripheral neuropathy in myeloma. Neurology 1981; 31:24–31.

169. Walsh JC. The neuropathy of multiple myeloma. An electrophysiological and histological study. Arch Neurol 1971; 25:404–414.

170. Kelly JJ, Kyle RA, Miles JM, Dyck PJ. Osteosclerotic myeloma and peripheral neuropathy. Neurology 1983; 33:202–210.

171. Ohi T, Kyle RA, Dyck PJ. Axonal attenuation and secondary segmental demyelination in myeloma neuropathies. Ann Neurol 1985; 17:255–261.

172. Bardwick PA, Zvaifler NJ, Gill GN, Newman D, Greenway GD, Resnick DL. Plasma cell dyscrasia with polyneuropathy,

organomegaly, endocrinopathy, M-protein and skin changes: The POEMS syndrome. Medicine 1980; 59:311–322.

173. Nakanishi T, Sobue I, Toyokura Y, Nishitani H, Kuroiwa Y, Satoyoshi E, Tsubaki T, Igata A, Ozaki Y. The Crow-Fukase syndrome: A study of 102 cases in Japan. Neurology 1984; 34:712–720.

174. Duston MA, Skinner M, Anderson J, Cohen AS. Peripheral neuropathy as an early marker of AL amyloidosis. Arch Intern Med 1989; 149:358–360.

175. Kelly JJ Jr, Kyle RA, O'Brien PC, Dyck PJ. The natural history of peripheral neuropathy in primary systemic amyloidosis. Ann Neurol 1979; 6:1–7.

176. Kyle RA, Dyck PJ. Amyloidosis and neuropathy. In: Dyck PJ, Thomas PK, Griffin JW, Low PA, Poduslo JF, eds., Peripheral Neuropathy, 3rd ed. Philadelphia: WB Saunders, 1993;1295–1309.

177. Kyle RA, Greipp PR. Amyloidosis (AL). Clinical and laboratory features in 229 cases. Mayo Clin Proc 1983; 58:665–683.

178. McLeod JC. Paraneoplastic neuropathies. In: Dyck PJ, Thomas PK, eds., Peripheral Neuropathy, 3rd ed. Philadelphia: WB Saunders, 1993; 1583–1590.

179. Trojaborg W, Frantzen E, Andersen I. Peripheral neuropathy and myopathy associated with carcinoma of the lung. Brain 1969; 92:71–82.

180. Lipton RB, Galer BS, Dutcher JP, Portenoy RK, Berger A, Arezzo JC, Mizruchi M, Wiernik PH, Schaumburg HH. Quantitative sensory testing demonstrates that subclinical sensory neuropathy is prevalent in patients with cancer. Arch Neurol 1987; 44:944–946.

181. Croft PB, Wilkinson M. Carcinomatous neuromyopathy. Its incidence in patients with carcinoma of the lung and carcinoma of the breast. Lancet 1963; 1:184–188.

182. Croft PB, Wilkinson M. The incidence of carcinomatous neuromyopathy in patients with various types of carcinoma. Brain 1965; 88:427–448.

183. McLeod JG. Peripheral neuropathy associated with lymphomas, leukemias and polycythemia vera. In: Dyck PJ, Thomas PK, Griffin JW, Low PA, Poduslo JF, eds., Peripheral Neuropathy, 3rd ed. Philadelphia: WB Saunders, 1993;1591–1598.

184. Denny-Brown D. Primary sensory neuropathy with muscular changes associated with carcinoma. J Neurol Neurosurg Psychiatry 1948; 11:73–87.

185. Croft PB, Wilkinson M. The course and prognosis in some types of carcinomatous neuromyopathy. Brain 1969; 92:1–8.

186. Croft PB, Henson RA, Urich H, Wilkinson PC. Sensory neuropathy with bronchial carcinoma: A study of four cases showing serologic abnormalities. Brain 1965; 88:501–514.

187. Horwich MS, Cho L, Porro RS, Posner JB. Subacute sensory neuropathy: A remote effect of carcinoma. Ann Neurol 1977; 2:7–19.

188. Anderson NE, Rosenblum MK, Graus F, Wiley RG, Posner JB. Autoantibodies in paraneoplastic syndromes associated with small-cell lung cancer. Neurology 1988; 38:1391–1398.

189. Fawcett DP, McBrien MP. Transitional cell carcinoma of the renal pelvis presenting with peripheral neuropathy. Brit J Urol 1977; 49:202.

190. Graus F, Elkon KB, Cordon-Cardo C, Posner JB. Sensory neuronopathy and small cell lung cancer. Antineuronal antibody that also reacts with the tumor. Amer J Med 1986; 80:45–52.

191. Graus F, Elkon KB, Lloberes P, Ribalta T, Torres A, Ussetti P, Valls J, Obach J, Agusti-Vidal A. Neuronal antinuclear antibody (anti-Hu) in paraneoplastic encephalomyelitis simulating acute polyneuritis. Acta Neurol Scand 1987; 75:249–252.

192. Chalk CH, Lennon VA, Stevens JC, Windebank AJ. Seronegativity for type 1 antineuronal nuclear antibodies ("anti-Hu") in subacute sensory neuronopathy patients without cancer. Neurology 1993; 43:2209–2211.

193. Hawley RJ, Cohen MH, Saini N, Armbrustmacher VW. The carcinomatous neuromyopathy of oat cell lung cancer. Ann Neurol 1980; 7:65–72.

194. Croft PB, Urich H, Wilkinson M. Peripheral neuropathy of sensorimotor type associated with malignant disease. Brain 1967; 90:31–66.

195. Harati Y, Niakan E. The clinical spectrum of inflammatory angiopathic neuropathy. J Neurol Neurosurg Psychiatry 1986; 49:1313–1316.

196. Vincent D, Dubas F, Hauw JJ, Godeau P, Ohermitte F, Buge

A, Castaigne P. Nerve and muscle microvasculitis in peripheral neuropathy: A remote effect of cancer? J Neurol Neurosurg Psychiatry 1986; 49:1007-1010.

197. Walsh JC. Neuropathy associated with lymphoma. J Neurol Neurosurg Psychiatry 1971; 34:42-50.

198. Sagar HJ, Read DJ. Subacute sensory neuropathy with remission: An association with lymphoma. J Neurol Neurosurg Psychiatry 1982; 45:83-85.

199. Schold SC, Cho ES, Somasundaram M, Posner JB. Subacute motor neuropathy: A remote effect of lymphoma. Ann Neurol 1979; 5:271-287.

200. Krendel DA, Stahl RL, Chan WC. Lymphomatous polyneuropathy. Biopsy of clinically involved nerve and successful treatment. Arch Neurol 1991; 48:330-332.

201. Cameron DG, Howell DA, Hutchinson JI. Acute peripheral neuropathy in Hodgkin's disease. Neurology 1958; 8:575-577.

202. Currie S, Henson RA, Morgan HG, Poole AJ. The incidence of non-metastatic neurological syndromes of obscure origin in the reticuloses. Brain 1970; 93:629-640.

203. Lisak RP, Mitchell M, Zweiman B, Orrechio E, Asbury AK. Guillain-Barré syndrome and Hodgkin's disease: Three cases with immunological studies. Ann Neurol 1977; 1:72-78.

204. Moore RY, Oda Y. Malignant lymphoma with diffuse involvement of the peripheral nervous system. Neurology 1962; 12:186-192.

205. Sumi SM, Farrell DF, Knauss TA. Lymphoma and leukemia manifested by steroid-responsive polyneuropathy. Arch Neurol 1983; 40:577-582.

206. Borit A, Altrocchi PH. Recurrent polyneuropathy and neurolymphomatosis. Arch Neurol 1971; 24:40-49.

207. Wells LE, Silver RT. The neurologic manifestations of acute leukemia: A clinical study. Ann Int Med 1957; 46:439-449.

208. Williams HM, Craver LF, Diamond HD, Parsons H. Neurological Complications in Lymphomas and Leukemia. Springfield, IL: Charles C. Thomas, 1959.

209. Schwab RS, Weiss S. The neurologic aspects of leukemia. Am J Med Sci 1935; 189:766-778.

210. Hunt WE, Bouroncle BA, Meagher JN. Neurologic complications of leukemia and lymphomas. J Neurosurg 1959; 16:135-151.

211. Krendel DA, Albright RE, Graham DG. Infiltrative poly-
      neuropathy due to acute monoblastic leukemia in hematologic
      remission. Neurology 1987; 37:474–477.
212. Vital C, Bonnaud E, Arne L, Barrat M, Leblanc M. Poly-
      neuritis in chronic lymphoid leukemia. Ultrastructural study of
      the peripheral nerve. Acta Neuropathol 1975; 32:169–172.
213. Powles RL, Malpas JS. Guillain-Barré syndrome associated
      with chronic lymphatic leukemia. Brit Med J 1967; 3:286–
      287.
214. Sandler SG, Tobin W, Henderson ES. Vincristine-induced
      neuropathy. A clinical study of fifty leukemic patients. Neu-
      rology 1969; 19:367–374.
215. Mcleod JG, Penny R. Vincristine neuropathy: An electrophy-
      siological and histological study. J Neurol Neurosurg Psychia-
      try 1969; 32:297–304.
216. LoMonaco M, Milone M, Batocchi AP, Padua L, Restuccia
      D, Tonali P. Cisplatin neuropathy: Clinical course and neuro-
      physiological findings. J Neurol 1992; 239:199–204.
217. Lipton RB, Apfel SC, Dutcher JP, Rosenberg R, Kaplan J,
      Berger A, Einzig AI, Wiernik P, Schaumburg HH. Taxol
      produces a predominantly sensory neuropathy. Neurology
      1989; 39:368–373.
218. Sahenk Z, Barohn RJ, New P, Mendell JR. Taxol neuro-
      pathy: An electrodiagnostic and sural nerve biopsy finding.
      Arch Neurol. 1994; 51:726–729.
219. Sahenk Z. Toxic neuropathies. Sem Neurol 1987; 7:9–17.
220. Schaumberg HH, Berger AR, Thomas PK. Pharmaceutical
      agents. In: Disorders of Peripheral Nerves, 2nd ed. Philadel-
      phia: FA Davis, 1992;257–273.
221. Le Quensne PM. Neuropathy due to drugs. In: Dyck PJ, Tho-
      mas PK, Griffin JW, Low PA, Poduslo JF, eds., Peripheral
      Neuropathy, 3rd ed. Philadelphia: WB Saunders, 1993;1571–
      1581.
222. Spring SB, Laughlin C, Arvin AM, Hay J, Straus SE,
      Whitley RJ, Gershon AA, Silverstein SJ. Workshop sum-
      mary. Ann Neurol 1994; 35:S2–S3.
223. Mahalingam R, Wellish M, Wolf W, Dueland AN, Cohrs R,
      Vafai A, Gilden D. Latent varicella-zoster viral DNA in hu-
      man trigeminal and thoracic ganglia. N Engl J Med 1990;
      323:627–631.

224. Thomas JE, Howard FM Jr. Segmental zoster paresis—a disease profile. Neurology 1972; 22:459–466.

225. Greenberg MK, McVey AL, Hayes T. Segmental motor involvement in herpes zoster: An EMG study. Neurology 1992; 42:1122–1123.

226. Ragozzino MW, Melton LJ III, Kurland LT, Chu CP, Perry HO. Population-bassed study of herpes zoster and its sequelae. Medicine 1982; 61:310–316.

227. Straus SE, Ostrove JM, Inchauspe G, Felser JM, Freifeld A, Croen KD, Sawyer MH. Varicella-zoster virus infections. Biology, natural history, treatment, and prevention. Ann Int Med 1988; 108:221–237.

228. Robertson DRC, George CF. Treatment of postherpetic neuralgia in the elderly. Brit Med Bull 1990; 46:113–123.

229. Hope-Simpson RE. Postherpetic neuralgia. J Roy Coll Gen Pract 1975; 25:571–575.

230. Miller AE. Selective decline in cellular immune response to varicella zoster in the elderly. Neurology 1980; 30:582–587.

231. Weksler ME. Immune senescence. Ann Neurol 1994; 35:S35–S37.

232. Wood MJ. Current experience with antiviral therapy for acute herpes zoster. Ann Neurol 1994; 35:S65–S68.

233. Watson CPN, Evans RJ, Watt VR. Post-herpetic neuralgia and topical capsaicin. Pain 1988; 33:333–340.

234. Bernstein JE, Korman NJ, Bickers DR, Dahl VM, Millikan LE. Topical capsaicin treatment of chronic postherpetic neuralgia. J Amer Acad Dermatol 1989; 21:265–270.

235. Max MB. Treatment of post-herpetic neuralgia: Antidepressants. Ann Neurol 1994; 35:S50–S53.

236. Nathan PW, Wall PD. Treatment of post-herpetic neuralgia by prolonged electric stimulation. Brit Med J 1974; 3:645–647.

237. Rowbotham MC. Managing post-herpetic neuralgia with opiods and local anesthetics. Ann Neurol 1994; 35:S46–S49.

238. Stewart JD. Focal Peripheral Neuropathies, 2nd ed. New York: Elsevier, 1993.

239. Wilbourn A, Aminoff MJ. Radiculopathies. In: Brown WF, Bolton CF, eds., Clinical Electromyography, 2nd ed. Boston: Butterworth, 1993; 177–209.

240. Parry GJ. Disease of spinal roots. In: Dyck PJ, Thomas PK, Griffin JW, Low PA, Poduslo JF, eds. Peripheral Neuropathies, 3rd ed. Philadelphia: WB Saunders, 1993; 899–910.

241. Epstein NE, Epstein JA. Individual and coexistent lumbar and cervical canal stenosis. Spine: State of the Art Reviews 1987; 1:401–420.

242. MacNab I. The pathogenesis of spinal stenosis. Spine: State of the Art Reviews 1987; 1:369–381.

243. Tsairis P, Dyck PJ, Mulder DW. Natural history of brachial plexus neuropathy. Report on 99 patients. Arch Neurol 1972; 27:109–117.

244. England JD, Sumner AJ. Neuralgic amyotrophy: An increasingly diverse entity. Muscle Nerve 1987; 10:60–68.

245. Wilbourn AJ. Brahcial plexus disorders. In: Dyck PJ, Thomas PK, Griffin JW, Low PA, Paduslo JF, eds., Peripheral Neuropathies, 3rd ed. Philadelphia: WB Saunders, 1993; 911–950.

246. Eisen AA. The electrodiagnosis of plexopathies. In: Brown WF, Bolton CF, eds., Clinical Electromyography, 2nd ed. Boston: Butterworth-Heinemann, 1993; 211–225.

247. Evans BA, Stevens JC, Dyck PJ. Lumbosacral plexus neuropathy. Neurology 1981; 31:1327–1330.

248. Chad DA, Bradley WG. Lumbosacral plexopathy. Sem Neurol 1987; 7:97–107.

249. Donaghy M. Lumbosacal plexus lesions. In: Dyck PJ, Thomas PK, Griffin JW. Low PA, Paduslo JF, eds., Peripheral Neuropathies, 3rd ed. Philadelphia: WB Saunders, 1993; 91–950.

250. Bradley WG, Chad D, Verghese JP, Liu HC, Good P, Gabbai AA, Adelman LS. Painful lumbosacral plexopathy with elevated erythrocyte sedimentation rate: A treatable inflammatory syndrome. Ann Neurol 1984; 15:457–464.

251. Verma A, Bradley WG. High-dose intravenous immunoglobulin therapy in chronic progressive lumbosacral plexopathy. Neurology 1994; 44:248–250.

252. Kori SH, Foley KM, Posner JB. Brachial plexus lesions in patients with cancer: 100 cases. Neurology 1981; 31:45–50.

253. Jaeckle KA, Young DF, Foley KM. The natural history of lumbosacral plexopathy in cancer. Neurology 1985; 35:8–15.

254. Stewart JD. Compression and entrapment neuropathies. In:

Dyck PJ, Thomas PK, Griffin JW, Low PA, Poduslo JF, eds., Peripheral Neuropathy, 3rd ed. Philadelphia: WB Saunders, 1993;961–979.

255. Dawson DM. Entrapment neuropathies of the upper extremities. N Engl J Med 1993; 329:2013–2018.

256. Kimura J. Median nerve. In: Brown WF, Bolton CF, eds., Clinical Electromyography, 2nd ed. Boston: Butterworth-Heinemann, 1993; 227–248.

257. Miller RJ. Ulnar nerve lesions. In: Brown WF, Bolton CF, eds., Clinical Electromyography, 2nd ed. Boston: Butter-worth-Heinemann, 1993;249–269.

258. Katirji MB, Wilbourn AJ. Common peroneal mononeuropathy: A clinical and electrophysiologic study of 116 lesions. Neurology 1988; 38:1723–1728.

259. Dawson DM, Hallett M, Millender LH. Entrapment Neuropathies, 2nd ed. Boston: Little, Brown and Co., 1990.

260. Dyck PJ, Lambert EH. Lower motor and primary sensory neuron disease with peroneal muscular atrophy. I. Neurologic, genetic and electrophysiologic findings in hereditary polyneuropathy. Arch Neurol 1968; 18:603–618.

261. Dyck PJ, Lambert EH. Lower motor and primary sensory neuron disease with peroneal muscular atrophy. II. Neurologic, genetic and electrophysiologic findings in various neuronal degenerations. Arch Neurol 1968; 18:619–625.

262. Harding AE, Thomas PK. The clinical features of hereditary motor and sensory neuropathy types I and II. Brain 1980; 103:259–280.

263. Verhagen WIM, Gabreels-Festen AAWM, van Wensen PJM, Joosten EMG, Vingerhoets HM, Gabreels FJ, de Graaf R. Hereditary neuropathy with liability to pressure palsies: A clinical, electroneurophysiological and morphological study. J Neurol Sci 1993; 116:176–184.

264. Chance PF, Alderson MK, Leppig KA, Lensch MW, Matsunami N, Smith B, Swanson PD, Odelberg SJ, Disteche CM, Bird TD. DNA deletion associated with hereditary neuropathy liability to pressure palsies. Cell 1993; 72:143–151.

265. Mendell JR. Sahenk Z. Recent advances in diagnosis and classification of Charcot-Marie-tooth disease. Current Opinion in Orthopedics 1993; 4(V):39–45.

266. Amato AA, Gronseth GS, Callerame KJ, Kagan-Hallet KS, Bryan WW, Barohn RJ. Tomaculous neuropathy: A clinical and electrophysiologic study in patients with and without deletions in chromosome 17p11.2. Muscle Nerve (in press).

267. Mendell, JR, Jiang XS, Warmolts JR, Nichols WC, Benson MD. Diagnosis of Maryland/German familial amyloidic polyneuropathy using allele-specific enzymatically amplified, genomic DNA. Ann Neurol 1990; 27:553–557.

268. Izumoto S, Younger D, Hays AP, Martone RL, Smith RT, Herbert J. Familial amyloidotic polyneuropathy presenting with carpal tunnel syndrome and a new transthyretin mutation, asparagine 70. Neurology 1992; 42:2094–2102.

269. Yasuda T, Sobue G, Doyu M, Nakazato M, Shiomi K, Yanagi T, Mitsuma T. Familial amyloidotic polyneuropathy with late-onset and well preserved autonomic function: A Japanese kindred with novel mutant transthyretin (Ala^{97}-Gln). J Neurol Sci 1994; 121:97–102.

8

Fatigue

Lauren B. Krupp, P. K. Coyle, and Martin Sliwinski
State University of New York at Stony Brook
School of Medicine
Stony Brook, New York

I. GENERAL ASSESSMENT AND TREATMENT OF FATIGUE

A. Introduction

Fatigue is common in a variety of neurologic disorders. It can affect patients of any age, but presents particular challenges in the elderly. Fatigue is defined as an overwhelming sense of tiredness, lack of energy, or feeling of exhaustion. It should be distinguished from symptoms of depression, which include lack of self-esteem, despair, or feelings of hopelessness. Fatigue is also distinct from limb weakness. It is most easily conceptualized as the feeling of exhaustion that transiently accompanies the flu in healthy individuals. Among many patients with certain neurologic and medical conditions, fatigue can be chronic and severe.

B. Fatigue in Medical Illness

Pathological fatigue is distinct from the fatigue healthy adults experience. Compared to the fatigue of healthy controls, patients with multiple sclerosis (1), systemic lupus erythematosus (2), chronic fatigue syndrome (3–5), or lyme disease (6) invariably rate their fatigue as more disabling. In these patients, fatigue negatively impacts on activities of daily living to a significantly greater degree than does fatigue for healthy controls.

New onset of fatigue in any patient may be an important sign of illness. Patients with undiagnosed conditions (thyroid disease, systemic lupus erythematosus, sleep disorders, diabetes, multiple sclerosis, or Parkinson's disease) may present with fatigue as their sole or chief complaint. In patients with known neurologic illness, fatigue may represent a change in disease activity. This may be true of postpolio syndrome, multiple sclerosis, or Parkinson's disease. Fatigue assessment in any patient includes evaluating such related factors as mood, level of physical activity, severity of the underlying disease, medication, sleep, cognitive dysfunction, and social support.

C. Fatigue Measurement

A variety of instruments have been developed to assess and measure fatigue for clinical and research purposes (2,5,7,8–11). Several fatigue scales and their relative advantages and disadvantages are shown in Table 1. Since fatigue is inherently a subjective experience analogous to pain, the most appropriate measure of the symptom is a self-report instrument that can quantify what the patient experiences. Measuring fatigue with a validated instrument and following its course is helpful in the evaluation and management of any patient with this complaint.

D. Evaluation of the Fatigued Patient

The patient who presents with a sole complaint of fatigue is usually initially seen in a primary care setting. As outlined in Table 2, the evaluation requires a complete medical and neurological history, examination, and laboratory screen including thyroid function test (TFT), electrolytes and liver function panel (SMA-23), complete blood cell count (CBC), antinuclear antibody (ANA), erythrocyte sedimentation rate (ESR), and urinalysis (UA). The estimated mean cost of a compre-

Table 1 Fatigue Scales

Scale	Pros	Cons
Visual analogue scale	Brief, simple	Prone to impulsive answers
Rand Index of Vitality (7)	Easy to score and administer	Limited range of aspects of fatigue
Medical Outcome Survey Fatigue Scale (11)	Assesses psychological aspects and disabilities	May take some time
Mental/Physical Fatigue Scale (8)	Characterizes mental and physical components	Forces patients into dichotomous thinking
Fatigue Severity Scale (2)	Assesses disabling features, has established reliability	Not quite as detailed as some scales

Table 2 Evaluation of Fatigue

History
  Assess for systemic and neurologic disease
  Review medications
    (beta blockers, antidepressants, anticonvulsants)
  Assess related symptoms
    (pain, sleep, memory, mood)
  General medical exam
  Neurologic exam
    Focal deficits
    Mental status
    Administer fatigue and depression measures
  Laboratory screen
    CBC, SMA-23, ANA, ESR, TFT, U/A
  Special studies (in selected cases)
    Neuropsychological testing
    Polysomnography
    EEG
    MRI
  Psychiatric referral (in selected cases)

hensive yet not overly exhaustive work-up for fatigue in a primary care setting is $131 (12). In 50% of fatigued patients in a primary care center this work-up yields a positive diagnosis (12). This approach can detect easily treatable etiologies of fatigue such as anemia, renal disease, hypothyroidism, or diabetes, and screens for inflammatory, autoimmune, neoplastic, or infectious etiologies. In addition to this work-up, it is also appropriate to evaluate other symptoms or problems that may be contributing to fatigue.

One symptom that can cause fatigue is pain. Pain can interfere with daily functioning, add stress, disrupt sleep, and make fatigue unmanageable that was previously mild. Among patients with cancer, pain is the most important correlate of fatigue (13). Pain also correlates with fatigue in patients with rheumatoid arthritis (14). A review of systems approach focusing on headache, muscle pain, radicular or back pain may reveal that these factors are contributing to a patient's lack of energy.

Sleep disorder may be experienced as fatigue. In a sample of patients referred for chronic fatigue syndrome, we and others identified a subset of patients with a variety of sleep disorders (15,16). Some of our findings on polysomnography and neurologic examination among subjects referred for chronic fatigue syndrome to our neurology practice are shown in Table 3. A relationship between fatigue and sleep disturbance has also been noted in multiple sclerosis (17,18). Careful assessment of a patient's sleep habits is helpful when evaluating fatigue. Questions regarding where they sleep best, observations by their partner on quality of sleep, number of nocturnal awakenings, and apneic episodes may help identify previously undiagnosed sleep disorders. Such disorders may be primarily responsible for fatigue or contribute to its severity. In patients in whom excessive sleepiness or disturbed sleep is a primary complaint, or in whom the general exam is suspicious for apnea, polysomnography may be appropriate.

Another factor that contributes to fatigue is cognitive loss. Short-term memory problems, slowed reaction times, and associated cognitive event-related potentials are correlated with fatigue in multiple sclerosis (19). Some chronic fatigue syndrome patients with cognitive complaints also have slowed reaction times and mild deficits on neuropsychological testing (20). In patients with fatigue and histories of major cognitive loss, neuropsychological evaluation may be helpful. As shown in Table 3, neuropsychological evaluation disclosed multi-infarct dementia and early Alzheimer's disease in two elderly patients we evaluated for chronic fatigue.

Assessment of mood is critical in patients with fatigue. It is important to ask about family history of psychiatric illness by either questionnaire or interview; examine the nature of the family unit and assess current support systems; and evaluate current level of self-esteem and anxiety. In addition to the history, a simple quick office approach is to use self-report depression questionnaires. Brief self-report instruments with demonstrated reliability and validity for depression measurement that have been widely used are the Beck depression inventory (21) and the Center for Epidemiologic Studies Depression Scale (CES-D) (22). Both scales provide cut-off scores that can identify a patient at risk for clinical major depression.

Table 3 Neurologic and Psychiatric Disorders Presenting with Severe Fatigue in 100 Patients Referred for Chronic Fatigue Syndrome

Narcolepsy	Migraine
Sleep apnea	Alzheimer's disease
Nocturnal myoclonus	Major depression
Multi-infarct dementia	Obsessive-compulsive personality disorder
Multiple sclerosis	Adjustment reaction
Lyme disease	Dysthymia

For patients in whom overwhelming fatigue is refractory to all forms of therapy, psychiatric referral may be of value even if depressive symptoms are not elevated. Psychiatric evaluation may disclose previously unrecognized psychosocial or psychiatric problems, or may simply rule out this possibility so that more aggressive medical treatment is pursued. Before considering treatment for fatigue with amphetamine-type medication, we routinely have patients assessed by a psychologist or psychiatrist.

The fatigued patient with a known neurologic or medical disorder should have his or her underlying condition assessed. For example, in multiple sclerosis or Parkinson's disease new neurologic symptoms or signs accompanying fatigue may signify a worsening of the underlying condition, impending exacerbation, or possible medication side effect. Assessing changes of prescribed medication such as dopaminergic agents, antihypertensive agents, tricyclic antidepressants, benzodiazepines, or anticonvulsants is appropriate. If there is no change in either medication or disease activity, evaluation should parallel that of a patient without known neurological disorder whose sole complaint is fatigue.

E. Treatment

Fatigue treatment requires a multidisciplinary approach. Many factors may contribute to fatigue severity, so that combined therapeutic modalities are the most effective. Nonpharmacologic treatments are an important part of therapy. Patients directly benefit when their symptom is recognized as genuine. They appreciate having the opportunity to discuss it with their physician. Not infrequently, family members will not appreciate the differences between the pathologic fatigue of medical disease (which is invariably more overwhelming, constant, and severe) and their own transient and mild "normal" fatigue. They may be less understanding toward the patient because there is not a visually obvious cause for disability. Education and reassurance are very useful in these situations.

In addition to reassurance, other nonpharmacologic treatments for fatigue are available but require an individualized approach. Depending on patients' emotional reaction to symptoms and level of activity, some individuals benefit from mild and limited exercise programs to combat the frequent deconditioning that occurs with fatigue. Others need to be cautioned that overexertion is not helpful, and that cutting back on activity is something they must learn to accept. In particular instances, rest periods during the workday and avoidance of conditions that worsen fatigue (such as heat in multiple sclerosis patients) are also beneficial.

Behavior modification therapy may reduce associated symptoms of depression and fatigue components caused by mood disorder (23). Behavioral therapies may be effective on an individual or group basis. They are structured in a format analogous to chronic pain treatment groups, and have been shown for some patients to provide a major benefit (23).

Often nonpharmacologic measures must be supplemented with drug therapy. Examples of medications used to treat fatigue are shown in Table 4. Most reports of drug therapy for fatigue have been concerned with multiple sclerosis or chronic fatigue syndrome (24–31). Amantadine (Symmetrel) and pemoline (Cylert) have been compared to placebo in double-blind randomized treatment studies (24,26–28). Murray found that among 32 multiple sclerosis patients treated for fatigue with 100 mg bid of amantadine, improvement was marked in 31%, moderate in 15.6%, and mild in 15.6% (27). In a larger subsequent study of multiple sclerosis patients with fatigue, using a crossover placebo-controlled design, a significant decrease in fatigue in the amantadine group was noted (24). However, the effect was small and side effects were numerous in the amantadine and placebo groups (24).

The mechanism of action of amantadine is unknown. Rosenberg and Appenzeller (25) found that fatigue responders had higher levels of beta-endorphin, beta-lipotropin, and lower levels of pyruvate and lactate. This may have been due to increased activity associated with less fatigue, or to a di-

Table 4 Medications to Treat Fatigue

	Side effects
CNS stimulants	
Pemoline (Cylert) 18.75–112.5 mg OD	Irritability, insomnia, palpitations
Methylphenidate (Ritalin) 2.5–20 mg	Insomnia, headache, restlessness
Dopaminergic	
Amantadine (Symmetrel) 100 mg bid	Livedo reticularis, insomnia
Selegiline (Eldepryl) 5 mg bid	Confusion
Antidepressants	
Desipramine (Norpramin) 25–200 mg	Insomnia, palpitations
Protriptyline (Vivactil) 5–10 mg tid	Insomnia, palpitations
Fluoxetine (Prozac) 20–60 mg	Anorexia, anxiety, insomnia
Sertraline (Zoloft) 50–200 mg	GI complaints, headache, insomnia

rect effect of amantadine. Cognitive function as measured by tasks of attention improved in one study of fatigued multiple sclerosis patients treated with amantadine (29). We have not been able to reproduce this finding in a sample of multiple sclerosis patients who underwent an extensive neuropsychological evaluation before and during treatment with placebo and amantadine (31).

Pemoline, a mild CNS stimulant, may also be of value in treating fatigue. Anecdotal experience suggests a positive effect with this medication. A double-blind randomized crossover trial of pemoline in multiple sclerosis fatigue noted a slight benefit over placebo (28). Forty-six percent of treated patients had excellent or good relief with pemoline compared to only 19.5% with placebo. Poorly tolerated side effects occurred in 25% of the pemoline group (28).

We recently completed a randomized study comparing pemoline, amantadine, and placebo in the treatment of multiple sclerosis fatigue using a parallel group design (26). A modest benefit of amantadine but not of pemoline was noted when each drug was compared to placebo (26). Similar to previous studies (24,28), a strong placebo effect was present.

Other medications used with some success on an anecdotal basis for fatigue, but not systematically studied, include selegiline and central nervous system (CNS) stimulants such as methylphenidate (Ritalin) or dextroamphetamine. CNS stimulants should be used with caution, but in selected cases have value. They are contraindicated in patients with abuse potential.

Another pharmacologic strategy for fatigue consists of antidepressant medication. This is clearly the treatment of choice for patients with coexisting major depression. However, even patients who deny depressive symptoms may have definite responses to antidepressant medication. Agents with the least sedating properties are preferable such as fluoxetine (Prozac), sertraline (Zoloft), desipramine (Norpramin), or protriptyline (Vivactil).

In patients in whom fatigue is associated with sleep disorder, improved sleep hygiene is important. Exercise 6 hours before sleep can help, and patients should be cautioned not to look at the time every few minutes. Medications for insomnia may also lower fatigue in selected cases. Occasionally fatigue is associated with anxiety. Alleviating anxiety or panic attacks with appropriate therapies has a beneficial impact on fatigue.

II. FATIGUE IN SPECIFIC DISEASES OF THE ELDERLY

A. At-Risk Patients

In the healthy elderly, fatigue is generally not a major problem. We assessed fatigue in 23 subjects aged 50 to 82 who were free of chronic medical conditions. Their mean fatigue score was not significantly different from younger healthy controls (32). Among healthy elderly persons with depressive symptoms, fatigue is more disabling. In elderly subjects with high depression scores (>16 on the CES-D) fatigue is significantly higher than similarly aged subjects with low depression ($p < 0.003$) (32). However, age does not significantly correlate with severity of fatigue in either depressed or nondepressed medically healthy subjects.

The combination of fatigue and depression can affect cognitive performance in the elderly. In a study of elderly subjects who rated their health as "good," depressed subjects did worse in experimental tests of visual-spatial short-term memory than did nondepressed subjects (33). Fatigue in these older depressed subjects was exacerbated to a greater degree by an experimentally produced effort-full condition than among nondepressed elderly subjects (33).

In the medically ill population fatigue is common, but it does not correlate with age. We examined the relationship between fatigue and age using a 9-item fatigue severity scale in patients with systemic lupus erythematosus, Lyme disease, multiple sclerosis, chronic fatigue syndrome, and major depression, or dysthymia (32). We found that fatigue did not significantly correlate with age in any of these disorders ($p > 0.25$ in all cases), and the median correlations between age and fatigue for all groups was 0.06 (NS) (32).

However, when an elderly patient presents with a chief complaint of fatigue, a comprehensive evaluation is critical. In elderly patients with chronic fatigue we have found specific etiologies for fatigue more often than we have in younger subjects. Diseases in which the elderly are at particular risk, such as cancer, chronic obstructive pulmonary disease or heart disease, may all produce fatigue and must be ruled out. Among older patients referred to a neurologist for persistent fatigue (see Table 3) we identified major depression, adjustment disorder, dysthymia, nocturnal myoclonus, sleep apnea, multi-infarct dementia, Lyme disease, and Parkinson's disease as primarily responsible for fatigue. Since major depression is frequent in the elderly, this must also be considered as a possible contributor to fatigue (34,35). This is particularly important if the medical work-up is unrevealing.

B. Postpolio Syndrome

Postpolio syndrome is a long-term sequela of acute poliomyelitis occurring in approximately 25–40% of survivors (36, 37). Most patients are over the age of 50 when they develop postpolio syndrome. The syndrome is characterized by new weakness, aches, pain, cold intolerance, and extreme fatigue. Weakness my involve limbs, trunk, or respiratory muscles. Pain may be muscular or involve joints. The fatigue is either systemic or muscle related. It is a symptom in 47–89% of the postpolio population (36,37). Before attributing fatigue to postpolio syndrome one should exclude things such as back injury, radiculopathy, compressive neuropathy, and other causes of fatigue. The fatigue is often described as a feeling of excessive tiredness, overwhelming exhaustion, or flu-like sensation (37). Among one group of postpolio patients studied, physical exertion exacerbated fatigue in 48%, while in 70% of healthy controls it had the opposite effect (36). Although postpolio fatigue is common in older patients who have polio, its severity is not associated with patient age (37).

Postpolio patients compared to age-matched controls with respect to health habits show no differences in sleep, alcohol use, or coffee use (36). Postpolio patients are more likely to report mild to moderately elevated depressive symptoms than controls. However, depressed and nondepressed postpolio patients do not differ in the progression of fatigue severity (36). The qualitative experience of fatigue differs between depressed and nondepressed postpolio patients in that lack of energy, inability to concentrate, and a heavy sensation in the muscles were more frequently reported among those postpolio patients with concurrent depressive symptoms (36). Fatigue in postpolio syndrome can be ameliorated by such measures as patient and family education, instruction in energy-conserving techniques, adequate provision of rest periods, stretching exercises, relaxation techniques, and treatment of depression if it is a coexisting symptom.

C. Parkinson's Disease

Patients with Parkinson's disease commonly experience fatigue (38,39). One-third report fatigue as the most disabling symptom, and over half consider fatigue among their three worst symptoms. Fatigue correlates with depressive symptoms, but nondepressed parkinsonian patients may suffer from fatigue as well (38).

Fatigue severity only weakly correlates with severity of Parkinson's disease as measured by the Parkinson's disease severity scale of Hohen and Yahr. Fatigue does not appear to vary significantly with time of day or diurnal motor activity (39).

The role of sleep and its effect on fatigue in Parkinson's disease has been studied (39). Parkinson's disease patients and age-matched healthy controls do not differ significantly in their subjective reports of sleep disturbance. However, Parkinson's disease patients with excessive daytime sleepiness, compared to similarly symptomatic controls, more frequently report altered dreams, waken during the night with pain and stiffness, and have problems turning in bed. In the Parkinson's group no clear relationship has emerged between fatigue severity and subjective problems with sleep maintenance, excessive daytime sleeping, diurnal fluctuations, or medication (39).

D. Head Trauma

Fatigue was a significant complaint for 63% of head-injured patients including some elderly subjects at Braintree Rehabilitation who responded to a survey (40). The frequency of fatigue showed no dependence on the location of neuropathology documented by neuroimaging, or the duration of posttraumatic coma and amnesia. Glasgow outcome scores at 6 and 12 months also did not predict fatigue (40). Nap requirement did not differ among patients with different sites of CNS injury. A history of substance abuse did not significantly increase the patient's risk of developing fatigue or its duration after head injury. In contrast, anticonvulsant use had a qualitative ameliorating effect on the subjective complaint of fatigue after medication was stopped. All centrally acting medications were noted to increase the incidence of subjective fatigue (40). Thus, in head injury the complaint of fatigue does not appear to be related to the severity of the neurologic illness but may be modulated by medication.

E. Multiple Sclerosis

Fatigue is a problem for 80–90% of multiple sclerosis patients (2,41). Although multiple sclerosis most commonly begins among patients 20–40 years of age, it is occasionally first diagnosed in patients aged 50 and older. Frequently multiple sclerosis causes continued problems in diagnosed individuals as they age. With improvements in medical care, a larger number of patients with multiple sclerosis now reach old age.

Multiple sclerosis fatigue is not correlated with patient's age, gender, or neurologic impairment (as measured by the Kurtzke disability scale) (1). Multiple sclerosis fatigue does overlap with depressive symptoms in multiple sclerosis, but is clearly a distinct problem. In one study of severely fatigued multiple sclerosis patients, less than 10% met criteria for current major depression (42).

Certain features distinguish multiple sclerosis fatigue from fatigue experienced by other medical patients or controls. Over 90% of multiple sclerosis patients report that heat dramatically worsens fatigue, while cool temperatures help relieve fatigue (1). This feature is not shared by fatigued patients with SLE (2), Lyme disease (6), or healthy controls (1). Multiple sclerosis patients frequently associate their fatigue with impaired physical rather than mental activity (27). In one study over 90% of patients picked activities such as walking, housework, going out, or grooming over mental activities such as concentration as most affected by fatigue (24).

Fatigue affects a variety of aspects of daily living. In response to a series of open-ended questions regarding their health, multiple sclerosis patients responded frequently that feeling tired accompanied activities such as using a wheelchair, moving about, or working. Feelings of tiredness also were associated with aching, feeling stiff, or new responsibilities such as childrearing (43).

F. Postoperative Fatigue

Fatigue is a major symptom of the postoperative period and is a particular problem for older patients. Among 38 patients undergoing abdominal surgery, the level of postoperative fatigue peaked after 1 week and returned to preoperative levels 1 month later (44). Three months later fatigue was significantly less than the preoperative period. Fatigue is not explained by total body protein or measures of muscle contractility (44). However, during certain portions of the postoperative period, change in fatigue is significantly associated with perceived motor effort and grip strength (45). Postoperative fatigue does significantly correlate with preoperative fatigue severity and is more common in subjects who are elderly, suffer from cancer, and are in pain (45). Studies have not linked fatigue to muscular defects (44). The mechanism of postoperative fatigue is judged to be central in origin.

G. Rheumatologic Disorders

Depressive symptoms and pain are frequent in chronic rheumatologic conditions and may exacerbate fatigue. Immunologic abnormalities in these disorders may also be important in the pathogenesis of fatigue. Depression has been correlated with fatigue in patients with rheumatologic disorders such as systemic lupus erythematosus (2,46), rheumatoid arthritis (14,47), and Lyme disease (6). However, the correlation between fatigue and depression was relatively weak, implying that variables other than depression contribute to fatigue. In older rheumatoid arthritis patients (aged 56–86), pain accounted for 19% of the variance of fatigue (14). The combination of pain with quality of sleep, comorbid conditions, duration of disease, physical activity, and functional status accounted for 42% of the variance of fatigue (14).

Lyme disease, a multisystem disorder that can cause peripheral and central neurologic complications, is associated with fatigue at all stages of the illness (6). Fatigue is most frequent in disseminated disease and in patients treated for late complications (6). In a subset of patients, fatigue persists for many months even after other Lyme disease manifestations have subsided (6).

H. Chronic Fatigue Syndrome

Chronic fatigue syndrome is a genuine but poorly understood illness (48). It is defined mainly by a set of symptoms out of proportion to identifiable pathology. Symptoms may be chronic or intermittent for days or weeks with periods of relative remission. There are no objective diagnostic tests for chronic fatigue syndrome, and it is a diagnosis of exclusion.

In 1988 the Centers for Disease Control and Prevention (CDC) published a case definition for chronic fatigue syndrome (49). To meet the case definition a patient must fulfill two major criteria, and either 8 of 11 symptom criteria, or 2 objective and 6 symptom criteria. The first major criterion is the new onset of severe and debilitating fatigue present for at least 6 months. The second major criterion is the absence of an identifiable medical or psychiatric etiology for fatigue. Minor symptom criteria include generalized headache, myalgia, arthralgia, fever, sore throat, painful lymph nodes, muscle weakness, prolonged fatigue after exercise, neuropsychological symptoms, sleep disturbance, and an abrupt onset of the fatigue problem. Objective criteria are docu-

mented low-grade fever, nonexudative pharyngitis, and palpable or tender cervical or axillary lymph nodes.

In 1992 the National Institutes of Health (NIH) published
recommended modifications of the definition (49). Patients
with specific psychiatric diagnoses and certain postinfectious
fatigue syndromes are excluded, while patients with selected
confounding diagnoses are included. This acknowledges that
certain psychiatric disorders (50–55) as well as fibromyalgia
syndrome (56) overlap with chronic fatigue syndrome.

Chronic fatigue syndrome is most commonly a disorder
of young and middle-aged adults (57). However, we have
seen some individuals over age 65 referred for this disorder.
Among the elderly referred for chronic fatigue syndrome it is
particularly important to evaluate for depression, dementing
disorders, sleep disorders, medication side effects, and systemic illness.

The most common symptoms in chronic fatigue syndrome
patients are cognitive loss, sleep, and psychological disturbances (56,57). Each problem must be specifically explored
in the history. Features that suggest underlying psychiatric
disease are (1) gradual onset of fatigue; (2) lack of somatic
symptoms; (3) prior psychiatric history with current psychiatric complaints; and (4) suicidal ideation.

The physical examination of the chronic fatigue syndrome
patient should evaluate for low-grade fever, nonexudative
pharyngitis, palpable cervical/axillary nodes, photophobia,
muscle tenderness, and crimson crescents on the anterior
pharynx (56). Minor abnormalities (positive Romberg, gait
ataxia) have been reported in the neurological examination,
but they are generally not striking and fairly nonspecific.

The cause of chronic fatigue syndrome is unknown (59–
64). Several etiologic factors have been suggested including
chronic infection by a specific agent or immunologic causes.
To date, however, no single virus or bacterium has been
consistently associated with chronic fatigue syndrome cases
(65–68) and several agents have been specifically excluded
(60,67–69). Immunologic factors associated with chronic fa-

tigue syndrome include cytokine abnormalities, impaired natural killer cell activity, T-cell dysfunction, and B-cell abnormalities (64,69–74). Unfortunately, many studies have not rigorously controlled for confounding factors (medications, mood, etc.) and have not used uniform assay techniques. Psychological factors have been the most consistently implicated in chronic fatigue syndrome. Psychiatric diagnoses (depression, anxiety, somatoform disorders) can be made in 42–82% of patients (51–53).

REFERENCES

1. Krupp LB, Alvarez LA, LaRocca NG, Scheinberg L. Clinical characteristics of fatigue in multiple sclerosis. Arch Neurol 1988; 45:435–437
2. Krupp LB, LaRocca NC, Muir-Nash J, et al. The fatigue severity scale applied to patients with multiple sclerosis and systemic lupus erythematosus. Arch Neurol 1989; 46:1121–1123
3. Krupp LB, Mendelson WB, Friedman R. An overview of CFS. J Clin Psychiatry 1991; 52:403–410.
4. Kroenke K, Wood DR, Mangels D, et al. Chronic fatigue in primary care. JAMA 1988; 260:929–934
5. Fisk JD, Ritvo PG, Ross L, et al. Measuring the functional impact of fatigue: Initial validation of the fatigue impact scale. Clin Infect Dis 1994; 18(suppl 1):S79–S83
6. Krupp LB, Schwartz JE, Jandorf L. Fatigue in Lyme disease. In: Coyle PK (ed.), Lyme Disease. St. Louis: Mosby Year Book, 1993
7. Brook RH, Ware JE, Davies A, et al. Overview of adult health status measures fielded in the Rand's Health Insurance Study. Med Care 1979; 71(suppl):1–55
8. Wessley S, Powell R. Fatigue syndromes: A comparison of postviral fatigue with neuromuscular and affective disorders. J Neurol Neurosurg Psychiatry 1989; 52:940–948
9. Piper BF, Lindsey AM, Dodd MJ, et al. The development of an instrument to measure the subjective dimension of fatigue. In: Funk SG, Tornquist EM, Champagne MT, et al. (eds.), Key Aspects of Comfort: Management of Pain, Fatigue, and Nausea. New York: Springer Publishing Co., 1989

10. Schwartz J, Jandorf L, Krupp LB. The measurement of fatigue: A new scale. J Psychosom Res 1993; 37:753–762

11. Stewart AL, Hays RD, Ware JE. The MOS Short Form General Health Survey—Reliability and validity in a patient population. Med Care 1988; 26:724–735

12. Elnicki DM, Shocklor WR, Brick JE, et al. Evaluating the complaint of fatigue in primary care: Diagnoses and outcomes. Amer J Med 1992; 93:303–306

13. Pickard-Holley S. Fatigue in cancer patients: A descriptive study. Cancer Nursing 1991; 14:13–19

14. Belza BL, Henke CJ, Yelin EH, Epstein WV, Gilliss CL. Correlates of fatigue in older adults with rheumatoid arthritis. Nursing Res 1993; 42:93–99

15. Krupp LB, Jandorf L, Coyle PK, Mendelson WB. Sleep in chronic fatigue syndrome. J Psychosom Res 1993; 37:325–331

16. Buchwald D, Pascualy R, Bombadier C, Kith P. Sleep disorders in patients with chronic fatigue. Clin Infec Dis 1994; 18(suppl 1):S68–72

17. Caruso LS, LaRocca NC, Tyron W, et al. Activity monitoring of fatigued and non-fatigued persons with MS. Sleep Res 1991; 20:368

18. Giancarlo T, Kapen S, Saad J. Analysis of sleepiness and fatigue in multiple sclerosis. Ann Neurol 1987; 22:187

19. Sandroni P, Walker C, Starr A. Fatigue in patients with MS. Arch Neurol 1992; 49:517–524

20. Scheffers MK, Johnson R Jr, Grafman J, et al. Attention and short-term memory in CFS patients. Neurology 1992; 42:1667–1675

21. Beck AT, Ward CH, Mendelson M. An inventory for measuring depression. Arch Gen Psych 1961; 4:561–571

22. Radloff LS. CES-D scale: A self-report depression scale for research in the general population. Appl Psychol Meas 1977; 1:385–401

23. Friedberg F, Krupp LB. A comparison of cognitive behavioral treatment for chronic fatigue syndrome and primary depression. Clin Infect Dis 1994; 18(suppl 1):S105–110

24. Canadian MS Research Group. A randomized controlled trial of amantadine in fatigue associated with multiple sclerosis. Can J Neurol Sci 1987; 14:273–278

25. Rosenberg GA, Appenzeller O. Amantadine, fatigue, and multiple sclerosis. Arch Neurol 1989; 45:435–437

26. Krupp LB, Coyle PK, Doscher C, et al. Fatigue therapy in multiple sclerosis: Results of a double blind randomized parallel trial of amantadine pemoline and placebo. Neurology (in press).

27. Murray TS. Amantadine therapy for fatigue in multiple sclerosis. Can J Neurol Sci 1985; 12:251–254

28. Weinshenker BG, Penman M, Bass B. A double-blind, randomized, crossover trial of pemoline in fatigue associated with multiple sclerosis. Neurology 1992; 42:1468–1471

29. Cohen RA, Fisher M. Amantadine treatment of fatigue associated with multiple sclerosis. Arch Neurol 1989; 46:676–667

30. Lloyd AR, Hickie, MD, Brockman A, et al. Immunological and psychological therapy for patients with chronic fatigue syndrome: A double-blind placebo controlled trial. Amer J Med 1993; 94:197–203.

31. Krupp LB, Sliwinski M, Masur D, et al. Impact of fatigue treatment on cognitive functioning in MS. Ann Neurol 1993; 34:248

32. Krupp LB. Unpublished data

33. Hayslip B, Kennelly KJ, Maloy RM. Fatigue, depression and cognitive performance among aged persons. Exp Aging Res 1990; 16:111–115

34. NIH Consensus Development Panel on Depression in Late Life: Diagnosis and treatment of depression in late life. JAMA 1992; 268:1018–1024

35. Burke WJ, Nitcher RL, Roccaforte WH, Wengel SP. A prospective evaluation of the geriatric depression scale in an outpatient geriatric assessment center. J Amer Geriatr Soc 1992; 40:1227–1230

36. Berlly MH, Strauser WW, Hall KM. Fatigue in postpolio syndrome. Arch Phy Med Rehab 1991; 72:115–118

37. Chetwynd J, Botting C, Hogan D. Post polio syndrome in New Zealand: A survey of 700 polio survivors. New Zealand Med J 1993; 106:406–508

38. Friedman J, Friedman H. Fatigue in Parkinson's disease. Neurology 1993; 43:2016–2018

39. Van Hilten JJ, Weggeman M, Van der Velde EA, et al. Sleep, excessive daytime sleepiness, and fatigue in Parkinson's disease. J Neural Transmission 1993; 5:235–244

40. Cowell LC, Katz DI. Manuscript in preparation

41. Freal JE, Kraft GH, Coryell SK. Symptomatic fatigue in multiple sclerosis. Arch Phys Med Rehabil 1984; 65:135–138

42. Pepper C, Krupp LB, Friedberg F, et al. Comparison of psychiatric characteristics in chronic fatigue syndrome, multiple sclerosis, and depression. J Neuropsychiatry and Clin Neurosci 1993; 5:1–7

43. Monks J. Experiencing symptoms in chronic illness: Fatigue in multiple sclerosis. Int Disabil Stud 1989; 11:78–85

44. Schroeder D, Hill GH. Postoperative fatigue: A prospective physiological study of patients undergoing major abdominal surgery. Aust N J Surg 1991; 61:774–779

45. Schroeder D, Hill GL Predicting postoperative fatigue: Importance of preoperative fatigue. World J Surg 1993; 17:226–231

46. Krupp LB, LaRocca NC, Muir J, Steinberg AD. A study of fatigue in systemic lupus erythematosus. J Rheumatol 1990; 17:1450–1452

47. Katon WJ, Buchwald DS, Simon GE, et al. Psychiatric illness in patients with chronic fatigue and those with rheumatoid arthritis. J Gen Intern Med 1991; 6:277–285

48. Holmes GP, Kaplan JE, Gantz NM, et al. CFS: A working case definition. Ann Intern Med 1988; 108:387–389

49. Schluederberg A, Straus SE, Grufferman S (eds.). Considerations in the design of studies of CFS. Rev Infect Dis 1991; 13:S1–S140

50. Wood GC, Bentall RP, Gopfert M, Edwards RH. A comparative psychiatric assessment of patients with chronic fatigue syndrome and muscle disease. Psychol Med 1991; 21:619–628

51. Hickey I, Lloyd A, Wakefield D, Parker G. The psychiatric status of patients with CFS. Br J Psychiatry 1990; 156:534–540

52. Lane TJ, Manu P, Matthews DA. Depression and somatization in CFS. Am J Med 1991; 91:335–344

53. Manu P, Matthews DA, Lane TJ. Panic disorder among patients with chronic fatigue. South Med J 1991; 84:451–456

54. Whelton CL, Salit I, Moldofsky H. Sleep, EBV infection, musculoskeletal pain, and depressive symptoms in CFS. J Rheumatol 1992; 19:939–943

55. Taerk GS, Toner BB, Salif IE, et al. Depression in patients with neuromyasthenia (benign myalgic encephalomyelitis). Int J Psychiatry Med 1987; 17:49–56

56. Goldenberg DL, Simms RW, Geiger A, Komaroff AL. High frequency of fibromyalgia in patients with chronic fatigue seen in a primary care practice. Arthritis Rheum 1990; 33:381–387

57. Klonoff DC. Chronic fatigue syndrome. Clin Infec Dis 1992; 15:812–823

58. Cunha BA. Crimson crescents—a possible association with CFS [letter]. Ann Intern Med 1992; 116:347

59. Demitrack MA, Dale JK, Strass SE, et al. Evidence for impaired activation of the hypothalamic-pituitary-adrenal axis in patients with CFS. J Clin Endocrinol Metab 1991; 73:1224–1234

60. Buchwald D, Cheney PR, Peterson DL, et al. A chronic illness characterized by fatigue, neurologic and immunologic disorders, and active human depressions, type 6 infection. Ann Int Med 1992; 116:103–113

61. Shafran SD. Review: The CFS. Amer J Med 1991; 90:730–739

62. White P. Fatigue syndrome: Neurasthenia revived. Brit Med J 1989; 298:1199–1200

63. Holmes GP, Kaplan JE, Steward JA, et al. A cluster of patients with chronic mononucleosis-like symptoms. JAMA 1987; 257:2297–2302

64. Klimas NG, Salvato FR, Morgan R, Fletcher MA. Immunologic abnormalities in CFS. J Clin Microbiol 1991; 28:1403–1410

65. Levine PH, Jacobson S, Pocinki AG, et al. Clinical, epidemiologic, and virologic studies in 4 clusters of the CFS. Arch Intern Med 1992; 152:1611–1616

66. Leventhal LJ, Naides SJ, Freundlich B. Fibromyalgia and parvovirus infection. Arthritis Rheum 1991; 34:1319–1324

67. Bode L, Komaroff AL, Ludwig N. No serologic evidence of Borna disease virus in patients with CFS. Clin Infect Dis 1992; 15:1049

68. Dale JK, DiBisceglie AM, Hoofnagle JH, Straus SE. CFS: Lack of association with hepatitis C virus infections. J Med Virol 1991; 34:119–121

69. Komaroff AL, Wang SP, Lee J, Grayston JT. No association of chronic chlamydia pneumoniae infection with CFS. J Infect Dis 1992; 165:184

70. Chao CC, Janoff EN, Hu S, et al. Altered cytokine release in peripheral blood mononuclear cell cultures from patients with the CFS. Cytokine 1991; 3:292–298

71. Gupta S, Vayuvegula BA: Comprehensive immunological analysis in CFS. Scan J Immunol 1991; 33:319–327

72. Ho-Yen DO, Billington RW, Urquehart J: NK cells and the post viral fatigue syndrome. Scan J Infect Dis 1991; 23:711–716

73. Keller RH, Lane JL, Klimas N. Association between HLA class II antigens and the CFIDS. Clin Infect Dis 1994; 18:S154–S156

74. Linde A, Andersson B, Svenson SB, et al. Serum levels of lymphokines and soluble cellular receptors in primary EBV infection and in patients with CFS. J Infect Dis 1992; 165:994–1000

9

Sleep in the Elderly: Overview and Selected Disorders

Cynthia L. Comella
Rush-Presbyterian–St. Luke's Medical Center
Chicago, Illinois

I. INTRODUCTION

A. Overview of Sleep

Sleep occupies approximately one-third of adult life. Although the function of sleep is not understood, the inherent necessity for sleep is widely recognized and is present in all mammals. The notion that sleep is a time of rest and brain inactivity persisted until the 20th century when electrophysiologic techniques were applied to the study of sleep. Sleep was found to be a dynamic process, with the cyclic recurrence of different stages. The discovery of rapid eye movement (REM) sleep by Aserinsky and Kleitman in 1953 (1,2) was a major advance in sleep research, stimulating physiologic and clinical studies of sleep. During sleep, periods of REM alternate with periods of non-REM (NREM) at intervals of approximately 90 minutes. REM sleep is a period of heightened brain activity, autonomic activation, rapid eye movements, phasic muscle jerks, and mentation in the form of dreams. The anatomic and neurochemical substrates of REM sleep have been partially elucidated through experiments in animals (3–12). Several brainstem nuclei have been identified as playing a critical role in the generation of REM sleep. The tonic and phasic com-

Table 1 Sleep Stages Defined and Percent of Normal Sleep Time of Each Stage

	Electroencephalographic and clinical features	Normal percentage of sleep
Rapid eye movement (REM)	EEG: Low voltage, mixed frequency Autonomic activation Skeletal muscle atony Rapid eye movements	20–25%
Stage 1	Low arousal threshold Slow rolling eye movements EEG: Low voltage, mixed frequency	2–5%
Stage 2	Higher arousal threshold EEG: K complexes and sleep spindles	45–55%
Stage 3	High arousal threshold EEG: 20–50%, high voltage (>75 microvolts), slow waves (frequency <2 cycles per second)	3–8%
Stage 4	High arousal threshold EEG: 50% high voltage (≥75 microvolts), slow waves (frequency <2 cycles per second)	10–15%

Source: Reference 13.

ponents of REM may be mediated by different neuronal populations. Although acetylcholine is a major neurotransmitter involved in REM sleep, other neurochemicals also have a role.

Less is known about the anatomic substrate and neurochemistry of NREM sleep. NREM sleep is comprised of four stages. Stage 1 is the transition period from wakefulness to sleep with a slowing of electroencephalographic waveforms often accompanied by slow rolling eye movements; stage 2 is marked by the occurrence of K complexes and sleep spindles, and stages 3 and 4 are marked by epochs of synchronous delta waves, also called slow-wave sleep (Table 1) (13).

B. Overview of Sleep in the Elderly

Normal sleep in young adults is comprised of 75–80% NREM sleep, with the first third of the night predominantly slow-wave sleep; REM sleep is present for 20–25% of the total sleep time and predominates in the last third of the night. Nocturnal awakenings occupy less than 5% of the night (14). A variety of sleep disorders have been associated with aging (15–18). However, characterizing normal age-related sleep alterations is hampered by deciding on the definition of normal aging. Factors that may independently affect sleep tend to occur with increasing frequency as individuals age. These include medical problems, medications, urologic disturbances, menopause, depression, and changing social circumstances (retirement, loss of a spouse) (19–22). In addition, some sleep disorders are more common in the elderly.

Survey studies of communities in Great Britain and the United States have shown that older people are more likely to report short sleep times, longer sleep latencies, and more frequent nocturnal awakenings (23–27). There is an increase in the use of medications specifically for sleep in the elderly population, with many continuing to use medications for greater than a 1-year period (28). Bixler and his group found that sleep disorders, specifically insomnia, occurred in 40% of those over the age of 50 in the metropolitan Los Angeles area (29). Bliwise conducted a survey in Sunnyvale, California, and observed a much reduced prevalence of approximately 3–4% in the same age group. He attributed this low prevalence to the relatively healthy condition of the inhabitants included in his survey, speculating that perhaps age-related increases in sleep disturbance were the result of increased health problems (27).

In contrast, the survey study in two Iowa counties conducted by Habte-Gabr and associates found that in those over the age of 65, the total hours of sleep actually increased, but the percentage of elderly subjects who reported feeling rested in the morning decreased (30). Kripke reported a 6-year follow-up on their population and found that mortality appeared to be increased in those individuals who reported sleep durations less than 7 hours or greater than 7.9 hours. Those using sleeping medications were also subject to increased mortality (31).

In some survey studies, the proportion of women complaining of sleep disturbance was greater than the number of men (27,30). The use of sedative hypnotics has also been observed to be greater among older women (28).

The increasing recognition by physicians of the importance of sleep in elderly is shown by a recent survey of 45 geriatricians (10 with university affiliations). This survey showed that sleep was considered to be clinically important by 73% of physicians interviewed. Although recognized as important, only half of these physicians reported that they specifically asked their elderly patients about sleep, and only 13% had received any specific training in at least one educational course (32).

C. Sleep Assessment Techniques

The patient history and history from the bed partner provide vital information about the quality of sleep and daytime functioning. The interview should include the usual bedtime, final awakening time in the morning, number of arousals during the night and duration of these arousals, presence of snoring or observed respiratory pauses, restlessness and movements during sleep, presence and severity of daytime sleepiness, and occurrence of daytime naps. The frequency, dosage, and duration of sedative hypnotics, as well as current intake of other medications, is also important information (33).

In studies addressing the problem of sleep in the elderly, several techniques have been used. Some of the more frequently used methods are listed in Table 2, with the advantages and drawbacks for each method. Subjective measures include self-report questionnaires and sleep logs. Objective measures include actigraphy (34,35) and polysomnography.

Polysomnography (PSG) is a continuous recording of sleep throughout the night, with the ability to monitor electro-encephalography, eye movements, respiratory and cardiac changes, blood oxygen saturation, and muscle activation. PSG is considered to be the optimal technique to objectively evaluate sleep. The terminology to describe sleep architecture measured by PSG is presented in Table 3. Although considered the gold standard for evaluating sleep, the difficulties encountered in staying the night in the sleep laboratory, especially for the older or demented patient, may limit the usefulness of this technique. The development of home monitoring techniques may provide additional ways to evaluate sleep, without the necessity of laboratory monitoring (36,37).

Comparing the PSG findings across age groups is hampered by the changes in waking electroencephalographic waveforms accompanying normal aging. Changes in alpha rhythm, a reduction of slow activity with augmentation of faster rhythms, most prominent in the temporal lobes have been described (38). During sleep, there may be additional age-related alterations. Stage 2 sleep is determined by the presence of sleep spindles and K complexes. With normal aging, there may be a normal reduction in the number and frequency of sleep spindles. This reduction does not appear to correlate with cognitive changes, but has been negatively correlated with sulcal enlargement on brain imaging (39,40). Changes in slow-wave sleep have also been observed. In order to define a stage of sleep as stage 3 or 4, the presence of delta waves with an amplitude of 75 microvolts or higher is required. In the elderly, there is a marked reduction in the amplitude of delta waves (41–44). Webb proposed that in PSG evaluations of the elderly, the amplitude criteria should be eliminated (45). Using this modified scoring technique, he found that the amount of slow-wave sleep in a group of 40 subjects aged 50–60 years did not differ from younger subjects (46). Ehlers and Kupfer, however, reported that using power spectral analysis, there was a reduction of delta activ-

Table 2 Techniques Used to Evaluate Sleep

Technique	Description	Advantages	Disadvantages
Sleep logs or diaries	A continuous subjective documentation of sleep and wake time over consecutive 24-hour periods usually for 2 weeks	Monitor long periods of time Do at home 24-hour record Inexpensive	Subjective report Not accurate in cognitively impaired Only allows self-report of sleep–wake
Sleep questionnaire	Different types: a subjective interview concerning sleep amount, quality, and daytime functioning	Monitor the desirable period of time Overall assessment of sleep Deals with quality as well as quantity of sleep Inexpensive	Subjective report Not accurate in cognitively impaired Not sensitive to day-to-day changes

Actigraphy	A computerized, objective record of activity over consecutive 24-hour periods	Convenient as a wristband Objectively records activity Correlates with sleep logs	Not validated in many elderly groups May over- or underestimate sleep time Cannot stage sleep or indicate respiratory function
Polysomnography	Recording of electroencephalography, eye movements, respiratory function, electromyography, electrocardiography, and other selected parameters during sleep	Objective assessment Complete sleep staging and other objective measures possible Necessary to diagnose some disorders and assess severity	Changes due to laboratory environment (may need adaptation night) Inconvenient Expensive

Source: References 33–37.

Table 3 Sleep Polysomnographic Measures Defined

Total time in bed (TBT)	Time from settling into bed until cessation of study in morning
Total sleep time (TST)	Time from sleep onset to final morning awakening minus wake time during the night
Wake time after sleep onset (WASO)	Time awake after initial sleep onset until final morning awakening
Sleep latency (SL)	Time from settling into bed until sleep onset
Sleep efficiency (SE)	Total sleep time divided by the sum of wake time after sleep onset plus total sleep time
Non-REM sleep (NREM)	Nonrapid eye movement sleep; conventionally divided into four stages
NREM sleep (percent)	Time in non-REM sleep divided by total sleep time
REM sleep (REM)	Rapid eye movement sleep
REM sleep (percent)	Time in REM sleep divided by total sleep time
REM latency	Time from sleep onset to first REM period
Stage shifts	Number of times sleep changes from one stage to another, or to arousal
Apnea Index	Number of apneic episodes occurring in 1 hour of sleep ($\geq$5 designated as abnormal)
Apnea/ Hypopnea Index (AHI)	Number of apnea and hypopneas occurring in 1 hour of sleep
Movement Index (MI)	Number of movements per 1 hour of sleep ($\geq$5 designated as abnormal)

ity and a shift toward higher frequencies regardless of amplitude criteria (47).

This chapter will first summarize changes in sleep that have been described with normal aging. The second part of the chapter will review disorder of sleep associated with aging, focusing on the clinical features.

II. SLEEP IN THE NORMAL ELDERLY

A. Cross-Sectional Studies of Sleep in the Elderly

Sleep patterns observed in normal, healthy elderly subjects have been summarized comprehensively in a recent review by Bliwise (48). The characterization of age-related changes in sleep is complex and is influenced by numerous factors, including gender, concomitant medical problems, neurologic and psychologic status, exposure to daylight, and social issues. The elderly are not a homogeneous population, and the definition of normal aging may be problematic (49).

Defining the changes that occur with normal aging has largely depended on cross-sectional studies comparing groups of young subjects to elderly subjects. A listing of selected cross-sectional studies is presented in Table 4 (42,50–54). Longitudinal studies evaluating the same group of subjects from youth to old age would be the ideal method to define when these changes occur, the rapidity of the changes, and the risk factors for development of clinically significant sleep disturbances. This type of study, however, is not possible. Longitudinal studies in older individuals over a 2- to 15-year time span have been done and will be described below.

Differences in subjective sleep reported between the young and the old show that the elderly may have the same amount of sleep over a 24-hour period as younger counterparts, but sleep in the elderly tends to be distributed across a 24-hour period with shorter nocturnal sleep, frequent awakenings during the night (29), and increased frequency of daytime napping (25,55,56). It was thought that this redistribution of sleep across the day arose from irregularities of lifestyle due to lack of a work schedule and organized daytime activities. Monk and colleagues tested this hypothesis by comparing the social rhythm metric in 42 elderly subjects with

Table 4 Cross-Sectional Studies Evaluating Polysomnographic Features of Sleep in the Elderly

Study	Ages compared and number of subjects	Differences in elderly
Feinberg (1967) (42)	Young (N = 15) (Ages 19–36) Aged (N = 15) (Ages 65–96)	Reduced sleep efficiency Reduction in sleep spindles Reduction in slow-wave sleep
Feinberg (1974) (50)	5 age groupings (N = 105) (Ages 4–96)	Reduced slow-wave sleep Increased nocturnal arousals Shortened first NREM-REM cycle with more prolonged first REM
Hayashi (1982) (51)	Young (N = 13) (Ages 19–22) Aged (N = 15) (Ages 73–92)	Increase in percentage of nocturnal wake time Increase in stage 1 Reduced percent of REM Prolonged first REM episode

Webb (1982) (52)	Young (Ages 19–31) Aged (Ages 50–60)	Increase in number of nocturnal awakenings, men greater than women No change in slow-wave sleep using reduced-amplitude criteria No change in REM sleep
Reynolds (1985) (53)	Ages 60–70 vs. Ages 70–80 ($N = 40$)	Older men with less slow-wave sleep (preservation of slow-wave sleep in women) Increase in nocturnal arousals Longer first REM with equal distribution over the night
Reynolds (1991) (54)	Age groupings into 3: 1. 62–69 ($N = 28$) 2. 70–79 ($N = 43$) 3. 80–91 ($N = 27$)	Stable REM sleep across groups With aging, greater sleep fragmentation with better preservation of slow-wave sleep in women

21 young controls. They found that older individuals in fact had a greater regularity in daily lifestyle than did younger individuals (57). In a series of related studies, they observed that the sleep schedule in the elderly group was inflexible compared to the young adult (58). When removed from environmental day/night cues, in the "free running" situation, the elderly spent more time in bed but slept less efficiently. They did, however, demonstrate an overall improvement in alertness (59). Hoch and colleagues demonstrated that nuns with restricted sleep periods slept better than age-matched women (60). Taken together, these observations suggest that inherent circadian rhythms are not as strongly set in the elderly, but that regular schedules and habitual sleep periods may improve sleep. Other factors, besides circadian factors, also may contribute to sleep fragmentation. Zepelin and colleagues found that the elderly have a reduced threshold for auditory awakening, leading to arousals from less intense stimulus (61).

Buysse and colleagues evaluated subjective sleep in 44 healthy individuals over the age of 80 years compared to 35 young adults between the ages of 20 and 30 (62). They used the Pittsburgh Sleep Quality Index (PSQI), a questionnaire that evaluates seven different components: subjective sleep quality, sleep latency, sleep duration, habitual sleep efficiency, sleep disturbance, use of sleeping medication, and daytime dysfunction. By adding up these individual components, a global score is obtained, with higher scores reflecting worse overall sleep quality (63). Their study showed that 97.1% of the young group compared to 68.1% of the elderly group were classified by PSQI as "good" sleepers. They found that the PSQI scores were higher for the elderly than the young, with significant age effects noted for subjective sleep quality, sleep duration, habitual sleep efficiency, and sleep disturbances. Polysomnographic features of the two groups were also compared, and showed that elderly subjects had significantly reduced sleep efficiency with frequent arousals, increases in stage 1 and 2 sleep with reductions in stages 3 and 4, and REM sleep. In addition, the elderly subjects had more apneas and hypopneas per hour and an increase in periodic limb movements during sleep. Correlation of the subjective questionnaire responses to objective PSG findings indicated that subjective and objective measures did not differ for sleep latency, but sleep duration and efficiency were overestimated subjectively in both groups. Global PSQI scores did not correlate with any PSG measure in the elderly, although several correlations were found for the young subjects.

Using a different method of subjective sleep assessment, Hoch and associates (64) found a greater degree of correlation between subjective and objective sleep evaluations. They compared subjective reports of sleep and objective polysomnographic records of sleep in healthy elderly. Included in their study were 10 men and 10 women between the ages of 59 and 79. Self-report of sleep was obtained through 14-day sleep–wake logs and postsleep questionnaires. Polysomnograms were obtained on three consecutive nights. Comparisons were made between men and women and between the objective and subjective measures. Overall, these investigators found that women had significantly greater amounts and percentages of slow-wave sleep than did men (73 min and 20% vs. 31 min and 8.5%) There were no significant sleep-related respiratory disturbances in their study group. Comparing subjective to objective measures, subjective estimates of sleep latency and total sleep time correlated in both men and women. Overall, women were more accurate in their self-report as correlated with polysomnographic findings. Men additionally had a significant correlation between percent of stage 1 and subjective restlessness during sleep. In women, there were more subjective/objective correlations, including subjective restlessness and nocturnal arousals and the wake time after sleep onset; and the perceived soundness of sleep with PSG-measured delta sleep. Overall, women showed a higher proportion of significant and stable correlations between subjective and objective measures. Neither men nor women had good correlations of any subjective sleep measure with PSG-defined REM sleep.

Other studies have described differences in sleep related to gender. Reynolds and his colleagues (53) evaluated polysomnography in 40 healthy seniors living in the community. He compared polysomnographic features of elderly women and men. He found that older men had more difficulty maintaining sleep with less stage 3 and an increase in number of awakenings compared to women. With advancing age, women have better preservation of slow-wave sleep than men, although from the seventh to the ninth decade, women have reductions in sleep maintenance not observed in men (65).

A meta-analysis of 27 studies evaluating gender differences in people over the age of 58 showed that men tended to have more objective changes from the patterns of youthful sleep than older women, but that these changes were not pronounced (66). Although REM sleep has been found to be preserved in most studies, the distribution of REM sleep across the night changes with aging. In young adults, there is a progressive lengthening of REM periods; the elderly tend to have an equal temporal distribution of REM (51,67).

B. Longitudinal Studies of Sleep in the Elderly

Only a few studies have evaluated changes in sleep over time in the same group (Table 5). Bliwise and associates reported that in their 25 elderly subjects evaluated twice, separated by 4–7 years, there was a reduction in slow-wave sleep and an increase in sleep apneas and hypopneas without any change in the occurrence of periodic limb movements (68).

Hoch and colleagues (69) evaluated the PSG features of 19 healthy seniors aged 60–82 after an average of 2.2 years (range 12.5–56.6 months) and found that most EEG sleep parameters were stable, including the extent of sleep apnea and periodic limb movements. There was an increase in the number of arousals lasting greater than 30 seconds and the phasic components of REM sleep increased in the 9 men while decreasing in the 10 women. The subjective assessment of sleep quality as measured by a postsleep evaluation questionnaire also remained stable in this group of subjects over the

Table 5 Selected Longitudinal Studies in Elderly Subjects Using Polysomnography

Study	Number of patients	Years of follow-up	Findings
Webb (1982) (71)	5	15 years	Increase in slow-wave sleep using reduced-amplitude criteria for scoring
Hoch (1988) (69)	19 (ages 60–82)	2.2 years	Stable except for increase in number of nocturnal arousals
Bliwise (1989) (68)	25	4–7 years	Increase in respiratory events Reduction in slow-wave sleep
Phoha (1990) (70)	11 (ages 60–72)	3 years	Slight worsening of respiratory events Increase in nocturnal arousals Stable amounts of slow-wave sleep and periodic limb movements
Hoch (1994) (72)	27 "young" old (60–74 years) 23 "old" old (>75 years)	2 years	Most measures stable Slight reduction in sleep efficiency with age, mental status, and medical burden as risks

2-year period, with the men rating their sleep quality as better than their women counterparts at both evaluation points.

Phoha and associates reported their findings in 11 healthy community residents aged 60–72 years following 3 years (range 34–38 months) (70). Their subjects were selected for the low initial movement index (MI) and respiratory disturbance index (RDI), which is a measure of the number of respiratory events per hour of sleep. After 3 years, there was little change in sleep pattern except that the number of stage changes increased. In particular, they observed no change in slow-wave sleep or REM sleep. They also found no change in the occurrence of periodic limb movements. There was, however, a small but significant increase in apneas and hypopneas with the RDI increasing from 3.4 to 5.5 and maximum oxygen desaturation increasing from 3% to 5%. This increase in apnea and hypopnea was not associated with an increase in body weight.

Webb (71), using his modified amplitude criteria for scoring slow-wave sleep (45), observed that slow-wave sleep increased in his group of 5 patients evaluated initially in their 50s following 15 years. His findings are otherwise similar to other studies, demonstrating a sharp increase in the number and duration of nocturnal arousals and a fragmentation of REM sleep, with a greater number of REM periods but of shorter duration such that the overall REM time did not change significantly.

Recently, Hoch and associates studied two groups of subjects at yearly intervals for 2 years. The first group was the "old old," comprised of 23 people older than 75. The second group was the "young old," comprised of 27 individuals aged 60–74. They found that PSG measures were quite stable over the observation period, with the exception of a decline in sleep efficiency in the "old old" group. REM sleep percent was the only sleep architecture component that differed between the two groups, being reduced in the "old old" but stable over the study period. Self-report of sleep as measured by sleep logs was stable. Sleep quality as measured by the PSQI declined over the 2-year period and was predicted by an increase in medical problems and a deterioration in cognitive status (72).

C. Effect on Daytime Functioning and Daytime Sleepiness

The clinical impact of these changes in sleep in normal aged individuals has not been established. One of the major functions of a good night's sleep is to allow for alertness, good functioning, and lack of sleepiness the following day. Carskadon and associates found that daytime sleepiness as measured by the multiple sleep latency test (MSLT) did not correlate with total sleep time or a specific sleep stage determined by polysomnography in their group of 24 elderly subjects, but significantly correlated with measures of sleep fragmentation and sleep-related respiratory events (73).

To determine whether the elderly are more susceptible to daytime dysfunction from disrupted nocturnal sleep, Hoch and associates compared elderly to young adults following a 36–40-hour sleep deprivation period and subsequent recovery. They found that the elderly had decrements in performance on all measures regardless of condition; however, the elderly were not sleepier than young adults following sleep deprivation and the degree of daytime sleepiness did not correlate with performance or vigilance measures (74).

Similar results were reported by Bonnet. He evaluated 12 normal elderly and 12 young adults following 2 nights of artificially interrupted sleep at approximately 14 times per hour. He found that both groups deteriorated on morning tests of performance, reaction times, and vigilance, and had an increase in morning sleepiness. The older subjects, however, tended to have less deterioration on morning tests and tolerated the sleep disturbances better than the young adults (75).

In a similar comparison of young and old subjects, Reynolds found that young adults were sleepier than an elderly group following a night of sleep deprivation. The young group, however, tended to recover more quickly than the older group, who still had residual sleepiness 2 days following the sleep loss (76).

III. SELECTED DISORDERS OF SLEEP IN THE ELDERLY

A. Sleep in Parkinson's Disease

Parkinson's disease is a chronic, progressive neurologic disorder estimated to affect 200 per 100,000 people in the United States (77). The clinical diagnosis of Parkinson's disease is based on the findings of tremor, rigidity, bradykinesia or akinesia, and in more advanced disease, postural reflex impairment (78). Associated with these motor signs, there are numerous subjective complaints including stiffness, pain, difficulty with fine motor movements, and balance impairment. Sleep disturbance related to Parkinson's disease can arise from different mechanisms. Some of the frequently occurring causes are listed in Table 6.

Sleep disturbance is a common complaint of patients with Parkinson's disease. A survey study in the United Kingdom of 220 patients with Parkinson's disease found that 215 of those interviewed reported nocturnal sleep disruption. In the survey group, 75% reported sleep latency of less than 1 hour,

Table 6 Sleep Disturbances in Parkinson's Disease

Due to Parkinson symptoms	Fragmentation due to tremor, stiffness, rigidity, pain, difficulty turning over in bed
Due to medications	Sleep fragmentation, nightmares, hallucinations, insomnia, daytime sleepiness
Due to associated conditions	Depression
	Dementia
May be associated	Sleep apnea, REM sleep behavior disorder

with a mean latency of 26 minutes. However, 76% noted that their sleep was disrupted during the night by frequent awak-enings. The most frequent disturbance during the night was the need to urinate, with 80% reporting at least two nightly visits to the bathroom, and 33% getting up at least three times per night. The most frequent motor symptom experienced during the night was the inability to turn over in bed. Pain-ful leg cramps associated with Parkinson's disease occurred during the night in 55 percent of the patients. The nocturnal occurrence of tremor and foot dystonia were also common complaints (79). The high prevalence of sleep disturbance associated with PD has been found by others (80).

1. *Sleep in untreated Parkinson's disease*

The survey studies cited above evaluated a heterogeneous group of PD patients. In contrast, a survey of a relatively homogeneous group of nondepressed, nondemented, untreated mild Parkinson's disease showed that in the earlier disease stages sleep quality may not differ form age-matched spouse controls (81). This survey observation was supported by Ferini-Strambi and associates who conducted 2 nights of poly-somnography in 26 untreated, mild-stage PD patients and age-matched healthy controls. Objective sleep measures showed that except for a prolonged sleep latency, there were no other differences between the two groups for any of the sleep pa-rameters measured except that PD patients did demonstrate some defective cardiac autonomic activity during sleep (82).

Sleep studies in more advanced, untreated PD demon-strate that there are a number of sleep abnormalities associ-ated with the disease. PD patients are reported to have less total sleep time than normal elderly controls, reductions in stages 3 and 4 sleep, and frequent nocturnal arousals (83–86). REM (rapid eye movement) measures have not been consis-tent. Some investigators report that the total duration of REM sleep was decreased (83,84,86), although the percentage of REM time may not be different than that of controls (83). In addition, many untreated PD patients are found to have ab-normal movements during sleep, including increased blinking, blepharospasm, and tremor. These movements can occur during any sleep stage (84,87), but are more common in the lighter stages of sleep. A third feature of sleep in untreated PD may be an increased occurrence of episodes of central and obstructive sleep apnea (88). This observation is not consistent (89). It appears that in PD patients receiving no drug treatment at all, there are sleep disturbances that relate to the disease process itself.

2. The effect of dopaminergic therapy on sleep in Parkinson's disease

With advancing PD, however, the number of factors that may affect sleep increases. These include depression, pain (90,91), dementia, worsening motoric function, and a variety of anti-Parkinson medications.

A recent study evaluating continuous electronic activity monitoring in 89 PD patients showed that compared to normal controls, PD patients had higher levels of activity during the night, reflecting more severe sleep disruption. Of the mild to moderate PD patients studied, the use of levodopa or a direct dopamine agonist best predicted increased nocturnal activity (92). Similar findings of increased activity with levodopa were described using a different activity monitoring technique, although in this study there were fewer movements measured in bed during sleep than seen in the non-Parkinson controls (93).

In contrast, some investigators have observed improvements in sleep following levodopa initiation. Askenasy and colleagues evaluated sleep in 5 PD patients using polysomnography. Baseline studies were conducted following withdrawal from anti-Parkinson medications. Follow-up studies were obtained after the reinstitution of anti-Parkinson agents. These authors found that levodopa improved sleep efficiency and normalized muscle activity. (85). Improved sleep has also been observed with the use of sustained-release levodopa preparations, which treat parkinsonian symptoms during the night. Long-acting preparations have been observed to improve nocturnal akinesia, tremor, and rigidity (94), and to increase sleep efficiency, with a reduction in sleep fragmentation (95). In some patients receiving the long-acting preparations, beneficial effects were still apparent the following morning (96,97).

Although in some PD patients nocturnal use of levodopa may improve sleep, the effect of chronic dopaminergic treatment on sleep architecture may offset this initial benefit. Parenteral infusions of dopaminergic agents have been shown to delay the onset of REM sleep, or acutely inhibit an ongoing REM period (98,99). With chronic dopaminergic treatment, some investigators observe that there continues to be a suppression of REM sleep, and that the discontinuation of dopaminergic therapy resulted in REM rebound lasting up to 10 days in some patients (100). Others report that in the period immediately following the initiation of levodopa, there is a suppression of REM that resolves to baseline levels with chronic treatment (83,101). And yet another group reports that REM time actually increases with prolonged therapy (102). The apparently contradictory reports of the effect of chronic levodopa on sleep may be due to differences in methods. In some studies, there was no control of concomitant drug therapy, including hypnosedatives or anticholinergic drugs (100,102). Other studies included patients who had thalamotomies for PD in the past (83). In many reports, the clinical staging of the patients and their motoric response to dopaminergic agents is not indicated.

3. *Sleep disturbance–hallucination syndrome in PD*
   patients on chronic dopaminergic therapy

As many as 33% of PD patients treated chronically with dopaminergic agents develop dopaminergic drug-induced visual hallucinations (103). Factors reported to be associated with the occurrence of hallucinations include duration of levodopa therapy, presence of dementia, use of anticholinergic drugs or amantadine, age of PD onset, PD duration, and abnormal MMPI (Minnesota Multiphasic Personality Inventory) scores

(103–110). Nausieda and associates observed that PD patients with dopaminergic-induced hallucinations had preexisting sleep complaints, in particular, awakenings during the night (111). These investigators postulated that sleep disturbance and hallucinations were on a continuum, with sleep disruption as the initial event (106,111).

A single report of quantitative sleep studies in PD patients with dysphoric dreams demonstrated an absence of K complexes and sleep spindles with no specific architectural abnormalities. There was a variable suppression of REM (112). In a subsequent study of 5 hallucinating and 5 nonhallucinating PD patients, matched for severity of PD and dosages of anti-Parkinson medications, polysomnographic comparisons showed that hallucinations were associated with a reduced sleep efficiency and a marked reduction in REM sleep (113).

4.   *Sleep benefit in Parkinson's disease*

The above sections have dealt with the effect of PD and anti-Parkinson medications on sleep. Conversely, the effect of sleep on PD has been studied. Sleep benefit in Parkinson's disease describes a clinical phenomenon in which symptoms of Parkinson's disease, following sleep, are improved before any medication doses. Factor and colleagues found that 43.6% of the 78 PD patients interviewed thought that the morning was the "best time of day" for motor performance. The morning-better patients had a shorter duration of disease (114). Clark and Feinstein described sleep benefit in 6 patients, with a follow-up evaluation in one showing a reduction in the duration of morning benefit with progression of PD (115). We have recently completed a questionnaire study of 117 PD patients and found that 25% experience sleep benefit, lasting 2–3 hours after nocturnal sleep. The duration of sleep benefit correlated with reported duration of improvement following a single dose of levodopa and was more frequent in milder PD taking less anti-Parkinson medications (116). These observations taken together suggest that sleep may improve symptoms of PD, although the mechanism remains to be elucidated.

5. *REM sleep behavior disorder in PD*

Rapid eye movement sleep has several features distinguishing it from the other sleep stages, including cortical desynchronization, hippocampal theta activity, ponto-geniculo-occipital spikes, rapid eye movements, phasic muscle twitches, cardiorespiratory alterations, and skeletal muscle atonia. The anatomic areas underlying the generation of REM sleep are localized to brainstem nuclei (117,118). These pontine nuclei, including the pedunculopontine tegmental nucleus and lateral-dorsal tegmental nucleus, are active predominantly during REM sleep and project to the nucleus magnocellularis in the rostral and the paramedian reticular nucleus in the caudal medulla. The activation of these medullary nuclei, in turn, results in the loss of muscle tone during REM sleep. In cats, lesions of pontine nuclei have resulted in REM sleep without muscle atonia, the extent of the lesion determining the behavioral pattern observed in these animals (119).

The loss of normal muscle atonia during REM sleep in humans was recently described by Schenk and his colleagues (120,121). These investigators described the occurrence of purposeful behaviors, such as kicking, hitting, and jumping out of bed, during REM sleep. This parasomnia was called REM sleep behavior disorder (RBD). RBD may be associated with other neurologic disorders. In the largest series of 70 patients with RBD, Schenk and Mahowald found that 37.5% had associated neurologic disorders, including dementia, narcolepsy, vascular disease, multiple sclerosis, and brainstem astrocytoma. Parkinsonian syndromes, including olivopontocerebellar degeneration, were found in 8.5% of their patients (122). Silber and Ahlskog described REM sleep behavior disorder in 5 patients with parkinsonian syndromes: one with multisystem degeneration, one following thalamotomy, and 3 with associated dementia (123). Subsequently, these same investigators reported that symptoms of RBD precede onset of PD symptoms in 27% and antedate levodopa used in 45% (124). We have observed RBD in 50% of 8 treated PD patients and found that the occurrence of RBD may relate to the severity and duration of PD (125).

Pathologic studies in moderate to severe PD have shown a 40% reduction of cholinergic neurons and Lewy body formation in the pedunculopontine tegmental nucleus (126). Taken together these observations suggest that certain REM abnormalities may reflect anatomic subcategories of PD.

B. Sleep in Dementia

The sleep disturbances associated with dementia have recently been comprehensively reviewed by Bliwise (48,127). The changes that have been described involve both disturbances in sleep–wake cycle and changes in sleep architecture as measured polysomnographically. Selected studies comparing sleep in Alzheimer's disease to age-matched normal controls are summarized in Table 7 (41,128–136). The findings of most, but not all (132), of these studies indicate that sleep in AD is marked by increased sleep fragmentation, with frequent nocturnal arousals. This may be offset by increased tendency toward daytime napping such that the total time asleep over a 24-hour period may be the same as in nondemented controls (127,136).

The loss of diurnal sleep–wake patterns may not be apparent in mild AD (137), and may be more pronounced in multi-infarct dementia. Using actigraphy, Aharon-Peretz and associates observed that mild to moderate AD patients did not differ in sleep–wake cycles from normal controls (137). Vitiello and colleagues found that patients with severe AD had sleep periods throughout a 24-hour day, with loss of the normal diurnal patterns of sleep–wake (136). This has also been demonstrated in behavioral studies assessing sleep patterns over 24 hours for 14 consecutive days (138), and using other techniques of body movement monitoring (139–141). The loss of circadian rhythms has been ascribed to both anatomic changes in AD as well as to reductions in exposure to light and regular daily activities.

Anatomically, several nuclei involved in the generation of sleep have been shown to be affected by AD. The suprachiasmatic nucleus is a nucleus thought to have a major role in circadian rhythmicity. This nucleus is profoundly affected by degenerative processes in AD (142–145). Neurofibrillary tangles have been described in the brainstem reticular formation, nucleus dorsalis raphe, and nucleus magnocellularis (146, 147). The pedunculopontine nucleus is involved in the generation of REM sleep. Microscopic examination of the PPN in AD patients has shown loss of cholinergic neurons with neurofibrillary tangles in some of the remaining cells (148, 149).

Environmental clues for regular sleep–wake patterns are also found to be disrupted in AD. AD patients have a significantly reduced exposure to light (150,151), which has been associated with sleep disturbance and behavioral aberrations, including agitation and "sundowning" (151). Administration of bright light in the morning for 2 hours improved nocturnal sleep and behavioral disturbances in two studies, suggesting that the sleep–wake cycles of some AD patients could be reset (152,153). Okawa and colleagues also found that demented patients did not have stable circadian rhythms (154). They reported that enforcement of regular daytime activities could improve day–night sleep–wake cycles in 30% of their patients.

Polysomnographic studies of sleep architecture in AD have shown that in addition to sleep fragmentation, features that characterize sleep in AD include alterations of NREM sleep. In most, but not all (132), studies there is a reduction in stages 3 and 4 sleep (41,127–129,131,134). The loss of slow-wave sleep has been observed in cross-sectional studies to be most profound in those with the greatest severity of cognitive impairment (127,128,136). Stage 2 NREM sleep is also affected, with reductions in spindle formation and K complexes (132,134).

Alterations in REM sleep have been variable. Bliwise and colleagues described one AD patient with abundant REM

Table 7 Selected Studies of Sleep in Alzheimer's Disease

Study	Patient number	Findings
Feinberg (1967) (41)	Young $N = 15$ Aged normal $N = 15$ Chronic brain syndrome $N = 15$	CBS had longest sleep latency, reduced sleep efficiency, lowest percent of REM sleep, with shortened REM periods, less stage 4.
Prinz (1982) (128)	Aged controls $N = 11$ Advanced AD $N = 10$	Decreased REM, decreased slow-wave sleep, increased sleep fragmentation, loss of sleep–wake cycle but no difference in sleep over 24 hours
Prinz (1982) (129)	Aged controls $N = 22$ Mild AD $N = 18$ Moderate AD $N = 16$ Severe AD $N = 10$	Appreciable changes even in mild AD Decreased slow-wave sleep correlating with AD severity Reduced REM% and increased WASO in moderate and severe
Loewenstein (1982) (130)	Aged controls $N = 8$ Mild to moderate AD $N = 9$	Reduction in slow-wave sleep No change in REM measures Trend toward reduced sleep efficiency

Vitiello (1984) (131)	Controls $N = 9$ Dementia $N = 9$ of each Mild moderate, severe	Measured REM only Moderate to severe AD with reduced REM and longer REM latency No changes in mild AD from controls
Martin (1986) (132)	Controls $N = 9$ Mild to moderate dementia $N = 8$	Less delta with trend to shortened REM latency
Allen (1987) (133)	Controls $N = 14$ Severely demented $N = 30$	50% reduction in REM sleep in stage 2 No differences in slow-wave sleep or circadian rhythms
Bliwise (1989) (134)	Mild dementia $N = 28$	No difference in REM latency
Vitiello (1990) (135)	Controls $N = 45$ Mild dementia $N = 44$	Shortened REM latency Increased WASO Decreased slow-wave sleep complexes in spindles and K

sleep, who was found to have neuritic plaques in the periaqueductal gray matter and dorsal raphe nucleus (155). Other studies, however, have shown variable reductions in REM sleep (127,132,136), or no change from controls (129). Vitiello and associates evaluated 9 patients in each category of mild, moderate, and severe AD and normal controls and found that in mild AD REM sleep changes may be minimal, and it is only with advancing disease that changes occur. (130).

The changes in sleep described in AD are not specific. Similar abnormalities have been described in other degenerative neurologic disorders, including PD as described above. Longitudinal studies are necessary to further clarify the progression of the sleep disturbance in AD and to define the associated factors.

C. Sleep Apnea in the Elderly

Obstructive sleep apnea is defined by the International Classification of Sleep Disorders as "repetitive episodes of upper airway obstruction that occur during sleep, usually associated with a reduction in blood oxygen saturation." The same manual defines central sleep apnea as a "cessation or decrease of ventilatory effort during sleep usually associated with oxygen desaturation" (156).

In most studies, the frequency of sleep apnea and hypopnea is observed to increase with advancing age (157, 158). Krieger and associates compared 20 young adults to 20 healthy elderly and found that older subjects had a decreased minute ventilation during sleep and a greater degree of hypopnea and apnea (158). Similar findings were reported by other investigators. One of the largest studies of sleep-related respiratory disturbances in the elderly was conducted by Ancoli-Israel and colleagues (159). These investigators found that 24% of elderly subjects had more than 5 apneas per hour. If hypopneas are included, 81% of the elderly subjects had an index greater than 5 and 18% had an index greater than 50.

The determination of the clinical importance of respiratory disturbances during sleep had been addressed in several studies. The impact of a mild to moderate increase in respiratory disturbance index on daytime functioning appears to be minimal (160–162). However, Berry and associates reported that even mild respiratory disturbances may be associated with increased blood pressure and irregular heartbeats (163). Dickel and Mosko suggest that the best measure of the severity of sleep apnea is nocturnal oxygen desaturation and duration of the apneic events rather than the number of events per hour (164). Hoch and associates reported an increasing number of respiratory events across three decades of elderly (the 7th, 8th, and 9th decades). These events were predominantly central apnea with obstructive and mixed types also increased. There was also an increase in oxygen desaturation in the older group (165). Naifeh and colleagues, however, found that despite an increase in respiratory events, their older population did not have significant changes in the degree of oxygen desaturation, although their study included a fewer number of subjects (157).

As observed in the middle-aged population (166), most studies have observed that men tend to have more sleep-related respiratory disturbances than women (167). This has been attributed to an increase in supraglottic resistance in men, which rises further with advancing age (168). Postmenopausal women, however, appear to have greater respiratory disturbances than premenopausal women, suggesting a beneficial effect from hormonal factors (169). Older men with a diagnosis of Alzheimer's disease have been observed to have the highest degree of respiratory disturbances (165,170). Cross-sectional studies have shown that the RDI increases over successive decades. Longitudinal studies over a 4.6-year period in a group of elderly adults did not show significant changes in respiratory parameters (171), suggesting that the changes with aging are gradual. Factors that have predicted the presence of significant sleep apnea in addition to advancing age include increased body mass, reports of nocturnal respiratory pauses, daytime sleepiness, and restlessness with nocturnal wandering (159). Some researchers have found that there is a positive correlation between the severity of the respiratory disturbance and the severity of dementia (172).

The presence of sleep apnea may predict an increased mortality in the aged population. Bliwise and associates prospectively evaluated 198 patients 12 years following polysomnography and found that sleep apnea was marginally related to mortality (173). Ancoli-Israel, however, found that in women there was a strong association between mortality and abnormal nocturnal breathing (174), particularly if the respiratory disturbance index was greater than 50. Longitudinal population studies are needed to clarify the adverse influence of sleep-disordered breathing on health in the elderly.

There are now effective treatments available for clinically significant sleep apnea. Accurate diagnosis requires nocturnal monitoring of respiratory function. Although only a single night of evaluation may be required (175,176) in milder cases, variability in the occurrence of respiratory events may necessitate further monitoring nights (175,176). Advances in home respiratory monitoring may provide easier access and more convenient methods to evaluate sleep apnea.

D. Periodic Limb Movement Disorder (PLMD)

1. *Clinical features*

The term *nocturnal myoclonus* was used by Charles Symonds in 1953 to describe a heterogeneous group of movements occurring during sleep (177). Included in his original description were hypnic jerks, which are sudden myoclonic jerks involving the whole body, usually occurring at sleep onset. Hypnic jerks are now recognized as normal phenomena, distinct from another syndrome included in his report, now called periodic movements in sleep (PLMD).

Polysomnographic examinations are pivotal in defining PLMD, a syndrome of characteristic leg movements occurring mostly during stage 2 sleep. The movements are repetitive and periodic, characterized by a dorsiflexion of the big toe and foot with flexion of the leg at the knee and hip. An individual movement usually lasts between 1.5 and 2.5 seconds. The interval between movements is about 30 seconds. The movements cluster into episodes lasting several minutes to hours at a time (178).

Unless severe, PLMD is asymptomatic. The history is obtained through interview with the spouse, who will complain of being kicked by the patient during the night. In fact, the contribution of PLMD to sleep disturbance is unclear. Polysomnographic studies in 200 insomniac patients and 100 controls without sleep complaints demonstrated that the frequency of PLMD is similar, affecting 5–6% of each group (179). As a result, some researchers speculate that PLMD does not contribute to subjective sleep disturbances. Others suggest that PLMD is the result, rather than the cause, of chronic sleep disturbance (180). For most patients, unless PLMD is severe or associated with restless legs syndrome (RLS), there is no symptomatic sleep disturbance, although there may be electroencephalographic evidence of subclinical nocturnal arousals.

The prevalence of PLMD correlates positively with increasing age. While PLMD is rare below age 30, it is present in up to 30–40% of those older than 60 (178,181). Ancoli-Israel and associates recently interviewed and examined 427 people over the age of 65. They found that 45% had sufficient number of leg movements to meet the diagnostic criteria for PLMS. Those with PLMS reported being less satisfied with their sleep and tended to sleep alone (182). Bliwise found that the mean number of movements found in 63 elderly insomniacs was 81.4. In the group with number of movements greater than 40, 80% experienced at least moderate difficulties with sleep (183).

2. *Pharmacology and pathophysiology*

The etiology of PLMS is unknown. Although an anatomic lesion has not been identified, electrophysiologic studies suggest the involvement of subcortical structures. Nocturnal electromyographic recordings from leg muscles in PLMD patients demonstrate bursts of activity occurring periodically with a duration of 2–4 seconds. Normal motor nerve conduction studies and somatosensory-evoked potentials suggest that a primary motor nerve or afferent sensory disturbance is unlikely (184–186). The marked periodicity and stereotypic nature of the movements suggests that an underlying central nervous system pacemaker may be involved. The absence of abnormal electroencephalographic activity associated with the movements as determined by back averaging techniques makes a cortical origin unlikely (187). Abnormal blink reflexes in a pattern consistent with hyperexcitability of pontine interneurons similar to the blink reflex abnormality reported in Parkinson's disease suggest a supraspinal origin (185).

A pharmacologic abnormality has not been identified. Clinical trials with different pharmacologic agents have implicated dopaminergic, GABAergic, and benzodiazepine systems (187–191). Clonazepam significantly reduced leg movements in an uncontrolled open study (187). A double-blind, placebo-controlled study of 20 patients with PLMD presenting with insomnia or excessive daytime sleepiness demonstrated a reduction in leg movements and improved sleep parameters during clonazepam treatment (188). Another study of 10 patients, however, found that although sleep parameters improved, clonazepam had no significant effect on actual leg movements (189).

In a double blind, placebo-controlled study, baclofen improved sleep parameters and reduced the amplitude of the leg movements, although the mean number of leg movements increased (191). Whether the efficacy of the benzodiazepines or baclofen reflects direct activity on benzodiazepine receptors, modulation of GABA activity, or some other action is unknown.

The response to oral levodopa has been the most dramatic (192,193), suggesting a decrease of dopaminergic activity. The observation that parkinsonian patients with PLMD treated with dopaminergic agents have an improvement in PLMD corresponding with an improvement in parkinsonism has suggested nigrostriatal dopaminergic system involvement (194, 195).

IV. TREATMENT OF SLEEP DISORDERS IN THE ELDERLY

The treatment of sleep abnormalities in the elderly population relies heavily on determining the underlying cause for the sleep disturbance. Sleep disruption in older individuals may arise from numerous factors, either as a primary sleep disturbance or secondary to other physical, psychiatric, or neurologic disorders. The increasing prevalence of sleep disturbance associated with aging and the various treatments now available oblige physicians treating elderly patients to develop an awareness of the factors that may contribute to sleep disturbance, and to either conduct an appropriate evaluation and treatment, or refer to a sleep disorders specialist.

The evaluation of sleep disturbances in the elderly has been addressed in the beginning of this chapter. In the elderly patient who complains of insomnia or sleep disturbance, the routine use of hypnotic agents to promote sleep is not often recommended (196). If insomnia is likely to be limited to a short period of time, then judicious use of sleeping medications over a 2–4-week period may be a reasonable approach. For chronic insomnia, hypnotic agents are unlikely to be helpful and may contribute to the problem (197). In these patients, evaluation for underlying conditions such as depression, anxiety, or other psychiatric, medical, or primary sleep disorders should be undertaken. For example, if the sleep disturbance arises from depression, treatment of the depression may alleviate the sleep complaints.

Treatment of the different sleep disturbances associated with Parkinson's disease depends on the cause (79). The sleep disturbance associated with the motor features of PD includes waking up as a result of tremor, stiffness, or difficulty turning over in bed. These symptoms may be remedied by administration of levodopa at bedtime. Askenasy and associates have shown that in untreated PD, nighttime symptom treatment with carbidopa/levodopa reduces muscle tone and allows for improved sleep consolidation. The controlled-release preparations of carbidopa/levodopa may provide the longest duration of nocturnal benefit (94–96). Therapy can be initiated with half of a Sinemet-CR 50/200 at bedtime, and increased if necessary. For patients awaking in the early-morning hours as a result of discomfort due to PD symptoms, the traditional formulation of carbidopa/levodopa, with its rapid onset of action, may be preferable to controlled-release preparations. Patients who use carbidopa/levodopa during the night may report that their dreams become more vivid. If nocturnal hallucinations or significant confusion occurs, nighttime carbidopa/levodopa may need to be reduced or discontinued.

Anti-Parkinson medications may interfere with sleep. Selegiline is a selective MAO-B inhibitor at doses less than 10 mg per day. One of the metabolites of selegiline is a weak amphetamine compound that may interfere with sleep onset, especially if taken in the late afternoon or evening. The administration of selegiline in the morning and early afternoon, or reducing the dose, may reduce the effect on nocturnal sleep.

Dopaminergic agents may have a disruptive effect on sleep. The chronic use of dopaminergic agents may in some patients cause sleep disruption and lead to hallucinations (111, 113). Reduction or elimination of nocturnal levodopa and/or agonists may improve the psychiatric manifestations but may also worsen the motor aspects of PD. Clozapine is an atypical neuroleptic that treats hallucinations without usually worsening motor symptoms of PD. Clozapine has been effective in the treatment of dopaminergic drug-induced hallucinations but requires careful hematologic monitoring.

REM sleep behavior disorder, with or without parkinsonian features, may respond dramatically to low doses of clonazepam, with doses as low as 0.25 mg per night being effective.

The sleep problems associated with Alzheimer's disease can be a therapeutic challenge. Management of "sundowning" often requires the use of dopamine receptor–blocking agents. The management of the day–night sleep reversal has been approached using bright lights (2000 lux or greater), which has been found to be effective in a few patients (152). Establishing consistent schedules with regular wake and bedtimes, avoidance of multiple daytime naps, and routinely scheduled daily activities may also be helpful. Sedative hypnotics are unlikely to be a successful treatment approach and may cause increased confusion.

The treatment of sleep apnea in the elderly is largely determined by the severity of the apnea at night and the impact on daytime functioning. In patients with positional obstructive sleep apnea, training the patient to sleep on his or her side rather than the back, by using position monitors or tennis balls inserted into a pocket on the back of a well-fitted t-shirt, may alleviate the apnea. Other patients may benefit by oral appliances such as the tongue-retaining device, which holds the tongue forward during sleep. Among the approaches to more severe apnea, continuous positive airway pressure (CPAP) has been shown to be an effective method to improve apnea (198). CPAP requires, however, a snug-fitting nasal mask and may not be tolerated by the more elderly or confused patients. The treatment of central sleep apnea is more difficult. The use of low-flow oxygen may prevent the oxygen desaturations. Drugs that may affect nocturnal respirations, including protriptyline and acetazolamide, and CPAP have been used with varying success (199).

Periodic limb movement disorder (PLMD) is often asymptomatic, requiring no therapy. Symptoms usually arise from fragmented sleep, disruption of the spouse's sleep because of the kicking, or as a result of restless legs syndrome (RLS), a disorder often associated with PLMD and characterized by uncomfortable sensations in the legs when at rest, relieved by standing or walking.

The treatment of PLMD has involved four different classes of medications. Levodopa has been reported to be markedly effective (200). In a double-blind study demonstrated with doses as small as one carbidopa/levodopa 25/100, there was a reduction in nocturnal leg movements (201). Similarly, Walters and associates showed that the dopamine agonist, bromocriptine, was effective (202). Becker and his associates evaluated the clinical response and complications of dopaminergic treatment in 47 patients over a mean of 283 days. They found that 91.5% had a good response, with 70% remaining on therapy after 6 months. The mean bedtime dose of levodopa was 160 mg. Nausea was the most frequent side effect, affecting 11.6%; rebound morning symptoms of RLS were reported in 18.6% (203).

Other treatments have included bedtime dosing of clonazepam (0.5–2.0 mg) and baclofen (20–60 mg). The opioid compounds have also been shown to be effective treatments for RLS and PLMD (200,204,205). Because of the possibility of developing tolerance to these agents and the need to increase the dose to treat the symptoms, the opioid medications are reserved for patients who fail to respond to other types of treatment.

REFERENCES

1. Aserinsky E, Kleitman N. Regularly occurring periods of eye motility and concomitant phenomena during sleep. Science 1953; 118:273–274.
2. Aserinsky E, Kleitman N. Two types of ocular motility occurring in sleep. J Appl Physiol 1955; 8:11–18.
3. Quattrochi JJ, Mamelak A, Binder DK, Williams J, Rittenhouse C, Hobson JA. Dynamic suppression of REM sleep by parenteral administration of the serotonin-1 agonist eltorazine. Sleep 1992; 15:125–132.
4. Luebke JI, Greene RW, Semba K, Kamondi A, McCarley RW, Reiner PB. Serotonin hyperpolarizes cholinergic low-threshold burst neurons in the rat laterodorsal tegmental nucleus in vitro. Neurobiology 1992; 89:743–747.

5. Pastel RH, et al. Effects of chronic treatment with two selective 5-HT2 antagonists on sleep in the rat. Pharmacol Biochem Behav 1993; 44:797–804.

6. Bafhdoyan, et al. Simultaneous pontine and basal forebrain microinjections of carbachol suppress REM sleep. J Neurosci 1993; 13:229–242.

7. Zoltoski RK, et al. The relative effects of selective M1 muscarinic antagonists on rapid eye movement sleep. Brain Res 1993; 608:186–190.

8. Shiromani, et al. Cholinergically induced REM sleep triggers Fos-like immunoreactivity in dorsolateral pontine regions associated with REM sleep. Brain Res 1992; 580:351–357.

9. Datta et al. Effect of specific muscarinic M2 receptor antagonist on carbachol induced long-term REM sleep. Sleep 1993; 16:8–14.

10. Siegel JM. Brainstem mechanisms generating REM sleep. In: Kryger, Bloom, and Roth (eds.), Principles and Practice of Sleep Medicine, 2nd ed. 1993.

11. Shiromani, et al. Distribution of choline acetyltransferase immunoreactive somata in the feline brainstem: Implications for REM sleep generation. Sleep 1988; 11:1–16.

12. Hendricks JC, Morrison AR, Mann GL. Different behaviors during paradoxical sleep without atonia depend on pontine lesion site. Brain Res 1982; 239:81–105.

13. Rechtschaffen A, Kales AA. A Manual of Standardized Terminology, Techniques and Scoring System for Sleep Stages in Human Subjects. Washington, DC: U.S. Government Printing Office, Public Health Service, 1968.

14. Carskadon MA, Dement WC. Normal human sleep. In: Kryger MH, Roth T, Dement WC (eds.), Principles and Practice of Sleep Medicine, 2nd ed. London: WB Saunders, 1994; 16–25.

15. Dement WC, Miles LE, Carskadon MA. White paper on sleep and aging. Am Geriatr Soc 1982; 30:25–50.

16. Vitiello MV, Prinz PN. Sleep disturbances in the elderly. In: Albert ML, Knoefel JE (eds.), Clinical Neurology of Aging, 2nd ed. New York: Oxford University Press, 1994; 637–650.

17. Moran MG, Thompson TL, Nies AS. Sleep disorders in the elderly. Am J Psychiatry 1988; 145:1369–1378.

18. Prinz PN, Vitiello MV, Raskind MA, Thorpy MJ. Geriatrics:

Sleep disorders and aging. New Eng J Med 1990; 323:520–526.

19. Hyypa MT, Kronholm E. Quality of sleep and chronic illnesses. J Clin Epidemiol 1989; 42:633–638.

20. Woodward S, Freedman RR. The thermoregulatory effects of menopausal hot flashes on sleep. Sleep 1994; 17:497–501.

21. Ballinger CB. Subjective sleep disturbance at the menopause. J Psychosomatic Res 1976; 20:509–513.

22. Kronholm E, Hyypa MT. Age-related sleep habits and retirement. Ann Clin Res 1985; 17:257–264.

23. Hammond E. Some preliminary findings on physical complaints from a prospective study of 1,064,004 men and women. Am J Public Health 1964; 54:11.

24. Karacan I, Thornby J, Anch M, Holzer CE, Warheit GJ, Schwab JJ, Williams LL. Prevalence of sleep disturbance in a primarily urban Florida county. Soc Sci Med 1976; 10:239.

25. McGhie A, Russell S. The subjective assessment of normal sleep patterns. J Ment Sci 1962; 108:642.

26. Thornby J, Karacan I, Searle R, Salis C, Ware C, Williams R. Subjective reports of sleep disturbance in a Houston metropolitan health survey. Sleep Res 1977; 6:180.

27. Bliwise DL, King AC, Harris RB, Haskell WL. Prevalence of self-reported poor sleep in a healthy population aged 50–65. Soc Sci Med 1992; 34:49–55.

28. Morgan K, Dallosso H, Ebrahim S, Arie T, Fentem PH. Prevalence, frequency and duration of hypnotic drug use among the elderly living at home. Brit Med J 1988; 296:601–602.

29. Bixler EO, Kales A, Jacoby JA, Soldatos CR, Vela-Bueno A. Nocturnal sleep and wakefulness: Effects of age and sex in normal sleepers. Int J Neurosci 1984; 23:33–42.

30. Habte-Gabr E, Wallace RB, Colsher PL, Hulbert JR, White LR, Smith IM. Sleep patterns in rural elders: Demographic, health, and psychobehavioral correlates. J Clin Epidemiol 1991; 44:5–13.

31. Kripke DF, Simons RN, Garfinkel L, Hammond EC. Short and long sleep and sleeping pills: Is increased mortality associated? Arch Gen Psychiatry 1979; 36:103–116.

32. Haponik EF. Sleep disturbances of older persons: Physicians' attitudes. Sleep 1992; 15:168–172.

33. Naylor MW, Aldrich MS. Approach to the patient with disordered sleep. In: Kryger MH, Roth T, Dement WC (eds.), Principles and Practice of Sleep Medicine, 2nd ed. Philadelphia: WB Saunders, 1994; 413–417.

34. Chambers MJ. A re-examination of wrist actigraphy in the evaluation of insomnia. Sleep Res 1992; 21:333.

35. Beck AA, Schmidt-Nowara WW, Jessop CA. Relation of actigraphy to sleep logs in insomniacs. Sleep Res 1992; 21:171.

36. Thoman EB, Acebo C, Lamm S. Stability and instability of sleep in older persons recorded in the home. Sleep 1993; 16:578–585.

37. Broughton RJ. Ambulant home monitoring of sleep and its disorders. In: Kryger MH, Roth T, Dement WC (eds.), Principles and Practice of Sleep Medicine, 2nd ed. Philadelphia: WB Saunders, 1994; 978–983.

38. Duffy FH, Albert MS, McNaulty G, Garvey AJ. Age-related differences in brain electrical activity of healthy subjects. Ann Neurol 1984; 16:430–438.

39. Guazzelli M, Feinberg I, Aminoff M, Fein G, Floyd TC, Maggini C. Sleep spindles in normal elderly: Comparison with young adult patterns and relation top nocturnal awakening, cognitive function and brain atrophy. Electroenceph Clin Neurophysiol 1986; 63:526–539.

40. Principe JC, Smith JR. Sleep spindle characteristics as a function of age. Sleep 1982; 5:73–84.

41. Feinberg I, Korseko RL, Heller N. EEG sleep patterns as a function of normal and pathological aging in man. J Psychiatric Res 1967; 5:107–144.

42. Feinberg I, Fein G, Floyd TC, Aminoff MJ. Delta (.5-3) EEG waveforms during sleep in young and elderly normal subjects. In: Chase MH, Weitzman ED (eds.), Sleep Disorders: Basic and Clinical Research. New York: Spectrum Publications, 1983; 449–462.

43. Smith JR, Karacan I, Yang M. Ontogeny of delta activity during human sleep. Electroenceph Clin Neurophysiol 1977; 43:229–237.

44. Feinberg I, March JD, Floyd TC, Fein G, Aminoff MJ. Log amplitude is a linear function of log frequency in NREM sleep EEG of young and elderly normal subjects. Electroenceph Clin Neurophys 1984; 58:158–160.

45. Webb WB, Dreblow LM. A modified method for scoring slow wave sleep of older subjects. Sleep 1982; 5:195-199.

46. Webb WB. The measurement and characteristics of sleep in older persons. Neurobiol Aging 1982; 3:311-319.

47. Ehlers CL, Kupfer DJ. Effects of age on delta and sleep parameters. Electroenceph Clin Neurophys 1989; 72:118-125.

48. Bliwise DL. Sleep in normal aging and dementia. Sleep 1993; 16:40-81.

49. Kaye JA, Oken BS, Howieson DB, Howeison J, Holm LA, Dennison K. Neurologic evaluation of the optimally healthy oldest old. Arch Neurol 1994; 51:1205-1211.

50. Feinberg I. Changes in sleep cycle patterns with age. J Psychiatry Res 1974; 10:283-306.

51. Hayashi Y, Endo S. All-night polygraphic recordings of healthy aged persons: REM and slow-wave sleep. Sleep 1982; 5:277-283.

52. Webb WB, Dreblow LM. A modified method for scoring slow wave sleep of older subjects. Sleep 1982; 5:195-199.

53. Reynolds CF, et al. Sleep of healthy seniors: A revisit. Sleep 1985; 8:20-29.

54. Reynolds CF, et al. Electroencephalographic sleep in the healthy "old old." J Gerontol 1991; 46:39-46.

55. Gerard P, Collins KJ, Dore C, Exton-Smith AN. Subjective characteristics of sleep in the elderly. Age and Ageing 1978; 7(suppl):55-63.

56. Buysse DJ, Browman KE, Monk TH, Reynolds CF, Fasiczka AL, Kupfer DJ. Napping and 24-hour sleep/wake patterns in healthy elderly and young adults. J Am Geriatr Soc 1992; 40:779-786.

57. Monk TH, Reynolds CF, Machen MA, Kupfer DJ. Daily social rhythms in the elderly and their relation to objectively recorded sleep. Sleep 1992; 15:322-329.

58. Monk TH, Reynolds CF, Buysse DJ, Hoch CC, Jarrett DB, Jennings JR, Kupfer DJ. Circadian characteristics of healthy 80-year olds and their relationship to objectively recorded sleep. J Gerontol 1991; 46:M171-M175.

59. Monk TH, Moline ML. Removal of temporal constraints in the middle-aged and elderly: Effects on sleep and sleepiness. Sleep 1988; 11:513-520.

60. Hoch CC, Reynolds CF, Kupfer DJ, Houk PR, Berman SR,

Stack JA. The superior sleep of elderly nuns. Int J Aging and Human Development 1987; 25:1–9.

61. Zepelin H, McDonald CS, Zammit GK. Effects of age on auditory awakening thresholds. J Gerontol 1984; 39:294–300.

62. Buysse DJ, Reynolds CF, Monk TH, Hoch CC, Yeager AL, Kupfer DJ. Quantification of subjective sleep quality in healthy elderly men and women using the Pittsburgh Sleep Quality Index (PSQI). Sleep 1991; 14:331–338.

63. Buysse DJ, Reynolds CF, Monk TH, Berman SR, Kupfer DJ. The Pittsburgh Sleep Quality Index: A new instrument for psychiatric practice and research. Psychiatry Res 1989; 28:193–213.

64. Hoch CC, et al. Empirical note: Self report versus recorded sleep in healthy seniors. Psychopathology 1987; 24.

65. Reynolds CF, Monk TH, Hoch CC, Jennings JR, Buysse DJ, Houk PR, Jarrett DB, Kupfer DJ. Electroencephalographic sleep in the healthy "old old": A comparison with the "young old" in visually scored and automated measures. J Gerontol 1991; 46:M39–46.

66. Rediehs MH, Reis JS, Creason NS. Sleep in old age: Focus on gender differences. Sleep 1990; 13:410–424.

67. Reynolds CF, Kupfer DJ, Taska LS, Hoch CC, Sewitch DE, Spiker DG. Sleep of healthy seniors: A revisit. Sleep 1985; 8:20–29.

68. Bliwise DL, Ingham RH, Nino-Murcia G, Pursley AM, Dement WC. Five-year follow-up of sleep related respiratory disturbance and neuropsychological variables in elderly subjects. Sleep Res 1989; 18:202.

69. Hoch CC, Reynolds CF, Kupfer DJ, Berman SR. Stability of EEG sleep and sleep quality in healthy seniors. Sleep 1988; 11:521–527.

70. Phoha RL, Dickel MJ, Mosko SS. Preliminary longitudinal assessment of sleep in the elderly. Sleep 1990; 13:425–429.

71. Webb WB. The sleep of older subjects fifteen years later. Psychol Rep 1982; 50:11–14.

72. Hoch CC, Dew MA, Reynolds CF, Monk TH, Buysse DJ, Houk PR, Machen MA, Kupfer DJ. A longitudinal study of laboratory and diary-based sleep measures in healthy "old old" and "young old" volunteers. Sleep 1994; 17:489–496.

73. Carskadon MA, Brown ED, Dement WC. Sleep fragmenta-

tion in the elderly: Relationship to daytime sleep tendency. Neurobiol Aging 1982; 3:321–327.

74. Hoch CC, Reynolds CF, Jennings R, Monk TH, Buysse DJ, Machen MA, Kupfer DJ. Daytime sleepiness and performance among healthy 80 year olds and 20 year olds. Neurobiol Aging 1992; 13:353–356.

75. Bonnet MH. The effect of sleep fragmentation on sleep and performance in younger and older subjects. Neurobiol Aging 1989; 10:21–25.

76. Reynolds CF, Jennings JR, Hoch C, Monk TH, Berman SR, Hall FT, Matzzie JV, Buysse DJ, Kupfer DJ. Daytime sleepiness in the healthy "old old": A comparison with young adults. JAGS 1991; 39:957–962.

77. Marttila RJ. Epidemiology. In: Koller WC (ed.), Handbook of Parkinson's Disease. New York: Marcel Dekker, 1992; 35–57.

78. Stern MB, Koller WC. Parkinson's disease. In: Stern MB, Koller WC (eds.), Parkinsonian Syndromes. New York: Marcel Dekker, 1993; 3–29.

79. Lees AJ, Blackburn NA, Campbell VL. The nighttime problems of Parkinson's disease. Clin Neuropharm 1988; 11:512–519.

80. Nausieda PA, Glantz R, Weber S, Baum R, Klawans HL. Psychiatric complications of levodopa therapy of Parkinson's disease. Adv Neurol 1984; 40: 271–277.

81. Carter J, Carroll S, Lannon MC. Sleep disruption in untreated Parkinson's disease. Neurology 1990; 40(suppl 1):220.

82. Ferini-Strambi L, Franceschi M, Pinto P, Zucconi M, Smirne S. Respiration and heart rate variability during sleep in untreated Parkinson patients. Gerontology 1992; 38:92–98.

83. Kales A, Ansel RD, Markham CH, Sharf MB, Tan T. Sleep in patients with Parkinson's disease and in normal subjects prior to and following levodopa administration. Clin Pharmacol Ther 1971; 12:397–406.

84. Mouret J. Differences in sleep in patients with Parkinson's disease. Electroenceph Clin Neurophysiol 1975; 38:653–657.

85. Askenasy JM, Yahr MD. Reversal of sleep disturbance in Parkinson's disease by antiparkinsonian therapy: A preliminary study. Neurology 1985; 35:527–532.

86. Friedman A. Sleep pattern in Parkinson's disease. Acta Med Pol 1980; 21:193–199.

87. Stern M, Roffwang H, Duvoisin R. The parkinsonian tremor in sleep. J Nerv Ment Dis 1968; 147:202–210.

88. Efthimiou J, Ellis S, Hardie R, Stern G. Sleep apnea in idiopathic and postencephalitic parkinsonism. Adv Neurol 1986; 45:275–276.

89. Apps M, Sheaff P, Ingram D, Kennard C, Empey D. Respiration and sleep in Parkinson's disease. J Neurol Neurosurg Psychiatry 1985; 48:1240–1245.

90. Goetz CG, Wilson RS, Tanner CM, Garron DC. Relations between pain, depression and sleep alterations in Parkinson's disease. Adv Neurol 1986; 45:345–347.

91. Kostic VS, Kusic V, Covickovic-Sternic N, Marinkovic Z, Jankovic S. Reduced rapid eye movement sleep latency in patients with Parkinson's disease. J Neurol 1989; 236:421–423.

92. Van Hilten B, Hoff JI, Middelkoop AM, Van Der Velde EA, Kerkhof GA, Wauquier A, Kamphuisen AC, Roos RAC. Sleep disruption in Parkinson's disease. Arch Neurol 1994; 51:922–928.

93. Laihinen A, Alihanka J, Raitasuo S, Rinne UK. Sleep movements and associated autonomic nervous activities in patients with Parkinson's disease. Acta Neurol Scand 1987; 76:64–68.

94. Jansen ENH, Meerwaldt JD. Madopar HBS in Parkinson patients with nocturnal akinesia. Clin Neurol Neurosurg 1988; 90:35–39.

95. Nausieda PA, Leo GJ, Chesney C. A comparison of conventional and Sinemet CR on the sleep of parkinsonian patients. Neurology 1994; 44(suppl 2):A219.

96. Lees AJ. A sustained-release formulation of L-dopa (Madopar HBS) in the treatment of nocturnal and early-morning disabilities in Parkinson's disease. Eur Neurol 1987; 27(suppl 1): 126–134.

97. UK Madopar CR Study Group. A comparison of Madopar CR and standard Madopar in the treatment of nocturnal and early-morning disability in Parkinson's disease. Clin Neuropharmacol 1989; 12:498–505.

98. Gillin JC, Post RM, Wyatt R, Goodwin FK, Snyder F, Bunney WE. REM inhibitory effect of L-dopa infusion during human sleep. Electroenceph Clin Neurophys 1973; 35:181–186.

99. Cianchetti C. Dopamine agonists and sleep in man. In: Wauquier A (ed.), New York: Raven Press 1985; 121–133.

100. Wyatt RJ, Chase TN, Scott J, Snyder F. Effect of L-dopa on the sleep of man. Nature 1970; 228:999–1001.

101. Greenburg R, Pearlman CA. L-dopa, parkinsonism, and sleep. Psychophysiology 1970; 7:314.

102. Schmidt HS, Knopp W. Sleep in Parkinson's disease: The effect of L-dopa. Psychophysiology 1972; 9:88–89.

103. Tanner CM, Vogel C, Goetz CG, Klawans HL. Hallucinations in Parkinson's disease: A population study. Ann Neurol 1983; 14:136.

104. Celesia GC, Barr AN. Psychosis and other psychiatric manifestations of levodopa therapy. Arch Neurol 1970; 23:193–200.

105. Sacks OW, Kohl MS, Messeloff CR, Schwartz WF. Effects of levodopa in parkinsonian patients with dementia. Neurology 1972; 22:516–519.

106. Moskovitz C, Moses K, Klawans HL. Levodopa-induced psychosis: A kindling phenomenon. Am J Psychiatry 1978; 135:669–675.

107. Goetz CG, Tanner CM, Klawans HL. Pharmacology of hallucinations induced by long-term drug therapy. Am J Psychiatry 1982; 139:494–497.

108. Pederzoli M, Girotti F, Scigliano G, Aiello G, Carella F, Caraceni T. L-dopa long-term treatment in Parkinson's disease: Age related side effects. Neurology 1983; 33:1518–1522.

109. Rondot P, De Recondo J, Coignet A, Zeigler M. Mental disorders in Parkinson's disease after treatment with L-dopa. Adv Neurol 1984; 40:259–269.

110. Glantz R, Bieliauskas L, Paleologos N. Behavioral indicators of hallucinosis in levodopa-treated Parkinson's disease. Adv Neurol 1986; 45:417–420.

111. Nausieda P, Weiner W, Kaplan L, Weber S, Klawans H. Sleep disruption in the course of chronic levodopa therapy: An early feature of the levodopa psychosis. Clin Neuropharmacol 1982; 5:183–194.

112. Nausieda PA, Glantz R, Weber S, Baum R, Klawans HL. Psychiatric complications of levodopa therapy of Parkinson's disease. Adv Neurol 1984; 40:271–277.

113. Comella CL, Tanner CM, Ristanovic RK. Polysomnographic sleep measures in Parkinson's disease patients with treatment-induced hallucinations. Ann Neurol 1993; 34:710–714.
114. Factor SA, McAlarney T, Sanches-Ramos JR, Weiner WJ. Sleep disorders and sleep effect in Parkinson's disease. Movement Dis 1990; 5:280–285.
115. Clark EC, Feinstein B. The on-off effect in Parkinson's disease treated with levodopa with remarks concerning the effect of sleep. Adv Exp Med Biol 1977; 90:175–182.
116. Comella CL, Boehme J, Jaglin J. Sleep benefit in Parkinson's disease (abstract). Neurology 1995 (in press).
117. Jones BE. Paradoxical sleep and its chemical structural substrates in the brain. Neuroscience 1991; 40:637–656.
118. Shiromani PJ, Siegel JM. Descending projections from the dorsolateral pontine tegmentum to the paramedian reticular nucleus of the caudal medulla in the cat. Brain Res 1990; 517:224–228.
119. Hendricks JC, Morrison AR, Mann GL. Different behaviors during paradoxical sleep without atonia depend on pontine lesion site. Brain Res 1982; 239:81–105.
120. Schenk CS, Bundie SR, Ettinger MG, Mahowald MW. Chronic behavioral disorders of human REM sleep: A new category of parasomnia. Sleep 1986; 9:293–308.
121. Schenk CS, Bundie SR, Patterson AL, Mahowald MW. Rapid eye movement sleep behavior disorder. JAMA 1987; 257:1786–1789.
122. Schenk CH, Mahowald MW. Polysomnographic, neurologic, psychiatric, and clinical outcome report on 70 consecutive cases with REM sleep behavior disorder (RBD): Sustained clonazepam efficacy in 89.5% of 57 treated patients. Clev Clin J Med 1990; 57(suppl):S9–S23.
123. Silber CH, Ahlskog JE. REM sleep behavior disorder in parkinsonian syndromes. Sleep Res 1992; 21:313.
124. Silber MH, Ahlskog JE. REM sleep behavior disorder and Parkinson's disease (abstract). Neurology 1993; 43(suppl 2):A338.
125. Comella CL, Ristanovic R, Goetz CG. Parkinson disease patients with and without REM behavior disorder (RBD): A polysomnographic and clinical comparison. Neurology 1993; 43.

126. Hirsch E, Graybiel AM, Duyckaerts C, Javoy-Agid F. Neuronal loss in the pedunculopontine nucleus in Parkinson disease and in progressive supranuclear palsy. Proc Natl Acad Sci 1987; 84:5976–5980.

127. Bliwise DL. Dementia. In: Kryger MH, Roth T, Dement WC (eds.), Principles and Practice of Sleep Medicine, 2nd ed. Philadelphia: WB Saunders, 1994; 790–800.

128. Prinz PN, Peskind ER, Vitaliano PP, Raskind MA, Eisdorder C, Zemcuznikov N, Gerber CJ. Changes in the sleep and waking EEGs of nondemented and demented elderly subjects. J Amer Geriatric Soc 1982; 30:86–93.

129. Prinz PN, Vitaliano PP, Vitiello MV, Bokan J, Raskind M, Peskind E, Gerber C. Sleep, EEG and mental function changes in senile dementia of the Alzheimer's type. Neurobiology of Aging 1982; 3:361–370.

130. Loewenstein RJ, Weingartner H, Gillin JC, Kaye W, Eberts M, Mendelson WB. Disturbances of sleep and cognitive functioning in patients with dementia. Neurobiology of Aging 1982; 3:371–377.

131. Vitiello MV, Bokan JA, Kukull WA, Muniz RL, Smallwood RG, Prinz PN. Rapid eye movement sleep measures of Alzheimer's-type dementia patients and optimally healthy aged individuals. Biol Psychiatry 1984; 19:721–734.

132. Martin PR, Loewenstein RJ, Kaye WH, Ebert MH, Weingartner H, Gillin JC. Sleep EEG in Korsakoff's psychosis and Alzheimer's disease. Neurology 1986; 36:411–414.

133. Allen SR, Seiler WO, Stahelin HB, Spiegel R. Seventy-two hour polygraphic and behavioral recordings of wakefulness and sleep in a hospital geriatric unit: Comparison between demented and nondemented patients. Sleep 1987; 10:143–159.

134. Bliwise L, Tinklenberg J, Yesavage JA, Davies H, Pursley AM, Petta DE, Widrow PL, Guilleminalult C, Zarcone VP, Dement WC. REM latency in Alzheimer's disease. Biol Psychiatry 1989; 25:320–328.

135. Vitiello MV, Prinz PN, Williams DE, Frommlet MS, Ries RK. Sleep disturbances in patients with mild-stage Alzheimer's disease. J Geriatrics 1990; 45:M131–M138.

136. Vitiello MV, Peceta JS, Prinz PN. Sleep in Alzheimer's disease and other dementing disorders. Can J Psychology 1991; 45:221–239.

137. Aharon-Peretz J, Masiah A, Pillar T, Epstein R, Tzishcinsky O, Lavie P. Sleep–wake cycles in multi-infarct dementia and dementia of the Alzheimer type. Neurology 1991; 41:1616–1619.

138. Regestein QR, Morris J. Daily sleep patterns observed among institutionalized elderly residents. J Am Geriatr Soc 1987; 35:767–772.

139. Satlin A, Teicher MH, Lieberman HR, Baldessarini RJ, Volicer L, Rheaume Y. Circadian locomotor activity rhythms in Alzheimer's disease. Neuropsychopharmocology 1991; 5:115–126.

140. Witting W, Kwa IH, Eikelenboom P, Mirmiran M, Swaab DF. Alterations in the circadian rest-activity rhythm in aging and Alzheimer's disease. Biol Psychiatry 1990; 27:563–572.

141. Bliwise DL, Tinklenberg JR, Yesavage JA. Timing of sleep and wakefulness in Alzheimer's disease patients residing at home. Biol Psychiatry 1992; 31:1163–1165.

142. Goudsmit E, Hofman MA, Fliers E, Swaab DF. The supraoptic and paraventricular nuclei of the human hypothalamus in relation to sex, age and Alzheimer's disease. Neurobiol Aging 1990; 11:529–536.

143. Swaab DF, Fliers E, Partiman TS. The suprachiasmatic nucleus of the human brain in relation to sex, age and senile dementia. Brain Res 1985; 342:37–44.

144. Swaab DF, Roozendaal B, Ravid R, Velis DN, Gooren L, Wiliams RS. Suprachiasmatic nucleus in aging, Alzheimer's disease, and Prader-Willi syndrome. Progress in Brain Research 1987; 72:301–310.

145. Mirmiran M, Swaab DF, Kok JH, Hofman MA, Witting W, Van Gool WA. Circadian rhythms and the suprachiasmatic nucleus in perinatal development, aging and Alzheimer's disease. Progress in Brain Res 1992; 93:151–163.

146. Ishii T. Distribution of Alzheimer's neurofibrillary tangles in the brainstem and hypothalamus of senile dementia. Acta Neuropathol 1966; 6:181.

147. Hirano A, Zimmerman H. Alzheimer's neurofibrillary changes: A topographic study. Arch Neurol 1962; 7:227.

148. Mufson EJ, Mash DC, Hersh LB. Neurofibrillary tangles in cholinergic pedunculopontine neurons in Alzheimer's disease. Ann Neurol 1988; 24:623–629.

149. Jellinger K. The pedunculopontine nucleus in Parkinson disease, progressive supranuclear palsy and Alzheimer's disease. J Neurol Neurosurg Psychiatry 1988; 51:540–543.

150. Campbell SS, Kripke DF, Gillin JC, Hrubovcak JC. Exposure to light in healthy elderly subjects and Alzheimer's patients. Physio Behav 1988; 42:141–144.

151. Bliwise DL, Carroll JS, Lee KA, Nikich JC, Dement WC. Sleep and "sundowning" in nursing home patients. Psychiatry Res 1993; 48:277–292.

152. Mishima K, Okawa M, Hozumi S, Hori H, Takahashi K. Morning bright light therapy for sleep and behavior disorders in elderly patients with dementia. Acta Psychiatr Scand 1994; 89:1–7.

153. Satlin A, Volicer L, Ross V, Herz L, Campbell S. Bright light treatment of behavioral and sleep disturbances in patients with Alzheimer's disease. Am J Psychiatry 1992; 149: 1028–1032.

154. Okawa M, Mishima K, Hishikawa Y, Hozumi S, Hori H, Takahashi K. Circadian rhythm disorders in sleep-waking and body temperature in elderly patients with dementia and their treatment. Sleep 1991; 14:478–485.

155. Bliwise DL, Nino-Murcia G, Forno LS, Viseskul C. Abundant REM sleep in a patient with Alzheimer's disease.

156. Diagnostic Classification Steering Committee. The International Classification of Sleep Disorders. Kansas: Allen Press Inc, 1990.

157. Naifeh KH, Severinghaus JW, Kamiya J. Effect of aging on sleep-related changes in respiratory variables. Sleep 1987; 10:160–171.

158. Krieger J, Turlot JC, Mangin P, Kurtz D. Breathing during sleep in normal young and elderly subjects: Hypopneas, apneas, and correlated factors. Sleep 1983; 6:108–120.

159. Ancoli-Israel S, Kripke DF, Klauber MR, Mason WJ, Fell R, Kaplan O. Sleep-disordered breathing in community dwelling elderly. Sleep 1991; 14:486–495.

160. Ingram F, Henke KG, Levin HS, Ingram PTF, Kuna ST. Sleep apnea and vigilance performance in community-dwelling older sample. Sleep 1994; 17:248–252.

161. Berry DTR, Phillips BA, Cook YR, Schmitt FA, Gilmore RL, Patel R, Keener TM, Tyre E. Sleep-disordered breathing

in healthy aged persons: Possible daytime sequelae. J Gerontol 1987; 42:620–626.

162. Phillips BA, Berry DT, Schmitt FA, Magan LK, Gerhardstein DC, Cook YR. Sleep-disordered breathing in the healthy elderly: Clinically significant? Chest 1992; 101:345–349.

163. Berry DTR, Phillips BA, Cook YR, Schmitt FA, Honeycutt NA, Edwards CL, Lamb DG, Magan LK, Allen RS. Sleep-disordered breathing in healthy aged persons: One year follow-up of daytime sequelae. Sleep 1989; 12:211–215.

164. Dickel MJ, Mosko SS. Morbidity cut-offs for sleep apnea and periodic leg movements in predicting subjective complaints in seniors. Sleep 1990; 13:155–166.

165. Hoch CC, Reynolds CF, Monk TH, Buysse DJ, Yeager AL, Houck PR, Kupfer DJ. Comparison of sleep-disordered breathing among healthy elderly in the seventh, eighth, and ninth decades of life. Sleep 1990; 13:502–511.

166. Young T, Palta M, Dempsey J, Skatruc J, Weber S, Badr S. The occurrence of sleep-disordered breathing among middle-aged adults. N Engl J Med 1993; 328:1230–1235.

167. Bliwise DL, Feldman DE, Bliwise NG, Carskadon MA, Kraemer HC, North CS, Petta DE, Seidel WF, Dement WC. Risk factors for sleep disordered breathing in heterogeneous geriatric populations. J Am Geriatr Soc 1987; 35:132–141.

168. White DP, Lombard RM, Cadieux RJ, Zwillick CW. Pharyngeal resistance in normal humans: Influence of gender, age and obesity. J Appl Physiol 1985; 58:365–371.

169. Block AJ, Wynne JW, Boysen PG. Sleep-disordered breathing and nocturnal oxygen desaturation in postmenopausal women. Am J Med 1980; 69:75–79.

170. Smallwood RG, Vitiello MV, Giblin EC, Prinz PN. Sleep apnea: Relationship to age, sex, and Alzheimer's dementia. Sleep 1983; 6:16–22.

171. Mason WJ, Ancoli-Israel S, Kripke DF. Apnea revisited: A longitudinal follow-up. Sleep 1989; 12:423–429.

172. Hoch CC, Reynolds CF, Kupfer DJ, Houck PR, Berman SR, Stack JA. Sleep-disordered breathing in normal and pathologic aging. J Clin Psychiatry 1986; 47:499–503.

173. Bliwise DL, Bliwise NG, Partinen M, Pursley AM, Dement WC. Sleep apnea and mortality in an aged cohort. Am J Public Health 1988; 78:544–547.

174. Ancoli-Israel S, Klauber MR, Kriipke DF, Parker L, Cobarrubias M. Sleep apnea in female patients in a nursing home: Increased risk of mortality. Chest 1989; 96:1054–1058.

175. Lord S, Sawyer B, O'Connell D, King M, Pond D, Eyland A, Mant A, Holland JT, Hensley MJ, Saunders NA. Night-to-night variability of disturbed breathing during sleep in an elderly community sample. Sleep 1991; 14:252–258.

176. Mosko SS, Dickel MJ, Paul T, LaTour T, Dhillon S, Ghanim A, Sassin JF. Sleep apnea and sleep-related periodic leg movements in community resident seniors. J Am Geriatr Soc 1988; 36:502–508.

177. Symonds CP. Nocturnal myoclonus. J Neurol Neurosurg Psychiatr 1953; 16:166–171.

178. Bixler EO, Kales A, Vela-Bueno A, Jacoby JA, Scarone S, Soldatos CR. Nocturnal myoclonic activity in a normal population. Res Comm Chem Path Pharm 1982; 36:129–140.

179. Kales A, Bixler EO, Soldatas CR, Vela-Bueno A, Caldwell AB, Cadieux RJ. Role of sleep apnea and nocturnal myoclonus. Psychosomatics 1982; 23:589–600.

180. Coleman RM, Pollak CP, Weitzman ED. Periodic movements in sleep (nocturnal myoclonus): Relation to sleep disorders. Ann Neurol 1980; 8:416–421.

181. Lugaresi E, Cirignotta F, Coccagna G, Montagna P. Nocturnal myoclonus and restless legs syndrome. In: Fahn S, Marsden CD, Van Woert MH (eds.), Myoclonus. New York: Raven Press, 1986; 295–307.

182. Ancoli-Isreal S, Kripke DF, Klauber MR, Mason WJ, Fell R, Kaplan O. Periodic limb movements in sleep in community-dwelling elderly. Sleep 1991; 14:496–500.

183. Bliwise D, Pette D, Seidel W, Dement W. Periodic leg movements during sleep in the elderly. Arch Gerontol Geriatr 1985; 4:273–281.

184. Martinelli P, Coccagna G, Lugaresi E. Nocturnal myoclonus, restless legs syndrome, and abnormal electrophysiological findings. Ann Neurol 1987; 21:515.

185. Wechsler LR, Stakes JW, Shahani BT, Busis NA. Periodic leg movements of sleep (nocturnal myoclonus): An electrophysiologic study. Ann Neurol 1986; 19:168–173.

186. Mosko SS, Nudleman KL. Somatosensory and brainstem

auditory evoked responses in sleep-related periodic leg movements. Sleep 1986; 9:399–404.

187. Ohanna N, Peled R, Rubin AE, Zomer J, Lavie P. Periodic leg movements in sleep: Effect of clonazepam treatment. Neurology 1985; 35:408–411.

188. Peled R, Lavie P. Double-blind evaluation of clonazepam on periodic leg movements in sleep. J Neurol Neurosurg Psychiatr 1987; 50:1679–1681.

189. Mitler MM, Browman CP, Menn SJ, Gujavarty K, Timms RM. Nocturnal myoclonus: Treatment efficacy of clonazepam and temazepam. Sleep 1986; 9:385–392.

190. Guilleminault C, Mondini S, Montplaisir J, Mancuso J, Cobasko D, Dement WC. Periodic leg movement, L-dopa, 5-hydroxytryptophan, and L-tryptophan. Sleep 1987; 10:35–38.

191. Guilleminault C, Flagg W. Effect of baclofen on sleep-related periodic leg movements. Ann Neurol 1984; 15:234–239.

192. Montplaisir J, Godbout A, Poirier G, Bedart MA. Restless leg syndrome and periodic movements in sleep: Physiopathy and treatment by L-dopa. Clin Pharm 1986; 5:456–463.

193. Guilleminault C, Cetel M, Phillip P. Dopaminergic treatment of restless legs and rebound phenomenon. Neurology 1993; 43:445.

194. Askenasy JJ, Weitzman ED, Pollack CP, Pakier A. Periodic movements in sleep and basal ganglia dysfunction. Sleep Res (abstract).

195. Askenasy JJM, Weitzman ED, Yahr MD. Are periodic movements in sleep a basal ganglia dysfunction? J Neural Trans 1987; 70:337–347.

196. National Institute of Mental Health, Consensus Development Conference. Drugs and insomnia: The use of medications to promote sleep. J Am Med Assoc 1984; 251:2410–2414.

197. Gillin JC, Spinweber CL, Johnson LC. Rebound insomnia: A critical review. J Clin Psychopharmacol 1989; 9:161–172.

198. Sullivan CE, Grunstein RR. Continuous positive airway pressure in sleep-disordered breathing. In: Principles and Practice of Sleep Medicine, 2nd ed. Philadelphia: WB Saunders, 1994; 694–705.

199. Sanders MH. Medical therapy for sleep apnea. In: Kryger MH, Roth T, Dement WC (eds.), Principles and Practice of Sleep Medicine, 2nd ed. Philadelphia: WB Saunders, 1994; 678–693.

200. Kaplan PW, Allen RP, Buchholz DW, Walters JK. A double-blind, placebo-controlled study of the treatment of periodic limb movements in sleep using carbidopa/levodopa and propoxyphene. Sleep 1993; 16:717–723.

201. Brodeur C, Montplaisir J, Godbout U, Marinier R. Treatment of restless legs syndrome and periodic movements during sleep with L-dopa: A double blind controlled study. Neurology 1988; 38:1845–1848.

202. Walters AS, Hening WA, Kavey N, Chokroverty S, Gido-Frank S. A double-blind randomized crossover trial of bromocriptine and placebo in restless legs syndrome. Ann Neurol 1988; 24:455–458.

203. Becker PM, Jamieson AO, Brown WD. Dopaminergic agents in restless legs syndrome and periodic limb movements of sleep: Response and complications of extended treatment in 49 cases. Sleep 1993; 16:713–716.

204. Walters AS, Wagner ML, Hening WA, Grasing K, Mills R, Chokroverty S, Kavey N. Successful treatment of the idiopathic restless legs syndrome in a randomized double-blind trial of oxycodone versus placebo. Sleep 1993; 16:327–332.

205. Montplaisir J, Lapierre O, Warnes H, Pelletier G. The treatment of the restless leg syndrome with or without periodic leg movements in sleep. Sleep 1992; 391–395.

10

Headache and Neuralgias

Brian E. Mondell
The Johns Hopkins University School of Medicine, Baltimore, and Baltimore Headache Institute, Lutherville, Maryland

Russell C. Packard
University of West Florida, Pensacola, Florida

I. GENERAL PRINCIPLES

A. Introduction

Head pain occurs in at least 80% of Americans and is more prevalent among women (1). The International Headache Society has provided the most recent classification of head pain detailing more than 100 syndromes or clinical conditions that cause it (2). To understand head pain, look to the brainstem where ascending and descending neuronal systems modulate pain perception and associated clinical characteristics. Neurotransmitters such as serotonin, noradrenalin, substance P, and endorphins play a key role within these systems. The differential diagnosis of head pain depends on a detailed history, a comprehensive physical examination, and clinical testing. Accurate diagnosis permits sucessful treatment.

B. Head Pain Epidemiology and Mechanisms

1. *Epidemiology*

Epidemiologic research demonstrates that head pain is a universal complaint. Population-based studies show that 95% of women and 91% of men experienced headache in the 12 months prior to interview, and 76% of women and 57% of men experienced their most recent headache in the 4 weeks preceding the interview. In spite of the fact that head pain is one of the most prominent causes of time lost from work or school, approximately 72% of female and 85% of male study respondents never consulted a physician (1,3).

2. *Mechanisms*

Multiple theoretic mechanisms may explain primary (functional) head pain: vascular theory, neurovascular inflammation, and central theory. In the vascular theory, painful vasodilation and perivascular inflammation and/or opening of arteriovenous anastomoses cause headache (4,5). In the neurovascular inflammation theory, stimulation of the trigeminovascular system produces neurogenic plasma extravasation and headache (6). In the central theory, unstable serotonergic neurotransmission precipitates increased firing rates of raphe neurons, resulting in head pain (7). The final common pathway may be the descending trigeminal tract in the brainstem where head and face pain are represented and where interconnections are found with cephalic vasomotor activation and cranial musculature (8).

C. Evaluating Head Pain

To evaluate the patient presenting with head pain, obtain a complete history, perform a thorough physical examination, and order appropriate diagnostic studies. The history will suggest a provisional diagnosis that must be substantiated by physical examination and allied diagnostic tests. The patient's carefully documented illness can provide the best insight into potential etiology (9).

Although a complete history may be difficult to obtain, direct and indirect questioning techniques will ensure the discovery of all pertinent facts. It is essential to permit patients to relate the story of their head pain in their own terms. It is the responsibility of the person taking the history to qualify and clarify the historical facts (9).

1. *Present illness*

The head pain particulars obtained through history taking should be recorded logically in order to uncover the pattern and enable the identification of the type(s) of head pain. The first step in approaching head pain is determining acuity. Head pain of acute onset may be ominous, suggesting an intracranial disorder such as meningitis or encephalitis, subarachnoid hemorrhage, subdural hematoma, or tumor, or alternatively extracranial pathology such as glaucoma, intra- or extraocular inflammation, optic neuritis, or acute sinusitis. A variety of systemic disorders, for example, hypertension or pheochromocytoma, can also be responsible for causing acute headache. Subacute headache may be the manifestation of subdural hematoma, cerebral abscess, tumor, intracranial sinus thrombosis, benign intracranial hypertension, giant cell arteritis, and hypo- or hyperthyroidism. Chronic headache typically represents migraine or tension-type headache, but it has occasionally been the result of metabolic, systemic, or malignant disease (9).

Factors important in the documentation of present illness include onset, frequency, intensity, location, quality, precipitators or exacerbators, ameliorators, associated symptoms, and neurologic accompaniments (9).

Onset.   Asking about the earliest memory of head pain determines whether the head pain occurred in childhood or later in life, or after a traumatic episode. Is head pain a new event or one of a recurring series? Is head pain present upon awakening, or does it occur at night, awakening the patient from sleep? Since onset, are the essential characteristics the same (9)?

Frequency.   The frequency of head pain should be determined. Look for patterns of occurrence and recurrence at regular intervals (9).

Duration.   The duration of head pain should be ascertained. Note the longest, shortest, and average length of an attack (9).

Intensity. The intensity of head pain should be quantitated. Distinguish between mild, moderate, severe, or incapacitating pain. It is appropriate to measure pain by its effect on the activities of daily living. Minimal restriction implies mild pain. Medium restriction implies moderate pain. Significant restriction implies severe pain. A total restriction implies incapacitating pain (9).

Location. The location of head pain should be specified. Record where the pain starts, where the pain radiates, and where the pain settles (9).

Quality. The quality of pain should be defined. Use a variety of adjectives such as aching, boring, burning, expanding, gnawing, piercing, pounding, pressing, squeezing, stabbing, and throbbing (9).

Precipitators or exacerbators. The precipitators or exacerbators of head pain should be listed. Note multiple factors such as alcohol ingestion, changes in barometric pressure, bending over, exposure to bright lights, chewing, coughing, dietary intake, exertion, fatigue, head jarring, hunger, loud noises, menarche, menopause, menstruation, odors, position, sexual activity, sleep habits, sneezing, straining, stress, and touching (9).

Ameliorators. The ameliorators of head pain should be recorded. Indicate what has been done to relieve or reduce pain, including previous treatments (9).

Associated symptoms. The associated symptoms of head pain should be enumerated, with mention of bruxism, chills, clicking jaw, cold hands or feet, conjunctival injection, facial edema, fatigue, fever, flushing, lacrimation, malaise, nasal congestion, nausea, pallor, polyuria, rhinorrhea, scalp tenderness, and vomiting (9).

Neurologic accompaniments. The neurologic accompaniments that occur in association with head pain either before, during, or after an attack should be described. Special inquiry should be made for the following: amnesia, ataxia, blindness, blurred vision, confusion, diplopia, dysarthria, dysphagia, dysphasia, hearing loss, hemianesthesia, hemianopic field defects, impaired thought processes, incoordination, lethargy, lightheadedness, loss of consciousness, loss of depth perception, mood changes, numb extremities, paresis, ptosis, pupillary changes, scintillating scotomata, seizure, sphincter disturbances, teichopsia, tinnitis, vertigo, and visual obscurations (9).

2. *Past medical history*

It is important to inquire about the past medical history, specifically general health and strength, childhood illnesses, major adult illnesses, immunizations, operations and other hospitalizations, serious injuries, current and recent medications (prescription and over-the-counter drugs), and allergies (9).

3. *Family history*

The family history may be very important. Do any family members have symptoms similar to the patient's? Is there a history of nervous and mental disease among relatives? What is the state of health of parents and siblings? Among blood relations, is there a history of head pain, heart disease, high blood pressure, stroke, diabetes, kidney disease, thyroid disease, asthma and other allergic states, blood dyscrasias, cancer, or tuberculosis (9)?

4. *Personal and social history*

Review the patient's personal and social history. Assess the patient's home environment as a youth, including abuse and neglect, and parental divorce or separation. A history of reinforcing reactions of family or friends to the disability of head pain is important. The responses of sympathy and attention may set the stage for future maladaptive behavior. Consider socioeconomic class, cultural and educational background, occupation, marital status, adjustment to family life, general life satisfaction, military service, travel, and other exposures. Review personal habits such as diet, regularity of eating and sleeping, exercise, quantity of coffee, tea, and other caffeine-containing beverages consumed, as well as the use of tobacco, alcohol, or illicit drugs (9).

Take into account the effect of life events on the patient. Equally important are major unfavorable events and frustrating or irritating demands posed by everyday events. The presence of less successful strategies for coping—avoidance or self-criticism—may be important in the evolution of head pain. Also important is the search for obsessionality, hostility, and hypochondriacal or neurotic worry. Depression and associated sleep disturbances above and beyond what is a reasonable response to head pain are also worth noting. An inability to deal with stress could cause a breakdown in coping mechanisms that can increase susceptibility to head pain, or, alternatively, maladaptive responses could be the result of the experience of head pain (9).

5. *Systems review*

To complete the head pain history, perform a comprehensive review of systems. Assess each of the following areas: general constitutional symptoms, skin, skeletal, eyes, ears, nose, throat, mouth, endocrine, respiratory, cardiac, hematologic, lymph nodes, gastrointestional, genitourinary, neurologic, and psychiatric. This review will help to fill in the gaps of a head pain history that could be vague, complicated, or even contradictory (9).

6. *Physical examination*

A careful history often suggests a specific diagnosis, but a complete physical and neurologic examination will confirm a suspected diagnosis. Characterize the patient's general condition with a description including evidence of pain, restlessness, and mental state. Record vital signs—temperature, pulse, respiratory rate, blood pressure, height, and weight. Inspect the skin for lesions, rashes, and areas of pigmentation. Look for positive findings in the chest, abdomen, and extremities (9).

Thoroughly examine the head. Check the size and shape of the head. Palpate the skull for tenderness, protuberances, or depressions. Auscultate the skull at various points. Additionally, palpate and auscultate the carotid, temporal, and occipital arteries. Listen for orbital bruits. Thoroughly examine the eyes. Examine the temporomandibular joints, focusing on tenderness on pressure, limited opening of the mouth, or malocclusion. Finally, see if the frontal or maxillary sinuses are tender (9).

Assess the cervical spine next. Test the neck for tenderness and range of motion with flexion, extension, and rotation. Measure the length of the cervical spine. Evaluate thyroid size and character as well (9).

Perform a neurologic examination. Include mental status examination assessing orientation, memory, mood, affect, speech and articulation, and thought processes and perceptions. Test all cranial nerves. Check motor system for power, muscle wasting, alterations in muscle tone, and abnormal movements. Note gait, posture, and coordination. Describe any reflex changes or pathologic reflexes. Complete the neurologic examination with a search for any disturbances in sensory functioning (9).

7. *Diagnostic studies*

Use appropriate diagnostic studies to conclude the initial evaluation of the patient presenting with head pain. Include a routine laboratory profile consisting of complete blood counts and chemistries, thyroid function, and urinalysis. Measurement of erythrocyte sedimentation rate and screening for collagen vascular disease may be necessary. Any evidence for infection or hemorrhage should prompt spinal fluid examination. Neuroimaging techniques such as computed axial tomography, magnetic resonance imaging, and cerebral angiography are indicated in cases in which history and examination suggest a structural lesion (9).

D.   Classification of Head Pain

In order to effectively treat the patient presenting with head pain, carefully question, examine, and study the complete patient as well as his or her complaint of head pain. Through direct and indirect questioning, a complete history explores present illness, past medical history, family history, personal and social history, and a systems review. A detailed medical and neurologic examination complements the historical information. A comprehensive screening laboratory profile should be employed and neurodiagnostic studies should be used judiciously. A combined medical and neurologic approach should permit appropriate diagnosis and treatment (9).

A rational system of classification of head pain comes from the International Headache Society. Following these classification guidelines, consistent diagnostic accuracy will be ensured (2).

1. *Migraine*
    1.1. Migraine without aura
    1.2. Migraine with aura
        1.2.1. Migraine with typical aura
        1.2.2. Migraine with prolonged aura
        1.2.3. Familial hemiplegic migraine
        1.2.4. Basilar migraine
        1.2.5. Migraine aura without headache
        1.2.6. Migraine with acute-onset aura
    1.3. Ophthalmoplegic migraine
    1.4. Retinal migraine
    1.5. Childhood periodic syndromes that may be precursors to or associated with migraine
        1.5.1. Benign paroxysmal vertigo of childhood
        1.5.2. Alternating hemiplegia of childhood
    1.6. Complications of migraine
        1.6.1. Status migrainosus
        1.6.2. Migrainous infarction

2. *Tension-type headache*
    2.1. Episodic tension-type headache
        2.1.1. Episodic tension-type headache associated with disorder of pericranial muscles
        2.1.2. Episodic tension-type headache unassociated with disorder of pericranial muscles

2.2. Chronic tension-type headache
- 2.2.1. Chronic tension-type headache associated with disorder of pericranial muscles
- 2.2.2. Chronic tension-type headache unassociated with disorder of pericranial muscles

3. *Cluster headache and chronic paroxysmal hemicrania*
- 3.1. Cluster headache
  - 3.1.1. Cluster headache periodicity undetermined
  - 3.1.2. Episodic cluster headache
  - 3.1.3. Chronic cluster headache
    - 3.1.3.1. Unremitting from onset
    - 3.1.3.2. Evolved from episodic
- 3.2. Chronic paroxysmal hemicrania

4. *Miscellaneous headaches unassociated with structural lesion*
- 4.1. Idiopathic stabbing headache
- 4.2. External compression headache
- 4.3. Cold stimulus headache
  - 4.3.1. External application of a cold stimulus
  - 4.3.2. Ingestion of a cold stimulus
- 4.4. Benign cough headache
- 4.5. Benign exertional headache
- 4.6. Headache associated with sexual activity
  - 4.6.1. Dull type
  - 4.6.2. Explosive type
  - 4.6.3. Postural type

5. *Headache associated with head trauma*
- 5.1. Acute posttraumatic headache
  - 5.1.1. With significant head trauma and/or confirmatory signs
  - 5.1.2. With minor head trauma and no confirmatory signs
- 5.2. Chronic posttraumatic headache
  - 5.2.1. With significant head trauma and/or confirmatory signs

5.2.2. With minor head trauma and no confirmatory signs

6. *Headache associated with vascular disorders*
   6.1. Acute ischemic cerebrovascular disease
      6.1.1. Transient ischemic attack (TIA)
      6.1.2. Thromboembolic stroke
   6.2. Intracranial hematoma
      6.2.1. Intracerebral hematoma
      6.2.2. Subdural hematoma
      6.2.3. Epidural hematoma
   6.3. Subarachnoid hemorrhage
   6.4. Unruptured vascular malformation
      6.4.1. Arteriovenous malformation
      6.4.2. Saccular aneurysm
   6.5. Arteritis
      6.5.1. Giant-cell arteritis
      6.5.2. Other systemic arteritides
      6.5.3. Primary intracranial arteritis
   6.6. Carotid or vertebral artery pain
      6.6.1. Carotid or vertebral dissection
      6.6.2. Carotidynia (idiopathic)
      6.6.3. Postendarterectomy headache
   6.7. Venous thrombosis
   6.8. Arterial hypertension
      6.8.1. Acute pressor response to exogenous agent
      6.8.2. Pheochromocytoma
      6.8.3. Malignant (accelerated) hypertension
      6.8.4. Pre-eclampsia and eclampsia
   6.9. Headache associated with other vascular disorder

7. *Headache associated with nonvascular intracranial disorder*
   7.1. High cerebrospinal fluid pressure
      7.1.1. Benign intracranial hypertension
      7.1.2. High-pressure hydrocephalus

8.5.1. Birth-control pills or estrogens

8.5.2. Other substances

9. *Headache associated with noncephalic infection*

   9.1. Viral infection

      9.1.1. Focal noncephalic

      9.1.2. Systemic

   9.2. Bacterial infection

      9.2.1. Focal noncephalic

      9.2.2. Systemic (septicemia)

   9.3. Headache related to other infection

10. *Headache associated with metabolic disorder*

    10.1. Hypoxia

       10.1.1. High-altitude headache

       10.1.2. Hypoxic headache

       10.1.3. Sleep apnea headache

    10.2. Hypercapnia

    10.3. Mixed hypoxia and hypercapnia

    10.4. Hypoglycemia

    10.5. Dialysis

    10.6. Headache related to other metabolic abnormality

11. *Headache or facial pain associated with disorder of cranium, neck, eyes, ears, nose, sinuses, teeth, mouth, or other facial or cranial structures*

    11.1. Cranial bone

    11.2. Neck

       11.2.1. Cervical spine

       11.2.2. Retropharyngeal tendinitis

    11.3. Eyes

       11.3.1. Acute glaucoma

       11.3.2. Refractive errors

       11.3.3. Heterophoria or heterotropia

    11.4. Ears

    11.5. Nose and sinuses

       11.5.1. Acute sinus headache

       11.5.2. Other diseases of nose or sinuses

12.8. Facial pain not fulfilling criteria in groups 11 or 12

13. *Headache not classifiable*

E. Types of Primary Headache

1. *Migraine*

Migraine, one of the most frequently experienced forms of head pain, does not represent a single entity. There are two primary variants and several less common variants. Migraine is a complex form of head pain whose mechanism or mechanisms remain incompletely understood. Recent epidemiologic studies in subjects between 12 and 80 years reveal that 17.6% of women and 5.7% of men had one or more migraine headaches per year (10). Projecting these data to the U.S. population, 18 million women and 5.6 million men currently suffer from severe migraine headaches. Typically, migraine is a disorder affecting young adults. First migraine attacks can be experienced at any age, but the peak incidence is between 25 and 34 years. The overwhelming majority of migraine sufferers experience their first attack before the age of 40 years (11).

The most common form of migraine is migraine without aura. Migraine with aura occurs in the minority of sufferers. It is not uncommon to find both of these primary forms of migraine in the same individual. The remaining types of migraine attacks include some unusual migraine variants: familial hemiplegic migraine, basilar migraine, migraine aura without headache, migraine with prolonged aura, ophthalmoplegic migraine, retinal migraine, childhood periodic syndromes that are felt to be precursors to or associated with migraine, and a variety of complications of migraine including migrainous infarction.

Migraine is a paroxysmal disorder. Clearly defined attacks of head pain occur but are separated by intervals of freedom from head pain. The clinical features representing diagnostic criteria are detailed in Table 1 (2).

Table 1 Migraine

Migraine without aura
Previously used term: *common migraine*
Description: idiopathic, recurring headache disorder manifesting in attacks lasting 4–72 hours.
Typical characteristics: unilateral location, pulsating quality, moderate or severe intensity, aggravation by routine physical activity, and association with nausea, photo- and phonophobia.

Migraine with aura
Previously used terms: *classic migraine, classical migraine, ophthalmic, hemiparesthetic, hemiplegic, or aphasic migraine, migraine accompagnée, complicated migraine*
Description: idiopathic, recurring disorder manifesting with attacks of neurological symptoms unequivocally localizable to cerebral cortex or brainstem, usually gradually developed over 5–20 minutes and usually lasting less than 60 minutes.
Migraine with typical aura: consisting of homonymous visual disturbances, hemisensory symptoms, hemiparesis or dysphasia or combinations thereof; gradual development, duration under 1 hour and complete reversibility of the aura associated with headache.
Migraine with prolonged aura: consisting of one or more aura symptoms lasting more than 60 minutes and less than a week; normal neuroimaging.
Familial hemiplegic migraine: migraine with aura including hemiparesis and where at least one first-degree relative has identical attacks.
Basilar migraine: formerly known as *basilar artery migraine, Bickerstaff's migraine, syncopal migraine;* migraine with aura symptoms clearly originating from the brainstem or from both occipital lobes, for example, visual symptoms in both the temporal and nasal fields of both eyes, dysarthria, vertigo, tinnitus, decreased hearing, double vision, ataxia, bilateral paresthesias, bilateral pareses, decreased level of consciousness.
Migraine aura without headache: formerly known as *migraine equivalents, acephalgic migraine;* migrainous aura unaccompanied by headache.
Migraine with acute-onset aura: migraine with aura developing fully in less than 5 minutes; extensive investigations usually necessary to rule out thromboembolic transient ischemic attack.

Table 1 Continued

Ophthalmoplegic migraine
Description: repeated attacks of headache associated with paresis of one or more cranial nerves (III, IV, VI) in the absence of demonstrable intracranial lesion.

Retinal migraine
Description: repeated attacks of monocular scotoma or blindness lasting less than 1 hour and associated with headache; ocular or structural vascular disorder ruled out.

Childhood periodic syndromes that may be precursors to or associated with migraine
Previously used terms: *migraine equivalents*
Benign paroxysmal vertigo of childhood
Description: probably a heterogeneous disorder characterized by brief attacks of vertigo in otherwise healthy children.
Alternating hemiplegia of childhood
Description: infantile attacks of hemiplegia involving each side alternately; associated with other paroxysmal phenomena and mental impairment.

Complications of migraine
Status migrainosus: attack of migraine with headache phase lasting more than 72 hours despite treatment; headache-free intervals of less than 4 hours (sleep not included).
Migrainous infarction: formerly known as *complicated migraine;* one or more migrainous aura symptoms not fully reversible within 7 days and/or associated with neuroimaging confirmation of ischemic infarction.

In spite of continuing research activity, the exact pathophysiology of migraine remains unknown. A strong genetic tendency has been noted that results in a predisposition for imbalance of neurochemical tone and cephalic blood flow (12).

Although the traditional theory to explain migraine states that the symptoms known as aura are a result of vasoconstriction and head pain is a result of painful vasodilation, multiple neurobiological changes set off a cascade of events leading to any or all of the symptomatology known as migraine. Neurotransmitters such as serotonin, dopamine, and noradrenalin in addition to a variety of neuropeptides, prostaglandins, estrogens, and other substances will undoubtedly be implicated. The exact contribution of each remains to be unraveled (13).

The International Headache Society treatment recommendations for migraine are outlined in an adapted form in Table 2. All patients diagnosed with migraine require an acute attack–aborting medication. Preventive therapy is indicated if migraine occurs more than two times per month and does not respond adequately to "instant relief" therapy (14).

2. *Tension-type headache*

Tension-type headache typically begins as a paroxysmal disorder closely related to tension or stress. Tension-type headache may progress into a chronic condition in which head pain is perceived nearly daily and lacks obvious association to psychological or other situational factors. Although tension-type headache and migraine have been debated to be a spectrum disorder of one illness, the International Headache Society views tension-type headache and migraine as distinct clinical entities. Tension-type headache and migraine can certainly coexist, but they require somewhat different management approaches (2).

The overwhelming majority of headaches fall into the category of tension type. Similar to migraine, the majority of patients with chronic tension-type headache are women. Research, however, has failed to provide any specific explanation for this clinical observation (15,16). The International Headache Society diagnostic criteria for tension-type headache are found in Table 3 and enumerate the clinical features (2).

Current research negates the simplistic understanding that tension-type headache is simply a psychological disorder. There is also little evidence that excessive muscle contraction is the primary cause of tension-type headache in the majority of persons diagnosed with this ailment. Muscle contraction

Table 2 Treatment Recommendations for Migraine

Migraine without aura: Treatment of attacks
Since migraine attacks do not usually occur more than once or twice a week, acute treatment medications should not be used more than six times per month.

Analgesics

Nonsteroidal anti-inflammatory drugs

Acetylsalicylic acid (aspirin) 900–1000 mg

Ibuprofen 1200–1800 mg

Naproxen sodium 550–1100 mg

Ketorolac 30–90 mg IM

Acetaminophen 1000 mg

Antiemetics: indicated for nausea/vomiting and for promoting normal gastrointestinal activity; should be combined with analgesics or ergotamine preparations to enhance efficacy and tolerability

Metoclopramide 10 mg

Ergotamine preparations

Tablets or suppositories: 1–2 mg, maximum 4 mg/24 hr, not to be repeated in less than 4 days; maximum 16 mg/month; for no more than 6 attacks/month

Dihydroergotamine preparations

Intranasal formulation: one metered spray = 0.5 mg dihydroergotamine

Initially one spray into each nostril, repeated once after 15–20 minutes if necessary; not to be repeated within 4 days; for no more than 6 attacks/month

Subcutaneous or intramuscluar injection, intravenous administration (slowly over 10 minutes): to 1 mg (1 mg/cc, 1 vial); not to be repeated in less than 4 days; for no more than 6 attacks/month

Sumatriptan

Subcutaneous injections of 6 mg by autoinjector; second dose only if headache recurs within 4–24 hours after the first dose; no second injection if the first one fails; maximum 2 injections within 24 hours; weekly or monthly maximum use not yet established

Table 2 Continued

Migraine without aura: **Prophylactic treatment**
Beta blockers
Propranolol 40–160 mg, metoprolol 100–200 mg (propranolol
or metoprolol in divided doses or propranolol LA once daily),
nadolol 40–120 mg
Calcium channel blockers
Verapamil 240–360 mg daily in 3–4 divided doses
Tricyclic antidepressants
May be combined with beta blockers or calcium antagonists; for
special indications as listed:
Migraine with very frequent attacks
Migraine and medication misuse
Migraine and sleep disorder
Migraine and tension-type headache
Migraine and depression (may require higher doses)
Amitriptyline or doxepin 10–75 mg at night; if both fail, nor-
triptyline or imipramine 10–75 mg at night
Note: Imipramine and amitriptyline, effective in chronic headache but
not well tolerated, may be replaced by less toxic antidepressants, as
in current psychiatric and pain management.

Migraine with aura: Treatment of attacks
Generally the same as with migraine without aura; the use of vaso-
constrictors such as ergotamine and sumatriptan is controversial
during the aura phase of migraine.

Migraine with aura: Prophylaxis
Generally the same as with migraine without aura.

Status migrainosus
Since this condition is rare, the correct diagnosis must be established
before treatment is initiated. Consider hospital admission if headache
is very severe and has lasted for longer than 5 days, in the absence
of medication overuse or misuse. Treatment may require intravenous
rehydration, antiemetics, and steroids (dexamethasone 4–16 mg per
day with subsequent tapering course); and/or repetitive dihydroergotamine. Simultaneously, initiate prophylactic treatment.

Note: These suggestions indicate common practice but are not intended to
represent a professional standard.

Table 3   Tension-Type Headache

Episodic tension-type headache
Previously used terms: *tension headache, muscle contraction headache, psychomyogenic headache, stress headache, ordinary headache, essential headache, idiopathic headache, and psychogenic headache*
Description: recurrent episodes of headache lasting minutes to days; typically pressing/tightening in quality, of mild or moderate intensity, bilateral in location and not worsened with routine physical activity; nausea absent but photophobia or phonophobia present. Increased levels of tenderness of pericranial muscles and positive EMG possibly present.

Chronic tension-type headache
Previously used terms: *chronic daily headache*
Description: headache present for at least 15 days each month for at least 6 months; headache usually pressing/tightening in quality, mild or moderate in severity, bilateral and not worse with routine physical activity; nausea, photophobia or phonophobia may occur; increased levels of tenderness of pericranial muscles and positive EMG possibly present.

---

is a possible headache mechanism for some patients only. The pathophysiology of tension-type headache remains a mystery (17,18).

The management of the individual diagnosed with tension-type headache is likely to involve a combination of approaches: psychological intervention, physiological activities aimed at bodily relaxation, and pharmacological approaches. The International Headache Society treatment recommendations are listed in an adapted form in Table 4. The successful management of tension-type headache is labor intensive but can be accomplished using the principles outlined. Most tension-type headaches respond to simple analgesics such as aspirin or acetaminophen in preparations with or without caffeine. There is a risk of habituation and transformation of episodic tension-type headache into the chronic form induced

Table 4 Treatment Recommendations for Tension-Type
Headache (Episodic and Chronic)

Treatment of attacks
Avoid symptomatic drug treatment. If analgesics are used,
ibuprofen or naproxen are preferred. If they are taken for more
than 8 days/month, replace them with prophylactic treatment.

Prophylaxis
Tricyclic antidepressants
   Amitriptyline or doxepin 10–75 mg at night; if both fail, nortri-
     ptyline or imipramine 10–75 mg; or other antidepressants

Note: These suggestions indicate common practice but are not intended to
represent a professional standard.

by "instant relief" medication overuse, otherwise known as
drug rebound headache. Sedative hypnotics have little value
in the long-term picture. Traditional antidepressants have
proved effective in patients with or without depression, demonstrating this class of medication's ability to enhance the
activity of the endogenous pain-control system (14).

3. *Cluster headache*

Cluster headache is the most debilitating of the three primary
headache types. The extreme pain of cluster headache and its
tendency to disrupt sleep cause distress and progressive emotional and physical suffering (19).

Cluster headache is not as common as migraine, and unlike migraine, it is predominantly a male disorder. Cluster
headache typically begins in the sufferer's 20s. No strong
genetic component has been identified, although cases of cluster headache occurring in sequential generations in specific
families have been observed. The rather strikingly consistent
clinical features of cluster headache make it one of the most
easily definable forms of primary headache (19). The International Headache Society criteria for cluster headache and
cluster headache variants are in Table 5 (2).

Table 5   Cluster Headache and Chronic Paroxysmal Hemicrania

Cluster headache

Previously used terms: *erythroprosopalgia of Bing, ciliary or migrainous neuralgia (Harris), erythromelagia of the head, Horton's headache, histaminic cephalagia, petrosal neuralgia (Gardner), sphenopalatine, Vidian and Sluder's neuralgia, hemicrania periodica neuralgiformis*

Description: attacks of strictly unilateral pain orbitally, supra-orbitally, and/or temporally, lasting 15–180 minutes and occurring from once every other day to 8 times a day. Associated with one or more of the following symptoms: conjunctival injection, lacrimation, nasal congestion, rhinorrhea, forehead and facial sweating, miosis, ptosis, eyelid edema. Attacks occurring in series lasting for weeks or months (so-called cluster periods) separated by remission periods usually lasting months or years. Chronic symptoms in about 10%.

Episodic cluster headache

Description: occurs in periods lasting 7 days to 1 year separated by pain-free periods lasting 14 days or more.

Chronic cluster headache

Description: attacks occurring for more than 1 year without remission or with remission lasting less than 14 days.

Chronic cluster headache unremitting from onset

Previously used term: *primary chronic*

Description: attacks occurring for more than 1 year without remission or with remission lasting less than 14 days from onset.

Chronic cluster headache evolved from episodic

Previously used term: *secondary chronic*

Description: attacks occurring initially in periods lasting 7 days to 1 year separated by pain-free periods lasting 14 days or more, followed by an unremitting course for at least 1 year.

Chronic paroxysmal hemicrania

Previously used terms: Sjaastad's syndrome

Description: attacks with largely the same characteristics of pain and associated symptoms and signs as cluster headache, but shorter lasting, more frequent, occurring mostly in females, and absolutely responsive to indomethacin therapy.

Although cluster headache is easy to define, pathogenesis remains speculative. The clinical features suggest symptomatic expression of a mixture of vascular and neurogenic dysfunctional mechanisms affecting the intracavernous carotid artery. Hypothalamic involvement is indisputable, but the exact details remain an enigma (19).

Successful management of cluster headache involves patient education and aggressive pharmacologic therapy. The International Headache Society treatment recommendations are in Table 6 (14).

II. PAIN, HEADACHE, AND NEURALGIAS IN THE ELDERLY

A. Pain

The majority of all neurologic patients seen in clinical practice are elderly (20). The U.S. Census Bureau has estimated that by the year 2000 there will be 31 million persons over the age of 65 in the United States, with 13 million being over age 75 (21). It is also recognized that the fastest-growing segment of the American population is the group aged 65 and older (20). In spite of such estimates, most researchers and clinicians are more interested in neurological disorders of childhood and young or middle adulthood than in neurological disorders of the elderly. Similarly, in the pain literature, most research has been conducted in adult or pediatric populations, with few investigators addressing the issue of pain, particularly headache, in the elderly.

This neglect may be due to the myth that aches and pains are a normal accompaniment of aging (22). It is vital that elderly patients who present with pain, however, not be dismissed as normal. Many of the degenerative disorders or diseases observed in elderly persons (arthritis, cancer, neuromuscular disorders, trigeminal neuralgia, postherpetic neuralgia, or degenerative disk disease) are associated with significant

Table 6 Treatment Recommendations for Cluster Headache

Treatment of attacks

Oxygen inhalation at 100% at 7 L/min for 15–20 minutes while seated leaning forward

Dihydroergotamine nasal spray (0.5 mg) into each nostril or dihydroergotamine injection (0.5–1 mg) subcutaneously or intramuscularly self-administered by patient

Sumatriptan: one 6 mg subcutaneous injection for each attack with a maximum of two 6 mg injections in any 24-hour period

Note: Acute attack therapy should usually be given in addition to prophylactic treatment.

Prophylactic treatment for episodic cluster headache

Verapamil 240–480 mg daily in divided doses

Lithium in divided doses to maintain a therapeutic level of 0.5–1.0 mmol/L

Prednisone in addition to verapamil and/or lithium to "break the cycle," although it can be used alone as first line: 40–80 mg daily to start and a tapering course over 2–3 weeks to follow

Ergotamine tartrate or dihydroergotamine mesylate 1–2 mg daily for a maximum period of 6 weeks (only if other treatments fail)—safety limits appear to be higher than with migraine

Note: Treatment should continue for usual duration of cluster before reducing over a period of 1 week.

Prophylactic treatment for chronic cluster headache

Verapamil as above

Lithium as above

Verapamil and lithium combined

Prednisone as above

Note: These suggestions indicate common practice but are not intended to represent a professional standard.

pain and abnormal function (23–25). It is also assumed that pain is less common in the elderly than in younger patients, although the age-associated morbidity of pain has been reported as twice as great in those >60 years when compared to those <60 years (26). In a survey of community-dwelling people over age 60, Ferrell noted that 25–50% reported having pain (27).

Although elderly persons may experience more chronic pain-producing conditions, they are usually less likely to report pain. Only 7–10% of patients seen in pain clinics are over age 65 (28). Elderly patients are less likely to present with pain because they do not wish to displease the physician (20); they tend to have multiple health complaints, and pain may be low on this priority list (21); they believe that one must endure pain as part of life (22); and/or they fear expressing the complaint of pain because of past experiences (23,29,30). Some individuals may be unable to provide an accurate pain history due to cognitive impairment.

In some acute pain conditions, the appearance of pain or the physiological response to pain may be modified by advanced age. For example, there is evidence that pain associated with myocardial infarction (MI) is less with advanced age (31). In a survey of 1474 middle-aged and elderly MI patients, 30% of those over age 70 did not experience pain as a major symptom (31). In other situations, the pain may be similar, but the body's response to inflammation may be altered due to the decrease in white cell response and vital sign changes (24). Cauna cautions that these assertions be viewed cautiously, since basic processes of nociception are influenced only minimally by age (32).

1. *Common painful conditions*

The painful conditions most often observed clinically in geriatric patients are joint disease and low back pain. As in other cases, musculoskeletal or joint disease is often taken as a normal accompaniment to aging. Relationships have been shown, however, between musculoskeletal conditions and disability (33). Hughes and colleagues reported that joint impairment is an important risk factor for disability (33).

Low back pain (LBP) occurs in 90% of the adult population (34). In aging patients, it accounts for approximately $20 million in medical and economic costs each year in the

United States (34,35). Low back pain, however, is not in itself a diagnosis, and it is important that the clinician determine the etiology of the patient's LBP problem. The majority of patients presenting with low back pain and/or sciatica have pathology primarily affecting the fourth and fifth lumbar vertebrae and lumbosacral joint (36,37). Discussion of appropriate LBP examinations in geriatric patients may be found in Ferrell and Swezey (27,34).

2. *Treatment for pain*

There are several conservative treatments for managing chronic pain in the elderly. Pharmacological therapy (used with caution) consisting of simple analgesics and, if necessary, low-dose antidepressants and muscle relaxants are often helpful. Some patients may benefit from short-term NSAIDs (nonsteroidal anti-inflammatory drugs). Many pharmacological treatments are controversial. The opiate analgesics Darvon, Talwin, and methadone should be avoided in the elderly because of their negative side effects in this group (27). (A review of drug therapy for geriatric patients may be found in Portenoy [22]). Transcutaneous electrical nerve stimulation (TENS), physical therapy (traction and manipulation utilizing stretching techniques), and rest and exercise are often effective nonpharmacological strategies for pain management (27,34). Psychotherapy may be indicated in many cases of geriatric chronic pain due to the significant depressive symptoms that occur (24). In most instances, an integration of treatments or a multimodal treatment approach provides the optimal management of geriatric chronic pain (22).

3. *Psychosocial factors*

Stress and depression are prevalent in the elderly. Thus, the opportunity for pain to intensify stress and depression (or vice versa) may be more increased in older individuals than in the general population (24). Although psychological factors are rarely the primary cause of chronic pain in the elderly, they commonly occur secondarily and impair functioning and response to therapy (22). Eighty-seven percent of patients in chronic pain clinics have depression; conversely, 59% of patients requesting treatment for depression have recurring pain (38). In a study by Chaturvedi comparing depressed and nondepressed pain patients, depressed patients were more often elderly as compared to nondepressed patients (39). In a similar study, Chaturvedi and colleagues reported that depressive symptoms such as depressed mood, loss of appetite, loss of weight, and irritability were significantly more often reported by older patients as compared to younger patients (40).

In addition, the many changes that occur in an individual's environment after age 60 often arouse anxieties, fears, and dysphoria. Retirement is often a source of significant stress and anxiety. The patient may be faced with a reduction in economic resources, changes in relationships (such as a decrease in social contacts with coworkers), and/or boredom (24,41). Many patients report increased loneliness during old age, due to the death of friends and family members. Other potential losses include changes in social environment or residence (leaving one's home of 25 years to move to a smaller home or a care facility), lack of close friends (particularly those who knew the older person as a child), and lack of love and excitement (41). The patients may also suffer from increased hospitalizations or chronic illnesses that may intensify pain behaviors.

B. Headache

Headache often begins during childhood and increases through adulthood, but there seems to be a point where headache symptoms begin to diminish and almost disappear. If headache frequency and age were graphed, the result would resemble an inverted U, with the very young and very old experiencing lower rates of headache, and young and middle-aged adults experiencing higher rates (42). Table 7 lists the prevalence of headache (occurring at least one time every two weeks) by age and gender (43).

In a large series of subjects over 65 years of age, approximately 17% reported having frequent headaches (44).

Table 7 Prevalence of Headache by Age and Gender

Age	% Male	% Female
16–19	8	13
20–29	9	22
30–39	13	26
40–49	8	23
50–59	7	13
60–69	3	11
70+	10	21

The correlates most strongly associated with increase in headache incidence included, more frequently, pain in the neck and back, depressive symptoms and the patient's self-reported state of health and, less commonly, impaired vision, history of myocardial infarction, joint pain, and sleep disturbances (44,45). Headache was the 10th most common symptom reported in 1922 women and the 14th most common symptom reported in 1136 men in another sample of individuals over age 65 (46). Table 8 lists the prevalence of headache in elderly patients in two investigations by Hale and colleagues (25,46).

1. *Headache types*

The onset of migraine is very rare after age 50 (2%), although some patients with migraine continue to have attacks well into

Table 8 Prevalence of Headache in Elderly by Age and Gender

Age group	Study 1 (1987)		Study 2 (1986)	
	% Women	% Men	% Women	% Men
65–69	0	0	14.9	10.5
70–74	10.8	3.5	14.8	5.4
75–80	11.8	4.8	14.0	7.5
81–84	11.6	8.9	13.0	5.7
85+	9.6	3.9	8.3	3.0

their later years (47). Waters reported that the prevalence of migraine in women age 75 and older was 10%, as opposed to 30% in women ages 21 to 34 (48). Migraine headaches are the most prevalent between ages 35 and 45 (10). Similar to the general population, elderly patients are more likely to present with migraine without aura than migraine with aura.

Complicated migraine (distinguished by the presence of prominent associated neurologic symptoms often including paresthesia and frequent prolongation of neurologic deficits beyond the duration of the actual headache) poses significant diagnostic dilemmas in elderly patients (49). In particular, hemiplegic migraine, ophthalmoplegic migraine, and basilar migraine must be diagnosed with caution. In elderly patients presenting with these types of symptoms, causes of transient ischemic attacks, syncope, or other significant processes should be investigated (49).

Temporal arteritis is a relatively common headache disorder in the elderly. It reaches its greatest incidence in patients over age 70. The cause is thought to be an autoimmune reaction of elastic tissue, which most commonly affects the superficial temporal, ophthalmic, vertebral, and external carotid arteries and occipital branches (50). Partial or complete visual loss occurs in at least 50% of patients (49). Symptoms include malaise, fatigue, weight loss, low-grade fever, jaw claudication, visual disturbances, and symptoms referable to brainstem dysfunction (51). Pain is usually described as throbbing and sharp, dull, and burning (51).

In a retrospective study of 24 patients with biopsy-proven temporal arteritis, only six had headaches exclusively in the temporal area. Seven had headache affecting the temple, frontal, vertex, and occipital areas; two had generalized headaches; seven had headaches not involving the temple; and two did not experience headaches (51). Confirmatory tests for this disorder include an elevated erythrocyte sedimentation rate and biopsy of a long segment of artery showing the classic pathology (49). It has been suggested that, unless there are strong contraindications, a short course of steroid therapy be given to patients even with normal erythrocyte sedimentation rates and a negative biopsied artery because of the potential for false negative results and the dangers of blindness or brain infarction when deferring treatment (52,53).

Solomon and colleagues conducted a computer search of outpatients with a diagnosis of headache or temporal arteritis seen during 1988 at the Cleveland Clinic Foundation (54). Of 9950 patients, 359 age 65 or older had a diagnosis of headache, and 64 more were diagnosed with temporal arteritis (54). Migraine was 56% less frequent in older patients (15% vs. 34%), but tension headache was more commonly diagnosed in older patients (27% vs. 20%) (54). Only 5% of tension headache sufferers, however, report that headaches began after age 60 (55). At the present time, the etiology of chronic tension headache is thought to be at least partially centrally mediated, rather than exclusively dependent on excessive muscle contraction (56). Recent research indicates that tension headaches may be a more mild form of migraine and that the two disorders are at opposite ends of a continuum (56).

Cluster headache has typically gone undiagnosed in the elderly, because many clinicians have felt that this type of headache disorder did not present in older age groups. It can, however, begin at any age (19). Although cluster headache is predominantly a male disorder at all ages, a higher percentage of women develop this type of headache after age 60 than at younger ages (45). Patients who have unremitting cluster headaches (chronic cluster) typically have an older age of onset (19).

X-ray findings of cervical spondylosis and other cervical arthropathies are common in elderly patients (57). Headache of cervical origin typically results from the spread of pain from noxious stimulation of structures in the cervical spine, adjacent musculature, and connective tissue (57). Another common problem in the elderly is malocclusion and resulting temporomandibular joint misalignment. This produces inflammation in and about the joint and frequently pain in front of and around the ear (57).

Some researchers have attempted to establish a relationship between Parkinson's disease (PD) and headache. In studies, headache was noted in 25 of 71 patients with PD (35.2%) (58), and it occurred in 41.2% of PD patients as opposed to 13.4% of controls (59). The nuchal, temporal, and occipital regions were the most common sites, and dull pain was reported more frequently than pulsating pain (58). No correlation was evident between rigidity in the nuchal region or extremities and headache. In a survey of 223 chronic PD sufferers and 291 sex and age-matched controls, Lorentz found little differences in the prevalence of headache between PD patients and controls (60). Male PD patients did show a higher prevalence of moderate to severe migraine than controls (60).

2. *Pathophysiology of headache in the elderly*

Many reasons may exist for the decreased incidence of headache, particularly migraine, in older individuals. One of the most powerful arguments is the biochemical changes that accompany aging. The neurotransmitter, serotonin, has been implicated in the headache process for many years. Urine levels of 5-hydroxyindoleacetic acid (5-HIAA), a serotonin metabolite, often increase and platelet serotonin levels decrease during migraine attacks. In 1987, Raskin reported that 15 previously headache-free patients, who underwent electrode implantation in the periaqueductal gray region for intractable pain, soon developed a jabbing pain in the eye on the same side as the procedure followed by a throbbing headache (61). It was proposed that unstable serotonergic neurotransmission leads to increased raphe neuronal firing rates, followed by cerebral circulatory alterations and symptoms of migraine (61).

As one ages, there is a reduction in serotonin or S2 receptors. This works similarly to medications used in treating migraine headaches (i.e., sumatriptan or dihydroergotamine), which are thought to reduce migraine by altering serotonin receptors (62). Hormones that alter serotonergic receptor activity (such as ovarian hormones, which may account for the higher prevalence of migraine in females and menstrual migraine symptoms) are also less abundant in the elderly. Finally, the arteriosclerotic aging process results in less compliant blood vessels; thus, there is a decrease in dilatation and constriction in response to the migraine attack (45).

3. *Headache and medical disorders*

In evaluating an elderly patient presenting with headaches, it is important to obtain a careful history and perform a detailed physical and neurologic examination (see Table 9). Based on the results of these evaluations, further diagnostic studies may be indicated (57). EEG (assess for focal, paroxysmal, or diffuse abnormalities), CT or MRI of the head (look for lesions, hematomas, hemorrhage, or infarction), topographic brain mapping or evoked potentials (examine deficits in concentration or memory), and/or lumbar puncture (rule out meningitis or subarachnoid hemorrhage) are often employed. Regular recurrence of headache for a number of years is suggestive of benign headaches, but the sudden onset of severe headaches

Table 9   Guidelines for Basic Evaluation of Headaches in the Elderly

---

1.   History of headache
      a.   location and character of pain
      b.   precipitating factors
      c.   longevity of pain
2.   Detailed physical examination
      a.   potential extracranial causes (i.e., disorders of the sinuses, temporomandibular joints, and dentition)
      b.   areas of local tenderness or trigger zones
      c.   possibility of cervical spine disease
3.   Detailed neurological examination
      a.   evidence of diffuse cerebral dysfunction
      b.   evidence of focal neurologic signs

Source: Reference 57.

is suggestive of a more serious etiology requiring additional diagnostic examination.

In the elderly, headaches have been associated with serious medical conditions (63). This accentuates the need for careful and thorough medical and neurologic evaluation. Headache may be a warning sign for a serious disorder such as stroke, vascular inflammation, Parkinson's disease, subdural hematoma, brain tumor, meningitis, glaucoma, or accelerated hypertension. Lavyne and Patterson reported that headache is the first symptom of brain tumor approximately 50% of the time (64). A unilateral orbital or frontal headache associated with Horner's syndrome may be evidence of dissecting aneurysm or occlusion of the ipsilateral carotid artery (65). Explosive headache is considered an omen of a threatening intracranial event, such as intracranial hemorrhage or mass lesions (66). Headache has been observed in approximately 50% of patients with vertebrobasilar stenosis or occlusion, in 35% of patients with involvement of the internal carotid artery, and in 33% of patients with middle cerebral artery involvement (57,63).

Many serious conditions in the elderly have associated headaches that are distinguishable from benign headaches. In glaucoma, in addition to complaints of failing vision or the appearance of halos around specular light sources, headache pain is often dull, with a mild pulsating component localized to the periorbital regions, the forehead, and the temporal area, possibly radiating to the occiput (57). Intracranial mass lesions usually produce headaches that are nonthrobbing and steady (deep, aching pain), with pain most intense in the morning and decreasing when the patient assumes an upright position for some length of time (67). The headache history is often described as initially intermittent, but fairly constant in location, progressing to a more continuous pattern. Intracranial aneurysms may result in headaches that are periodic and uniformly localized to a single head region, typically involving the frontal and sometimes periorbital head regions (57). Extraocular muscle palsies and visual field deficits provide extra credence to this diagnosis (57). Subarachnoid hemorrhage may be indicated by explosive episodes of severe headache, with or without alterations of neurologic function (67).

Some studies have found that headache sufferers have higher diastolic blood pressure (42). Although hypertensive headache has no specific diagnostic features, the pain is usually localized in the occipital region, with the headache most pronounced during awakening and often diminishing 2–3 hours after arising (57). A relationship appears to exist between intensity of headache and degree of hypertension; a reduction of blood pressure often results in a decrease in headache (42).

The increased incidence of falls in the elderly often results in trauma or injury to the head and neck. Headaches associated with head or neck injuries are termed posttraumatic headaches (PTH). PTH is often associated with a host of other symptoms including impaired memory and concentration, dizziness, depression, anxiety, tinnitus, and visual disturbances (68). Posttraumatic symptoms may be compounded by the presence of age-related cognitive deficits or other age-related disturbances. The situation is made even more difficult when elderly patients present with headaches, but do not remember a bump to the head. The physician may need to enlist the help of family members or those close to the patient when working with this population (22).

In a retrospective study of geriatric headache patients, eight types of head and face pain were identified (see Table 10a) (Riebman TL. Geriatric headaches: A retrospective review. Personal communication). Various major stressful life events were reported as being associated with headache by many patients (see Table 10b). Treatment consisted of medication, biofeedback, psychotherapy, occipital nerve blocks, or combination therapy. Patients with posttraumatic headaches were least likely to respond to treatment. Also, the presence of hypertension and/or poor eating habits was associated with

Table 10a Most Common
Headache Types in Elderly Patients

Headache Type	Percentage
Vascular	30
Mixed	26
Tension	18
Posttraumatic	16

worse treatment outcome (69). Others have reported that medical problems such as hypertension, vertigo and dizziness, peptic ulcer, gastroesophageal reflux, and depression and anxiety were more common in recurrent idiopathic headache patients than age- and sex-matched nonheadache controls (69).

4. *Psychosocial factors*

In addition to hormonal and biochemical influences, psychosocial factors may also lead to a decrease in headaches in the elderly. Stress, while not directly causing headache or pain, is known to exacerbate a preexisting painful condition. Most individuals report that a primary source of stress is their occupation. Through retirement, elderly patients often find relief from a principal source of stress. Other sources of stress

Table 10b Major Stressful Life Events Associated with Headache

Stressful Life Event	Percentage
Chronic illness	31
Family problems	10
Caring for an invalid	6
Death of a spouse	5
Work-related stress	5
Alcohol/drug abuse	4
Death of a child/relative	3
Displaced from residence	2

for many younger individuals are increased responsibilities, particularly parenting duties, with subsequent losses of time for relaxation and pleasurable activities. In the vast majority of elderly individuals, there is a cessation of parenting duties and a decrease in responsibilities. Thus, elderly individuals often have more time for leisure activities or other hobbies.

In some geriatric patients, stressful life events such as boredom, alcoholism, lack of love and excitement, depression, illness, and poor relations with children may result in increased headache (41). Patients suffering from chronic headaches also may become depressed because of the continuous head pain. Ziegler and colleagues (70) found levels of depression were significantly greater among subjects reporting a history of severe headaches as compared to those without a headache history. Cox and Thomas observed that the reduction of headaches in 14 headache sufferers led to the reduction of depression (71).

5. *Treatment of headache*

Similar treatments as described previously for general pain may be used in managing headaches in elderly patients (see Tables 2, 4, and 6). Analgesics used in moderation, low-dose antidepressants, or muscle relaxants are often useful in this population. Nonpharmacological treatments should be employed where appropriate. Proper rest and exercise, dietary changes, and physical therapy are often beneficial (67). Psychotherapy or cognitive behavioral therapy is necessary for some patients. Recently, research has indicated that biofeedback may be effective in managing headaches in many elderly patients. Although for many years biofeedback has been considered an impressive nonpharmacological treatment for headache (72,73), it has been used less often with geriatric patients. Several investigators have reported that biofeedback may be useful in older patients if it is individualized and if the patient is motivated and able to cognitively appreciate the mechanisms involved (74,75).

C. Neuralgia

Neuralgias involve areas of facial pain (or related structures) associated with one or more branches of the cranial nerves. At times, neuralgias may overlap and resemble each other. It is likely that the mechanism of pain in all neuralgias is the same (76). Trigeminal neuralgia is the most common and well-known type.

Trigeminal neuralgia (TN) is a condition which, in approximately 90% of cases, occurs in individuals over 40 years of age (57). The incidence increases with age, and rates are slightly higher for women than men (77). TN involves branches of the trigeminal nerve, with only one division (most frequently the second) typically involved. The pain is often of such intensity that the whole side of the face is in pain. It occurs in sharp lancinating paroxysms that may last for several seconds or minutes, but usually from 20 to 30 seconds (76). It is often initiated by stimulating trigger zones located around the mouth, nares, or eyes. Activities such as touching, washing, chewing, swallowing, air blowing on the face, or talking can stimulate the trigger zones and initiate severe, high-intensity jabs of pain (76). The pain is usually described as sudden, intense, sharp, superficial, stabbing, or burning (77). The patient is asymptomatic between paroxysms.

The etiology of this disease is undetermined at the present time. A theory by Fromm and colleagues suggests that the peripheral trigeminal nerve is in an excitatory state due to chronic irritation from an external pressure or irritant (78). Action potentials then become disinhibited (due to failure of segmental inhibition in the trigeminal nucleus), resulting in a hyperactive sensory circuit and paroxysmal discharges in the trigeminal nucleus (78). In younger individuals, trigeminal neurlagia may be a manifestation of other neurologic disease. Disturbances in the trigeminal nerve are relatively common in multiple sclerosis, but this is usually only in younger patients (76). Cerebellopontine angle tumors have been reported in a small number of patients diagnosed with trigeminal neuralgia (79). Hypertension also appears to be a risk factor (80).

Medical therapy is indicated as the first line of treatment for TN (76) (Table 11a). The medications used are typically anticonvulsants (carbamazepine, phenytoin, chlorphenesin, baclofen) that inhibit or reduce synaptic neurotransmission (45). Analgesics and narcotics have little role in the treatment of TN. See Table 11a for a list of the most commonly used drugs in treating TN and their mechanism of action (77). Side effects include sedation, tremor, and nausea. Approximately 25–50% of patients receiving medical therapy will relapse in the long term. For patients who fail or cannot tolerate drug therapy, surgical treatment should be considered (see Table 11b) (77). A radiofrequency rhizotomy or glycerol injection should be considered before microvascular decompression.

Glossopharyngeal neuralgia (GN) is characterized by severe, burning pain in the tonsil and ear. It may be initiated by yawning, swallowing, or contact of food with the tonsillar region, and it almost always occurs on the left side. GN is rare; it is only 1% the incidence of TN. Ninety percent of

Table 11a Mechanisms of Medical Therapy for Trigeminal Neuralgia

	Carbamazepine (Tegretol)	Phenytoin (Dilantin)	Chlorphenesin (Maolate)	Baclofen (Lioresal)
Anticonvulsant activity	+ + +	+ + +	+	+
Muscle relaxant effect	+	+	+ + +	+ + +
Sedative effect	+ +	+	+ +	+ +
Analgesic effect	–	–	–	0

+ = degree of activity
0 = no activity
– = equivocal

Table 11b Comparison of Operative Procedures for Trigeminal Neuralgia

Type	Description	Complications
Radiofrequency rhizotomy	90% effective; minor percutaneous needle procedure; brief hospital stay	Facial sensory loss often quite severe; corneal hypesthesia (10%–15%) possible
Glycerol injection	85% effective; minor percutaneous needle procedure; brief hospital stay	Facial sensitivity loss is slight; persistent corneal hypesthesia; masseter weakness rare
Microvascular decompression	90% effective; major craniotomy; 4–10-day hospital stay	+4% serious post-operative complications 1% mortality

patients are over age 40 (77). The pain usually begins in the throat or ear but may radiate to the posterior third of the tongue, tonsils, pharynx, larynx, eustachian tube, or external auditory canal (77). If the patient does not respond to carbamazepine, baclofen, or clonazepam, the treatment of choice is intracranial section of the nerve (76,77).

Occipital neuralgia (ON) is often related to tension headaches and/or cervical spine disease. The pain is usually located in the occipital, suboccipital, and/or posterior parietal areas. Examination of the head may reveal marked tenderness over the occipital region at the origin of the greater occipital nerve (57). The pain is typically described as severe, sharp, unilateral, and radiating in an anterior position from the occipital regions. Trigger zones are activated by wearing a hat, use of a comb, or direct touching. The treatment consists of amitriptyline, local steroid and anesthetic injections and, lastly, C2 dorsal rhizotomy (77). ON may occur secondary to cervical spondylosis, craniocervical malformations, syringomyelia, and Arnold-Chiari malformations; it is often associated with nuchal muscle spasms (77). The pain may be in the same location, but is usually present for hours, days, or longer.

Postherpetic neuralgia (PN) occurs after a segmental herpes zoster eruption, due to activation of the varicella zoster virus in the trigeminal, geniculate, and dorsal root ganglion (81). To be diagnosed with PN, pain must have persisted for 1 month following the eruption. Approximately 25% of cases of PN occur in the trigeminal dermatomes, the vast majority in the first division (82). The incidence has been reported as 50% at age 60, 75% at age 70, and 10–15% in all cases (81).

A wide range of treatments with limited consistent success are avilable for PN. Some report that the disorder remits spontaneously (81). Corticosteriods during the acute infection appear to reduce the incidence of PN (45). In the acute phase, an elderly group treated with amantadine hydrochloride achieved total pain relief in half the time taken by a placebo group (83). The most extensively studied treatments for PN are tricyclic antidepressants. Amitriptyline (10–150 mg dosage) often provides moderate relief of pain in the majority of cases (84). Other treatments include topical capsaicin creams, nerve blocks, ethyl chloride spray, epidural injections, and TENS.

REFERENCES

1.   Ziegler DK. Headache: Public health problem. Neurol Clin 1990; 8:781–791.
2.   Headache Classification Committee of the International Headache Society. Classification and diagnostic criteria for headache disorders, cranial neuralgias, and facial pain. Cephalalgia 1988; 8(suppl 7):1–96.
3.   Linet MS, Stewart WF, Celentano DD, Ziegler DK, Sprecher M. An epidemiologic study of headache among adolescents and young adults. JAMA. 1989; 261:2211–2216.
4.   Wolff HG. Personality features and reactions of subjects with migraine. Arch Neurol Psychiatry 1937; 37:895–921.
5.   Heyck JRS. Pathogenesis of migraine. Res Clin Studies Headache 1969; 2:1–28.

6. Moskowitz MA. The neurobiology of vascular head pain. Ann Neurol 1984; 16:157-168.

7. Raskin NH. Headache, 2nd ed. New York: Churchill Livingstone, 1988;99-133.

8. Olesen J. Clinical and pathophysiological observations in migraine and tension-type headache explained by integration of vascular supraspinal and myofascial inputs. Pain 1991; 46:125-132.

9. Mondell BE. Evaluation of the patient presenting with headache. Med Clin North Am 1991; 75:521-524.

10. Stewart WF, Lipton RB, Celentano DD, Reed ML. Prevalence of migraine headache in the United States: Relation to age, income, race, and other sociodemographic factors. JAMA 1992; 267:64-69.

11. Selby G, Lance JW. Observations on 500 cases of migraine and allied vascular headache. J Neurol Neurosurg Psychiatry 1960; 23:23-32.

12. Russell MB, Hilden J, Sorenson SA, Olesen J. Familial occurrence of migraine without aura and migraine with aura. Neurology 1993; 43:1369-1373.

13. Diamond S. Migraine headaches. Med Clin North Am 1991; 75:545-566.

14. International Headache Society Education Committee. Treatment Recommendations, 1993.

15. Celentano DD, Linet MS, Stewart WF. Gender differences in the experiences of headache. Soc Sci Med 1990; 30:1289-1295.

16. Rasmussen BK, Jensen R, Schroll M, Olesen J. Epidemiology of headache in a general population—a prevalence study. J Clin Epidemiol 1991; 44:1147-1157.

17. Haynes SN, Cuevas J, Gannon LR. The psychophysiological etiology of muscle contraction-type headache. Headache 1982; 22:122-132.

18. Pikoff H. Is the muscular model of headache still viable? A review of conflicting data. Headache 1982; 24:186-198.

19. Kudrow L. Cluster headaches: Mechanisms and management. New York: Oxford University Press, 1980.

20. Adams RD, Victor M. The neurology of aging. In: Principles of Neurology. New York: McGraw Hill, 1993;526-536.

21. U.S. Bureau of the Census. Statistical Abstract of the United States—1988. Washington DC: U.S. Government Printing Office, 1988;108.

22. Portenoy RK, Farkash A. Practical management of non-malignant pain in the elderly. Geriatrics 1988; 43:29–47.

23. Forman WB, Stratton M. Current approaches to chronic pain in older patients. Geriatrics 1991; 46:47–52.

24. Kwentus JA, Harkins SW, Lignon N, Silverman JJ. Current concepts of geriatric pain and its treatment. Geriatrics 1985; 40:48–57.

25. Hale WE, Perkins LL, May FE, Marks RG, Stewart RB. Symptom prevalence in the elderly. JAGS 1986; 34:333–340.

26. Crook J, Rideout E, Browne G. The prevalence of pain complaints among a general population. Pain 1984; 18:299–314.

27. Ferrell BA, Ferrell BR. Principles of pain management in older people. Compr Therapy 1991; 17:53–58.

28. Sherman ED, Robillard E. Sensitivity to pain in relationship to age. In: Hansen PF, ed., Age with a Future: Proceedings of the Sixth Annual Congress of Gerontology. Philadelphia: F.A. Davis, 1964; 325–333.

29. Donovan MI. An historical view of pain management. Cancer Nursing 1989; 12:257–261.

30. Cleeland C. Barriers to cancer pain management. Oncology 1987; 1:19–26.

31. MacDonald JB. Coronary care in the elderly. Age Ageing 1983; 12:17–20.

32. Cauna N. The effects of aging on the receptor organs of the human dermis. In: Montaga W (ed.), Advances in Biology of the Skin, vol. 6. New York: Pergamon Press, 1965;63–94.

33. Hughes SL, Edelman PL, Singer RH, Chang RW. Joint impairment and self-reported disability in elderly persons. J Gerontol 1993; 48:S84–S92.

34. Swezey RL. Low back pain in the elderly: Practical management concerns. Geriatrics 1988; 43:39–44.

35. Hall HA. Back to school. Clin Orthop 1983; 179:10–17.

36. Grabias SL, Mankin HJ. Pain in the lower back. Bull Rheum Dis 1980; 30:1040–1045.

37. Porter RW, Hibbett C, Evans C. The natural history of root entrapment syndrome. Spine 1984; 8:418–421.

38. Lindsay PG, Wyckoff M. The depression-pain syndrome and

its response to antidepressants. Psychosomatics 1981; 22:571–577.

39. Chaturvedi SK. Depressed and non-depressed chronic pain patients. Pain 1987; 29:355–361.

40. Chaturvedi SK, Varma VK, Malhotra A. Depression in patients with non-organic chronic intractable pain. NIMHANS J 1985; 3:121–128.

41. Bana DS, Graham JR, Spierings ELH. Headache patients as they see themselves. Headache 1988; 28:403–408.

42. D'Allessandro R, Benassi G, Lenzi PL, Gamberini G, Sacquegna T, De Carolis P, Lugaresi E. Epidemiology of headache in the Republic of San Marino. J Neurol Psychiatry 1988; 51:21–27.

43. Paulin JM, Waal-Manning, HJ, Simpson FO, Knight RG. The prevalence of headache in a small New Zealand town. Headache 1985; 25:147–151.

44. Cook NR, Evans DA, Funkestein HH. Correlates of headache in a population-based cohort of elderly. Arch Neurol 1989; 46:1338–1344.

45. Baumel B, Eisner LS. Diagnosis and treatment of headache in the elderly. Med Clin North Am 1991; 75:661–675.

46. Hale WE, May FE, Marks RG, Moore MT, Stewart RB. Headache in the elderly: An evaluation of risk factors. Headache 1987; 27:272–276.

47. Wilkinson M. Clinical features of migraine. In: Vinken PJ, Bruyn GW (eds.), Handbook of Clinical Neurology, vol. 4. New York: American Elsevier Publishing Company, 1986.

48. Waters WE. Community studies of the prevalence of migraine. Headache 1970; 9:178–186.

49. Warner JJ. Headaches in older patients: Ddx and Tx of vascular and inflammatory pain. Geriatrics 1985; 40:30–44.

50. Houston K, Hunter G. Giant cell (cranial) arteritis: A clinical review. Am Heart J 1980; 100:99–105.

51. Solomon S, Cappa KG. The headache of temporal arteritis. JAGS 1987; 35:163–165.

52. Brownstein S, Nicolle DA, Codere F. Bilateral blindness in temporal arteritis with skip areas. Arch Ophthalmol 1983; 101:388–391.

53. Cohen DN. Temporal arteritis: Improvement in visual prognosis and management with repeat biopsies. Trans Am Acad Ophthalmol Otolaryngol 1973; 77:74–85.

54. Solomon GD, Kunkel RS, Frame J. Demographics of headache in elderly patients. Headache 1990; 30:273–276.

55. Langemark M, Olsen J, Poulsen DL, et al. Clinical characterization of patients with chronic tension headaches. Headache 1988; 28:290–296.

56. Mathew NT, Stubits E, Nigam M. Transformation of migraine into daily headache: Analysis of factors. Headache 1982; 22:66–68.

57. Warner JJ. Headaches in older patients: Ddx and Tx of common nonvascular causes. Geriatrics 1985; 40:69–76.

58. Indo T, Naito A, Sobue I. Clinical characteristics of headache in Parkinson's disease. Headache 1983; 23:211–212.

59. Nishikawa S, Harada H, Takahashi K, Shimomura T. Clinical study on headache in patients with Parkinson's disease. Clin Neurol Neurosurg 1982; 22:403–408.

60. Lorentz IT. A survey of headache in Parkinson's disease. Cephalalgia 1989; 9:83–86.

61. Raskin NH. On the origin of head pain. Headache 1988; 28:254–257.

62. Callahan M, Raskin NH. A controlled study of dihydroergotamine as therapy for intractable migraine. Neurology 1986; 36:995–997.

63. Friedman AP. Clinical approach to the patient with headache. Neurol Clin 1983; 1:361–368.

64. Lavyne MH, Patterson RH. Headache associated with brain tumor. In: Dalessio DJ (ed.), Wolff's Headache and Other Head Pain, 5th ed. New York: Oxford University Press, 1987; 343–351.

65. Mokri EE, Leviton A, Caplan L. Severe headache after carotid endarectomy. Headache 1975; 15:207–210.

66. Day JW, Raskin NH. Thunderclap headache: Symptom of unruptured cerebral aneurysm. Lancet 1986; 2:1247–1248.

67. Dhopesh V, Anwar R, Herring C. A retrospective assessment of emergency department patients with complaint of headache. Headache 1979; 19:37–42.

68. Packard RC. Mild head injury. Headache Quart 1993; 4:42–52.

69. Featherstone HJ. Headaches and heart disease: The lack of a positive association. Headache 1986; 26:39–41.

70. Ziegler DK, Rhodes RJ, Hassanein RS. Association of psychological measurements of anxiety and depression with headache

history in a non-clinic population. Res Clin Study Headache 1978; 6:123–125.

71. Cox D, Thomas D. Relationship between headaches and depression. Headache 1981; 21:261–263.

72. Andrasik F, Omaya ON, Packard RC. Biofeedback therapy for migraine. In: Diamond S (ed.), Migraine Headache Prevention and Management. New York: Marcel Dekker, 1990;213–238.

73. Diamond S, Montrose D. The value of biofeedback in the treatment of chronic headache: A four-year retrospective study. Headache 1984; 24:59–69.

74. Arena JG, Hannah SL, Bruno GM, Meador KJ. Electromyographic biofeedback training for tension headache in the elderly: A prospective study. Biof Self Regul 1991; 16:379–390.

75. Mannarino M. The present and future roles of biofeedback in successful aging. Biof Self Regul 1991; 16:391–397.

76. Dalessio DJ. Diagnosis and treatment of cranial neuralgias. Med Clin North Am 1991; 75:605–615.

77. Elkind AH. Management of atypical facial pain and the cranial neuralgias. In: Diamond S (director), The Practicing Physician's Approach to the Difficult Headache Patient. Lake Buena Vista, FL, 1993.

78. Fromm GH, Terrence CF, Maroon JC. Trigeminal neuralgia. Concepts regarding etiology and pathogenesis. Arch Neurol 1984; 41:1204–1207.

79. Raskin NH. Facial pain. In: Headache, 2nd ed. New York: Churchill-Livingstone, 1988; 333–373.

80. Katusic S, Beard CM, Bergstralh E, Kurland LT. Incidence and clinical features of trigeminal neuralgia, Rochester, Minnesota, 1945–1984. Ann Neurol 1990; 27:89–95.

81. Demorgas JW, Kierland RR. The outcome of patients with herpes zoster. Arch Dermatol 1957; 75:193–196.

82. Watson CPN. Post herpetic neuralgia. Neurol Clin North Am 1989; 7:231–248.

83. Galbraith AW. The treatment of acute herpes zoster with amantadine hydrochloride (Symmetrel). Br Med J 1983; 4:693–695.

84. Max MB, Schafer SC, Culnane M. Amitriptyline, but not lorazepam, relieves postherpetic neuralgia. Neurology 1988; 38: 1427–1432.

11

The Interpretation of Neurophysiologic Studies in the Elderly

Sudhansu Chokroverty
Veterans Administration Medical Center
Lyons, New Jersey,
St. Vincent's Hospital and Medical Center
New York, New York,
University of Medicine and Dentistry of New Jersey
Robert Wood Johnson Medical School
Piscataway, New Jersey, and
New York Medical College
New York, New York

I. INTRODUCTION

Beginning with electroencephalography (EEG) and electromyography (EMG) in the early part of this century, clinical neurophysiologic investigations have expanded considerably to study disturbances of functions of the central and peripheral nervous systems, including neuromuscular junctions and muscles, and the autonomic nervous system. Such studies may also include sensory and motor evoked potential (EP), autonomic neurophysiologic tests, sleep neurophysiologic study, electronystagmography (ENG), electro-oculography (EOG), posturography and other vestibular testing, tests to detect dysfunction of the voluntary movements, and tests to characterize involuntary movements. The importance of the clinical neurophysiologic tests is that they can evaluate the dynamic functions of the entire neuraxis in contrast to the morphologic evaluation by the neuroimaging studies (e.g., CT, MRI) and by biopsy of a nerve or muscle in a live patient. In addition, clinical neurophysiologic tests can quantitate the functional deficits, which is important not only for the diagnosis and differential diagnosis but also for following progress of the disease and for monitoring the effect of treatment (1).

Elderly persons are often afflicted with a variety of neurological and nonneurological disorders for which clinical neurophysiologic tests may play a vital role. The interpretation, however, of such tests in the elderly is fraught with pitfalls and fallacies that must be clearly understood for meaningful conclusions. There are many age-related changes clinically, morphologically, and physiologically in the nervous system and the neuromuscular apparatus of the elderly. Therefore, what is abnormal in the young may be considered normal in a disease-free elderly person. An understanding of such aberrations in the physiologic tests in the elderly is important and is the subject matter of this chapter.

Before beginning to address the interpretation of neurophysiologic tests in the elderly we are immediately faced with the difficulty of defining an elderly individual and particularly a normal elderly person. I will arbitrarily define an elderly person as an individual aged 65 years or older and a "normal" elderly person as one free of obvious diseases involving the neurological system, including the neuromuscular system, and free of general systemic diseases (e.g., cardiovascular, renal, metabolic, hematological, skeletal, or muscular diseases). The neurological signs of normal aging are mostly noted after age 60; around this age, results of many neurophysiologic tests begin to deviate from the normative data obtained from younger individuals.

According to best estimates, individuals over 65 will comprise 13% of the population in the year 2000 and 21% in the year 2050, contrasting with 4% in the year 1900 (2). This reflects increasing life expectancy resulting from modern advancement in the prevention and treatment of diseases. It should, however, be noted that it is the life expectancy that has been extending rather than the human life span, which is determined biologically and genetically and remains fixed (3).

What determines aging and the changes associated with aging are not known. For an understanding of this topic the readers are referred to Behnke et al (4) and Comfort (5). Beginning with the seminal papers by Critchley (6,7) there have been several accounts of neurological changes found in normal elderly individuals (8–12). Concomitant morphological and physiological correlates of the clinical signs have also been described. The problem again is in the definition of "normal" in this age group. Many studies did not rigorously exclude diseases and only a few studies carefully excluded disorders of the neuromuscular or other systems, finding genuine "abnormal" signs on neurological examination. Even in these cases, without a careful longitudinal study the significance of these signs remains somewhat questionable (8).

Another fallacy is the inclusion of subclinical neurological diseases in the normal population (8). In an autopsy survey, subclinical cerebral infarction was noted in 50% of the postmortem brains examined (13). There is also an increasing incidence of both the neurological and nonneurological disorders in the elderly. Some examples of common diseases found in the elderly are atherosclerotic cerebrovascular and cardiovascular disease, brain tumor, degenerative diseases of the nervous system, joints, and ligaments, falls and gait disorder, vertigo, cataract, sensorineural hearing impairment, infections, seizures, peripheral neuropathies, and acquired myopathies. Clinical neurophysiologic tests are important in many of these disorders.

II. NEUROLOGY OF AGING

A variety of neurological signs in the central and peripheral nervous system have been described in the normal elderly (7,8,10–13). Some common signs comprising neurology of aging are discussed below.

A. Higher Mental Functions

There is impairment of recent memory, particularly in learning new information or in recalling names, and slowing of central processing and reaction time. The morphological counterpart of these changes is thought to be the presence of age-related degenerative changes, such as senile plaques and neurofibrillary tangles in the aged brain as well as reduction of cortical neurons. The cognitive impairment of the normal elderly is often termed benign forgetfulness of senescence (14) or age-associated memory impairment (15). The more severe impairment of memory and cognition is associated with widespread senile plaques, neurofibrillary tangles, and granulovacuolar degeneration as found in the common dementing illness of old age, namely Alzheimer's disease. The boundary between the benign forgetfulness of senescence and the early stage of malignant cognitive impairment of Alzheimer's disease, and the distinction between the amount of plaques and tangles in Alzheimer's and normal brain in the senium, are often blurred.

B. Gait and Posture

Gait and postural abnormalities are common in the elderly (8,16,17). The elders often find it difficult to stand on one leg with one eye closed (12,13,17). The so-called senile gait is characterized by stooped posture with flexed attitude accompanied by short steps, reduced arm swings, shortening of the stride, and impaired speed and balance (3). Posturography detects distinct difference between the old and the young, and this will be described later.

C. Cranial Nerve Functions

Impairment of near vision (presbyopia) and sensorineural hearing loss (presbycusis) are common in many normal elders who may also have pupillary and oculomotor changes. Pupils may be miotic, showing impaired responses to light and convergence. The upward gaze is often restricted. In many normal elderly individuals there may also be impairment of taste and smell.

D. Motor and Sensory Systems

Grip strength and muscle bulk decrease with age. The important findings in the sensory system consist of impairment of vibration, particularly in the lower extremities, and raised threshold to pain sensation and possibly also to touch.

E. Reflexes

Ankle reflexes are often absent or markedly decreased with diminution of knee jerks. Polysynaptic reflexes (e.g., glabellar tap, snout and palmomental reflexes) show abnormalities in the elderly.

F. Morphological Correlates of Sensorimotor Changes

Morphological correlates of sensorimotor changes in old age include reduction of ventral horn cells, dorsal root ganglion cells, dorsal and ventral roots, and large-diameter myelinated sensory motor axons in the peripheral nervous system (3).

III. CLINICAL NEUROPHYSIOLOGIC TESTS AND THEIR INTERPRETATION IN THE ELDERLY

A. Tests to Detect Dysfunction of the Peripheral Somatic Nervous System

The two most important tests to detect impairment of the peripheral sensorimotor axons are nerve conduction studies (NCS) and electromyography (EMG). A number of NCS and EMG characteristics show significant changes with increasing age. It is beyond the scope of this chapter to discuss the techniques of NCS and EMG, and the readers are referred to standard text (18). Briefly, for NCS the nerves are stimulated usually by conventional electrical stimulation (sometimes by magnetic stimulator), and then compound muscle action potentials (CMAPs) in the case of motor nerves, and compound sensory action potentials (CNAPs) in the case of sensory nerves, are analyzed. The latencies to CMAPs and CNAPs, and the distance between the two stimulating points, are measured and the conduction velocities (CVs) are computed by dividing the distance by the conduction time. The amplitudes, phases, and other morphological characteristics of the CMAPs and CNAPs are also analyzed. These measures are able to detect whether the nerve conduction is normal or abnormal. For this purpose normative data or reference values must be obtained using similar techniques and under similar conditions from a group of normal individuals free from neuromuscular disorders. Generally parametric statistics (e.g., mean and two standard deviations) are used to consider a value as within the normal range (approximately 95% of the population) (19–21). This is somewhat arbitrary and inclusion of a larger number of standard deviations may reduce sensitivity (i.e., the percentage of population with diseases who have an abnormal test result) but increase specificity (i.e., the percentage of disease-free people who have a normal result) (19,20). There may be both false positive results (i.e., an abnormal result in an individual without disease) and false negative results (i.e., a normal value in a person with disease) (19,20). Hence, all electrophysiologic measures must be considered in light of the clinical findings.

Other methods of analyzing data include nonparametric statistics by collecting the range of values in a group of normative population and percentile measures (19–21). There are fallacies in both methods depending on the sample size, technical errors, and inclusion of individuals with subclinical diseases (19,21). Finally, if normative data in the elderly are not readily available, comparisons between two neighboring nerves (e.g., ulnar and median) can be used when evaluating focal entrapment (e.g., carpal tunnel syndrome) as studies have shown no substantial age-related difference between median and ulnar sensory latencies in this age group (19).

Besides the statistical methodology, other important factors that significantly influence the electrophysiologic data must be considered during testing in the elderly. In addition to the factor of age, which is the subject matter for discussion in this chapter, height and temperature must also be controlled while collecting normative data (22–24). Many of the electrophysiological characteristics change linearly after age 50 and particularly after 60, and ideally normative data should be obtained for each decade after this age. Height is an important consideration in distal nerve conduction, H reflex, F response, and somatosensory evoked potential studies, and nomograms based on height should be constructed (22).

Temperature must be considered in both young and old (24) subjects, particularly in the elderly, who often have cold extremities because of circulatory insufficiency and reduction of subcutaneous fat (25). NCS and EMG data show significant changes if the limb temperature is low (24). Limb temperature should be maintained around 1°C during NCS and EMG studies to avoid confounding factors during electrophysiologic tests. Nerve conduction velocities slow by 1–2 meters/second/degree centigrade of lowering of limb temperature. Cooling of the limb is associated with prolonged distal sensory motor latencies, reduction of CVs, increased duration and amplitude of CMAPs and CNAPs (24). Cooling also alters the motor unit morphology by increasing the duration of CMAP and causing an excess of polyphasic potentials (26). In addition, in a cool extremity, spontaneous potentials (e.g., fibrillations and positive sharp waves) during needle EMG examination may be reduced (27). Hypothermia of the limb may also partially correct the myasthenic decremental responses on repetitive nerve stimulation tests (28).

1.   *Effects of age on nerve conduction*

In order to interpret the results of NCS in the elderly it is essential to know the effects of age on nerve conduction. Certain aspects of nerve conduction changes are noted consistently whereas others have been inconsistent. Besides the age-related changes the clinical neurophysiologists must take precautions against other confounding factors during the study. These factors may include accurate placement of active, reference, and ground electrodes; optimal temperature and position of the limbs; supramaximal rather than submaximal stimulation during motor nerve conduction study; avoidance of coactivation of the neighboring nerves; selection of correct stimulating points; accurate measurement of the distance; obtaining consistent CMAP morphology while stimulating at two different points on the same nerve; and recognition of normal variation (e.g., median-ulnar anastomosis, presence of accessory deep peroneal nerves).

Significant changes in CV, distal latency, and the amplitudes of CMAP and CNAP occur after age 60 (29). Plantar sensory, sural, and superficial peroneal sensory responses, and H reflexes, are sometimes not obtained in asymptomatic subjects after age 60 (29). Lower limb motor CVs and CMAP amplitudes are often mildly reduced or remain in the lower range of normal values. All these changes, therefore, have been considered normal for the age by some authors unless there is significant asymmetry in the values between the two sides (29), whereas others may consider these changes as evidence of a pathological process. Intrinsic foot muscles including the extensor digitorum brevis (EDB) muscles are often atrophic in normal elderly subjects. Thus, interpretation of peroneal nerve (PN) motor conduction slowing in the elderly may be problematic because of inability to obtain adequate CMAP from EDB after PN stimulation at the ankle. In such cases, CMAP should be obtained from proximal tibialis anterior muscles, but this makes it difficult to make a diagnosis of distal neuropathy (29).

According to MacDonnell and Shahani (25), the sensory motor decline in CVs is parabolic and not linear. On the other hand, Oh and others (30–35) stated that there is linear decrease of conduction velocities of motor, sensory, and mixed nerves with age after about 20 years. This age-related decrement is found in both proximal and distal nerve segments. An approximate decrement of 0.4 to 2.3 meters per second per decade is noted in the upper and lower limb motor studies

(33), whereas the rate of decline for median and ulnar sensory studies varies from 2 to 4 meters per second per decade (31,32). Oh (35) found a marked slowing of CV of the interdigital plantar nerves in subjects over 50, which may indicate the presence of a subclinical neuropathy of the plantar nerves in the elderly. Wagman and Lesse (36) and Taylor (37), in contrast, found nonlinear effects of age on the nerve conduction indices. Age-related mild prolongation of distal latency of motor nerves is noted by most authors, but Taylor (37) found no such changes. The amplitude of CMAP also shows gradual decline with age, but because of wide variability of these values in all ages this factor may not be of much significance in practice. Sensory amplitude also declines with age. According to LaFratta (31), sensory CNAP amplitude drops by 36% around the age of 60. Buchthal and Rosenfalck (38) noted an increase in temporal dispersion of the sensory potentials. Age must, therefore, be considered when interpreting nerve conduction data and age-specific normative data should be obtained to enhance the diagnostic sensitivity (37). Oh (30) suggested an age-related correlation value for NCV: 1 meter per second per decade for motor and 2 meters per second per decade for sensory conduction studies. Lascelles and Thomas (39) and Troghi et al. (40) provided some histological data (e.g., loss of large myelinated nerve fibers, segmental demyelination, and short internodal segments in the sural nerve biopsy samples obtained from normal subjects over 65) to explain minor electrophysiological "aberrations" or abnormalities in the elderly.

In comparing the studies of peroneal and tibial motor conduction and sural conduction in 52 young individuals, ages 10 to 40 years, and 52 older subjects, ages 41 to 84 years, Kimura (18,41) found that the amplitudes were significantly reduced in the older group, but found no change in conduction measurements except a reduction of peroneal velocity and a prolongation of H latency. Aging also affects the shape of the evoked potential, particularly at the sites of common entrapment (42). General consensus is that after 30–40 years conduction velocities begin to decrease. Usually there is less than a 10-meter-per-second decline between years 60 and 80 (37,43,44). A study by Meyer (45) showed a reduction of about 10% at 60 years. There is also an increase of latencies of the F waves with aging.

Horwitz and Krarup (46) studied the sural nerve orthodromically using the near-nerve technique in 273 normal subjects ages 5 to 90. They found an inverse relationship between the amplitude of the sensory potential and the age of the subject. The decline in amplitude of the sensory potential in the sural nerve is most likely related to the combination of decreased number and density of the myelinated fibers in the sural nerve and subcutaneous tissue atrophy seen with aging. Stetson et al. (47) studied the median, ulnar, and sural nerve conduction in 105 healthy asymptomatic adults. They found a decrease of 1.3 meters per second in the median sensory distal conduction velocity and 0.8 meters per second in motor conduction velocity per decade of aging and these values are similar to previous reports (48,49). They also found a decrease of sensory amplitude. They agreed with Buchthal and Rosenfalck (48) that a prolonged latency in a young age group will be missed if normal values based on the older age group are used.

Litchy et al (50) studied 323 individuals without neuromuscular diseases and took into consideration several variables such as the site, age, gender, height, weight, body surface area, and body mass index amongst several other factors that might influence nerve conduction studies. They included median, ulnar, tibial, and peroneal motor nerves as well as median (antidromic and palmar), ulnar (antidromic and palmar) and sural sensory nerves. They used an algorithm to determine Z scores and concluded that there are more independent physical variables, including age, affecting nerve conduction than is generally appreciated. They suggested that an approach taking into consideration all these physical variables would be a better predictor of abnormality in epidemiologic surveys, controlled clinic trials, and medical practice.

The above survey summarizes some of the pitfalls for electrodiagnostic studies of peripheral neuromuscular disorders in the elderly. A failure to adjust nerve conduction data to age, sex, skin temperature, and other variables will decrease the diagnostic specificity and sensitivity of the measures, and may result in misclassification of the individuals (46,50).

2. *Effect of age on needle EMG*

Needle EMG records electrical activities in the voluntary muscles by inserting either a monopolar or concentric needle into the muscle. Insertion and resting potentials, recruitment and firing patterns, and the morphology of the motor unit potentials (MUPs) are then studied. Normally the muscles are silent at rest, but in denervating conditions spontaneous potentials in the form of positive sharp waves, fibrillations, or fasciculations are seen accompanied by reduced recruitment and increased firing rate of the remaining motor units. Chronic denervation is associated with high-amplitude, long-duration potentials including excessive amounts of polyphasic potentials. In contrast, myopathy is associated with earlier recruitment and low-amplitude, short-duration potentials. Some indications for NCS and EMG in the elderly subjects include cervical and lumbosacral radiculopathies associated with degenerative disk diseases, entrapment neuropathy, polyneuropathies, amyotrophic lateral sclerosis, myasthenia or myasthenic syndrome, polymyositis and other acquired myopathies, and diseases causing myalgia, muscle cramps, and fatigue.

Age-related changes in the EMG characteristics must be considered for correct interpretation in the elderly. The duration of MUP increases with advancing age (51,52). Amplitude of MUPs sometimes also increases. These findings in a young subject would suggest a chronic neurogenic lesion, but in elderly the findings must be interpreted with caution and in light of the clinical findings. Aging alone does not give rise to spontaneous potentials unless there is denervation. Fasciculations limited to the gastrocnemius or any single muscle may be seen in an older person, but in absence of changes in motor unit morphology and fasciculations in other muscles this finding should be considered benign. Aging is associated with loss of motor axons and subsequent collateral reinnervation, causing enlargement of the motor unit size and formation of new immature motor endplates (25). These changes cause an increase in the duration of the MUP and lead to an excess of polyphasic potentials. In the elderly, loss of motor units often accompanied by an increase in the size of many of the surviving motor units both in standard (53–56) and in macro-EMG (57) study is noted. Brown (53) suggested that in the elderly healthy motor units are mixed with a few dysfunctional or degenerative motor units. In the elderly a reduction in strength is accompanied by slowing of the contraction time and half relaxation times in some (58,59) but not all muscles (54,60). Some of these electrophysiological changes may be related to the muscle biopsy findings in the elderly subjects of reduced cross-sectional area of the muscles, fiber type grouping, and presence of atrophic angular fibers.

3. *Single-fiber EMG*

SFEMG measures the characteristics of single fiber by insertion of a special needle and measures the jitter (variability) between the firing rates of two muscle fibers belonging to the same motor unit (61). In subjects over 50–60 years increased jitter (more than 50 microseconds), blocking, and increased fiber density (i.e., increased number of muscle fibers within 200 microns of the recording surface of the SFEMG needle) are found in the EDB and tibialis anterior muscles. These findings seem to be related to the age-related loss of motor axons with subsequent collateral sprouting.

4. *Quantitative EMG*

Quantitative EMG has recently been introduced to assess electrophysiologically the functions of the muscle in a quantitative manner. The methods include measurement of the MUP, analysis of the interference pattern, and turn-amplitude analysis. The characteristics of the various quantitative EMGs show age-related changes and, therefore, normative data obtained from the young cannot be applied to the older population. Howard et al (62) studied motor unit action potentials (MUAPs) from the biceps brachii, triceps, and tibialis anterior muscles in 30 normal subjects, ages 20–80 years, using an automated decomposition method of EMG (ADEMG) interference pattern. They found that the MUAP amplitudes, duration, and number of turns all increased linearly with age in both low-threshold and high-threshold MUAPs, suggesting an ongoing process of denervation and reinnervation. Mean MUAP firing rates, however, decreased with age. Clinical details are not provided. These findings support the SFEMG data of increased fiber density in the elderly.

5. *Mechanism of neuromuscular changes*

Brown (53) suggested that a multitude of factors are responsible for the neuromuscular regressive and degenerative changes in the aging. These factors include degeneration of the cells; cumulative effects of repeated trauma and compression or ischemia in the nerves and nerve roots; superimposed diseases (e.g., diabetes mellitus, neoplasm, metabolic and nutritional disorders); excitotoxic injury (e.g., glutamate toxicity causing intracellular transfer of calcium); oxidative stress due to free-radical accumulations causing mitochondrial dysfunction; inactivity of old age; errors in transcription and translation due to errors in the nuclear DNA or mitochondrial RNA, which may occur by chance or in response to environmental trauma; and finally, run-down of the biological clock (63).

B. Tests to Detect Dysfunction of the Central Somatic Nervous System

In the clinical neurophysiology laboratory the tests available to evaluate functions of the central somatic nervous system include somatosensory (SEP), brainstem auditory (BAEP) and visual (VEP) exogenous evoked potentials, endogenous event-related potentials (ERP), and motor evoked potentials (MEP).

For details of these techniques readers are referred to standard text (64). Each of these has important indications in geriatric neurology and each has age-related changes that are important to know for proper interpretation of the tests. In clinical practice, identification and measurement of evoked potential peaks and interpeak latencies are important. The limits of normality are usually set at a mean value and 2.5 standard deviations above the mean values measured in a group of healthy controls for each particular component of the evoked response. If the potentials change with age, careful considerations must be given to changes noted in different age groups. It is often difficult to collect such data from a large number of individuals encompassing all age ranges. To alleviate this problem it may be possible to compute the regression lines with confidence limits for each component of the evoked response obtained from fewer subjects (65). Goodin et al. (66–68) used this method to describe prolonged P300 latency in event-related potential in demented and normal aged subjects (68). The regression line technique cannot be used for discontinuous data (65).

1. *Effect of age on SEPs*

Somatosensory evoked potentials (SEPs) record responses after stimulation of the median, ulnar, or radial nerves in the upper extremities (commonly after stimulation of the median nerve in the standard neurophysiology laboratory) and after stimulation of the peroneal nerve at the knee or tibial nerve at the ankle. These evoked potentials in response to afferent stimulation are very small in amplitude (usually a few microvolts) and are recorded after upper limb nerve stimulation over Erb's point, C5 or C7 cervical vertebral column, and contralateral somesthetic area (C3 or C4 of the International electrode placement system), using both scalp-scalp and noncephalic references. Following lower limb nerve stimulation these responses are recorded over the popliteal fossa or the sciatic notch, lumbar, midthoracic, or cervial vertebral column, and Cz referred to Fz (the International system). Some

common conditions in geriatric neurology where SEP testing
may be useful include neurodegenerative diseases, cervical
and lumbosacral radiculopathy, involuntary movement disorders such as myoclonus, stroke, and myelopathy. SEP peak
latencies sometimes show an increase with aging, but this is
partly related to slowing of the peripheral nerve conduction
(69). An important interpeak latency in SEP is N13–N20,
which measures the central conduction in the ascending pathways from the highest cervical spinal cord or lower medulla
to the somesthetic cortex. There is a minimal increase in the
order of 0.3 milliseconds of central conduction time comparing subjects in the 40s with those in the 70s (2,5,70–72). SEP
amplitudes are extremely variable and show a nongaussian
distribution, and hence are not generally used in the routine
SEP study. Some investigators found an increase whereas
others found a decrease in SEP amplitudes with increasing
age. Most of the investigators found minimal changes in the
latencies and amplitudes of SEPs. Desmedt and Cheron (72)
reported slightly longer latencies for all cortical peaks in a
group of octogenarians and they ascribed these findings to
slowing of peripheral nerve conduction, but central conduction slows only slightly, and there is minor change in the scalp
topography. SEP amplitude decreases proportionately after age
40. In the lower limb SEP study, spinal cord conduction velocity does not change much before age 60, but after that age
it decreases significantly.

Lueders (73) found no difference in the absolute latencies
of N19 (N20) or P23 (P25) in 40 normal men between 19 and
70 years. Dorfmann and Bosley (69) studied 15 young adults
and 15 elderly subjects. They found a slowing of the median
nerve conduction velocity at a rate of 0.16 meters per second
per year for sensory fibers and slightly increased median and
tibial SEP latencies with advancing age as a result of slowing in both the central and peripheral segments of somatosensory pathways.

Evoked potentials may change with age and, therefore, an
equal number of normal subjects must be tested and included

in young adults, middle-aged, and elderly (over 60 years) subjects. In cortical myoclonus there is an enchancement of amplitude of the cortical SEPs (e.g., giant N20 and P25 amplitudes). Hence, normative data for amplitude are needed.

2. *Effect of age on BAEPs*

In clinical practice of all the auditory evoked potentials the short latency (within first 10 milliseconds) brainstem auditory evoked potentials (BAEPs) are the most useful and available in most of the neurophysiology laboratories. These responses are usually recorded from Cz connected to ipsilateral and contralateral ears following application of rarefaction or condensation clicks given to the ipsilateral ears. Besides age there are many important nonpathological factors that must be considered before using the data for clinical purpose (64,74). This test may be very useful in the elderly in the following conditions: cerebellopontine angle tumors; patients complaining of vertigo, dizziness, tinnitus, or hearing impairment; degenerative central nervous system diseases; and brainstem vascular or space-occupying lesions.

There are reports of prolongation of both the absolute and interpeak latencies of BAEPs with advancing age, but these findings in the literature have been inconsistent (75). Because of the inconsistent findings, age-specific normative data in the adults and elderly have not been generally in use (75).

The absolute latency of wave I increases with age and this has been attributed to the sensorineural high-frequency hearing loss (presbyacusis) of the elderly due to degenerative changes in the cochlea. The clinical utility of middle latency auditory evoked response and long latency cortical auditory potentials is limited.

Several investigators noted a minor increase in interpeak latencies in older normal subjects (71,74–76). Chiappa (64) stated that in clinical practice such minor changes do not require separate age-specific normative data if the laboratory uses a mixed gender group of normal subjects. Amplitude of BAEP waveforms also shows inconsistent changes with aging.

Rowe (75) found increased I–III and I–V but normal III–V interpeak latencies in 25 subjects after 50 years. These findings suggested slowing of conduction of the brainstem auditory pathways in the pontomedullary region in aged subjects. Rosenthal et al. (77) found delayed latencies of all the BAEP components with normal I–V interpeak latencies, suggesting peripheral auditory nerve dysfunction. The effect of aging on central or brainstem auditory pathways is thus minimal.

3.   *Effect of age on visual evoked potentials (VEPs)*

The most useful test for VEP in clinical practice is pattern-reversal visual evoked response (PVER). This cannot be studied in elderly subjects who are demented, uncooperative, or cortically blind, and in such patients flash-evoked visual evoked response study may be useful. The PVER study is usually performed after using a pattern-reversal checkerboard pattern and recording the responses from the occipital and frontal electrodes. Some important factors related to the stimulus, such as check size, contrast, luminance, rate of pattern reversal and filters, must be taken into consideration before obtaining the data for clinical use. The VER study may be useful in the following conditions in elderly patients: visual problems or visual field defects related to stroke, tumors, or trauma; ischemic optic neuropathy; Parkinson's disease; Alzheimer's diesase; and cortical blindness. Bodis-Wollner and Yahr (78) first showed an increase in VEP latency in Parkinson's disease using grating stimulus and improvement of this finding following L-dopa treatment. Later it was shown that the increase in VEP latency is proportional to the spatial frequency of the stimulus in these patients (79). Patients with Alzheimer's disease also show VEP changes (80–82). The VEP abnormalities in Alzheimer's disease are thought to be related to the cortical changes resulting from depletion of acetylcholine (83).

Shaw and Cant (84) reported an increase of P100 latency throughout the adult life. This has not been confirmed by the majority. The general consensus is that P100 latency remains stable in adult life until about 60 years after which it increases. Hence in the elderly population age-dependent normative data are needed to interpret PVER values. There are inconsistent changes in the amplitude of P100 in the elderly. It is to be noted that small check size and low luminance levels more severely affect the age-related P100 latency prolongation. Celesia and Daly (85) found an increase of 2 milliseconds per decade of P100 latency from the end of the second decade onward. In contrast, Asselman (86), Hennerici (87), Allison (88), Stockard (89), and coinvestigators found an increase of P100 latency by 2–5 milliseconds per decade beyond the 5th decade but no significant changes were seen before that age. Sokol et al. (90) and Celesia et al. (91) confirmed that P100 latency increase with age was more marked with smaller than larger check sizes. These age-related changes are due to alterations in the entire visual system including the retina.

In a study of 74 normal volunteers, using low luminance and small check sizes, Celesia and Daly (85) found a linear increase of mean P100 latency with age. In contrast, Allison et al. (88) found little or no increase in latency up to the age of 50 years after which there was progressive increase of P100 latency, thus agreeing with the data of Halliday et al. (92) and Faust et al. (93). Stockard et al. (89) found no significant age effect on P100 latency between 20 and 55 years, but in those over 60 years there was an increase in the mean latency. According to Halliday et al. (94), an increase in mean latency from the age of 50 onward was seen only in the female group. In the male group the data were inconclusive. Halliday (95) suggested that there may be minor visual defects in the elderly subjects related to mild lens opacities, discoloration of the lens, and retinal lesions, which should be carefully excluded by ophthalmological screening before including the subjects in the normal control group.

Tobimatsu et al. (96) recorded PVER in 109 normal subjects, ages 19–84 years, using three check sizes (15′, 30′, and 50′), high and low luminance, and high and low contrast. They found a curvilinear relationship between P100 latency and age. P100 latency was greater for low luminance and low contrast than for high luminance and high contrast for all check sizes. The age-latency function was similar between high and low luminance irrespective of the check size, but was different between high and low contrast. With small check size (e.g., 15′) there was no significant difference in P100 latency between the young and middle aged, whereas with larger check size (e.g., 30′ and 50′) a significant difference in P100 latency was detected with low contrast but not with high contrast. There was, however, a significant difference between the middle-aged and older individuals with both low and high contrast. There seems to be a decreased contrast sensitivity in old age. The authors concluded that these findings suggested a differential effect of age on multiple parallel channels (e.g., luminance channels, contrast channels) processing different visual information.

All flash-evoked VEP interpeak latencies increase after age 65 (97). Because of variability and inconsistency in flash-VEP peaks, PVER study has replaced flash-VEP study in clinical practice. However, in certain circumstances it is not possible to obtain PVER: e.g., patients with cortical blindness, hysterical blindness, moderately to severely demented and other incompetent patients who cannot focus on pattern stimuli.

4. *Effect of age on endogenous event-related potentials*

The long-latency ERPs are related to cognitive processing and consist of a series of negative and positive waves: e.g., N_1, N_2, P_2, P_3 (98,99). The best known is P_3 or P300 potential. Clinical application is limited, but there is some evidence that these waves may be useful in the diagnosis of some cases of dementia, e.g., Alzheimer's disease and Parkinson's disease with dementia, and they may be able to differentiate between dementia and depression (98,99). Other utility may be in patients with chronic alcohol abuse and chronic renal failure (98,99). There are several physiological factors that must be taken into consideration before ascribing the results as normal, e.g., aging (98,99). A direct positive correlation has been noted between aging and P300 obtained after auditory, visual, and somatosensory stimuli. P300 latency increases by about 1 to 1.5 milliseconds per year after age 20 (98). Therefore, for clinical usefulness a normative database must be aged matched.

5. *Effect of age on motor evoked potentials*

The recently introduced technique of magnetic stimulation, a noninvasive and relatively painless technique, has brought a new dimension into the electrophysiological armamentarium in the clinical neurophysiology laboratory (100). By this technique it is possible to assess the function of the corticospinal tract noninvasively by stimulating the motor cortex with the magnetic coil placed over the scalp. One can, therefore, determine central motor conduction by measuring conduction time from the motor cortex to the onset of CMAP in the hand or the leg muscles and subtracting from this the motor latency obtained after magnetic coil root stimulation over the cervical or lumbosacral vertebral column. Using this technique it is possible to determine abnormalities both in motor conduction and in the stimulus threshold (excitability) in patients with stroke, Parkinson's disease, motor neuron disease, as well as in demyelinating disorders (100–102). An important recent application of this technique is in the root stimulation and in the diagnosis of lumbosacral and cervical radiculopathy, and intercostal radiculoneuropathy (103–105). In addition, diabetic neuropathies affecting the proximal roots and nerves can be diagnosed. In the peripheral nerve conduction study the conventional electrical stimulation remains the standard technique, except in occasional uncooperative patients who cannot tolerate electrical shock, magnetic coil can be used to stimulate the peripheral nerves to study their functions. MEP obtained by magnetic coil stimulation of the motor cortex can also be used in patients with myelopathy, Guillain-Barré syndrome, and hereditary spastic paraplegia (100–102).

MEP indices are significantly altered by aging (102,106) and hence this factor must be considered before interpreting the results as normal or abnormal. An increase of MEP latency to onset of CMAPs may result from peripheral conduction delay and central motor delay. The influence of aging on central conduction time remains controversial (102,107). Eisen et al. (102) reported linearly increased latencies to MEPs in the thenar and tibialis anterior muscles in the 2nd to 9th decades. They also reported significiant linear reduction of MEP amplitude with age (102,106). Eisen et al. (106) measured peak-to-peak maximum amplitude of MEP obtained from the thenar and hypothenar muscles after transcranial magnetic cortical stimulation in 41 volunteers without neurological or other diseases aged 23 to 82 years. They found a linear decrease of the amplitude with age and stated that maximum MEP amplitude related to age is more meaningful than the MEP/CMAP ratio, and this is proportional to the number of fast-conducting cortical motor neurons excited. According to these authors, this situation parallels the amplitude reduction of CMAP and CNAP that characterizes axonal degeneration affecting the peripheral nervous system. Their study (106) also included 18 patients with Parkinson's disease whose ages ranged from 44 to 77 years. In 7 of these 18 patients, they found that the maximum MEP amplitudes were larger than normal for their age, whereas in 2 others the amplitude of the maximum MEP was smaller than normal for their age. The MEP latency in central motor conduction, however, was normal in PD patients. The authors suggested that it is possible that larger than normal MEPs in PD patients reflected spinal disinhibition. In this context it is notable that Delwaide (108) also found evidence of increased spinal disinhibition as indicated by enhanced F waves.

Prout and Eisen (109) also noted changes in the mean cortical threshold and cortical silent period (CSP) in the elderly. The range (difference between the maximum and the minimum values) of CSP interval was inversely related to age, and this age-dependent decline is linear (109). Also, the mean cortical threshold was significantly higher in older subjects (over 55 years) than in the younger individuals (109). Rossini et al. (107) described changes in the excitability threshold with increasing age. There are changes in the cortical threshold and CSP in patients with PD, ALS, and stroke. In PD the cortical threshold is decreased (i.e., increased excitability) and CSP is shortened (110). These findings may suggest motor cortical disinhibition due to dopamine deficiency and decreased nigrostriatal projections. These findings are altered after L-dopa treatment. In ALS, there is a significant linear relationship between cortical threshold and duration of the disease (109). The threshold is normal or even reduced early in the disease, but as the disease progresses threshold continues to rise, and with time the motor cortex can no longer be stimulated. These findings may have resulted from glutamate excitotoxicity. Similarly CSP in ALS is shorter early in the disease with cortical hyperexcitability that lengthens progressively with the progression of the disease and decrement of excitotoxicity (109).

C. EEG: Usefulness and Changes in the Elderly

EEG records the spontaneously occurring electrical activities from the surface of the brain using surface electrodes and 10–20 International Electrode Placement Technique. Both bipolar and common referential montages are used. The recording usually lasts about 45 minutes and standard guidelines are used in the clinical neurophysiology laboratory to record EEG. EEG is an important noninvasive test to diagnose a variety of conditions in the elderly population. The single most important test for the diagnosis of seizures and epilepsy (recurrent seizures) is EEG obtained in wakefulness and sleep (111). It should be noted that there is an increased incidence of epilepsy and seizures in the elderly population (112). In fact, the two highest incidence groups are children and the elderly. The most common cause of recurrent seizures in the elderly is cerebrovascular disease. In addition, in the elderly EEG is indicated as a noninvasive test in patients with stroke as the EEG findings precede positive findings in the CT scan.

In Alzheimer's and other types of dementias, EEG often shows slowing of the background rhythm. By directing attention to a focal abnormality, sometimes EEG would help in the diagnosis of a focal lesion, such as cerebral tumor. A distinctive and characteristic EEG pattern is noted in patients with Creutzfeldt-Jakob disease. EEG is also indicated in patients with cortical myoclonus and other degenerative diseases accompanied by dementia. In the differential diagnosis between syncope and seizure, EEG is an excellent screening test. To interpret an EEG in the elderly, its limitations and changes must be understood. In this section the discussion will be limited to the EEG in wakefulness, and in the next section the EEG changes in sleep will be described.

In the normal elderly person several EEG changes have been described in the past. It is, however, not certain whether such EEG changes are maturational or are related to pathological alterations of the nervous system. It is a common observation that many elderly individuals suffer from a variety of dementing illnesses, cerebral vascular disease, or systemic medical disorders that may cause metabolic encephalopathy (113). In addition, many elderly persons use a variety of medications that may affect the EEG. Many of the changes described in the past literature are now thought to be due to associated pathological processes or secondary to a variety of medications. Use of quantitative EEG, including brain electrical activity mapping and screening by neuropsychological tests to assess mental functions, has clarified the true EEG changes in the elderly. Except for some minor changes, the awake EEG in the normal disease-free elderly does not differ significantly from healthy young adults (114). Katz and Horowitz (115) recorded EEG in a group of healthy septuagenarians after carefully screening them by neurologic and neuropsychological examination. They found an average alpha frequency of 9.8 Hz and the EEG was normal, and similar to that of the young and middle-aged adults. In contrast, Obrist (116,117) described slowing of the alpha rhythm, an increase of fast activities, an excess of 6–7 Hz theta waves and focal temporal slow waves in many normal older individuals. The question, however, arises of how rigorously the patients had been screened for underlying pathological process.

In their quantitative EEG in 63 men between ages 30 and 80, including 34 over 60 years, Duffy et al. (118) failed to find any difference in the frequency bands of theta-delta activities between young and old. Similarly Giaquinto and Nolfe (119) did not find any difference in the amount of slow waves between the elderly (47 patients with a mean age of 75 years) and middle-aged individuals (16 patients with a mean age of 49 years). Recently, Oken and Kaye (120) analyzed the EEG using both conventional and quantitative methods in 22 extremely healthy subjects between 84 and 98 years. They found a posterior peak frequency of about 8 Hz in subjects younger then 84 and 7–8 Hz in 5 of 22 subjects older than 84 years. Niedermeyer (121) concluded that alpha slowing in old age may be related to the decline in mental function that may represent an early stage of progressive dementia of old age. Alpha blocking and impaired photic driving response in old age found by Kelley et al. (122), as well as alpha slowing, may be secondary to possible structural CNS alterations in the elderly.

An important finding in the EEG literature of the old has been intermittent focal temporal slowing (theta-delta, often more marked on the left side), which has been noted in 17–59% of healthy elderly individuals (116,120,123–126). Sometimes sharp transients accompany this temporal slow activity and these findings may be related to cerebral vascular disease causing asymptomatic small infarction of the temporal lobe (121), ventricular enlargement with cerebral atrophy (127), or white-matter hyperintensities on magnetic resonance imaging (120). Some recent findings correlated such focal slowing with abnormal neuropsychological scores (127–130). These observations suggest that the presence of focal left temporal slowing in the elderly is abnormal. Quantitative EEG study in mildly to moderately demented patients with Alzheimer's disease disclosed similar left temporal slowing (129,131,132).

Such focal left temporal EEG slowing in the early stage of Alzheimer's disease may suggest temporal hypometabolism as defined by positron emission tomography (PET) study (133).

Bussey and Obrist (134) noted an increase of fast activity in elderly volunteer community subjects, especially women. A similar increase in fast activity with increasing age was reported by Kugler (135), who suggested that the presence of such excessive fast activity in old age may correlate with preserved mental functioning.

Sleep-onset frontal intermittent rhythmic delta activity (FIRDA) in normal elderly subjects has been noted by Katz and Horowitz (136). Such FIRDA should be differentiated from that associated with a variety of neurological disorders. FIRDA is highly stimulus sensitive and disappears in deeper stages of sleep.

The relationship between cerebral blood flow and EEG changes in the elderly remains undetermined. No correlation has been noted between areas showing maximum blood flow reduction and those showing prominent EEG slowing, or between blood flow changes and alpha frequency changes in normal elderly subjects (137,138). The loss of choline acetyltransferase, the enzyme for synthesis of acetylecholine (8), has been thought to be associated with alpha slowing.

D. Clinical Neurophysiologic Study of Sleep in the Elderly

Sleep disturbances in the elderly are very common and often go unreported. According to the National Commission on Sleep Disorders Research (NCSDR) report (139), about 40 million Americans suffer from sleep disturbances, including a large number of those over 65. In addition to history and physical examination, tests in a modern clinical neurophysiology laboratory are essential for confirmation of specific diagnosis. The two most important tests to study sleep are overnight polysomnography (PSG) and the multiple-sleep latency test (MSLT). PSG (140) includes the following: EEG;

electro-oculogram (EOG); electromyogram of the chin and sometimes the limb muscles; respiration by oronasal thermistor and by abdominal and thoracic strain gauges or respiratory inductance plethismographic bands (Respitrace); electrocardiography; and continuous recording of oxygen saturation by pulse oximetry. MSLT (141,142) is essential for documenting pathologic sleepiness and for diagnosing narcolepsy, and is performed in the daytime. MSLT consists of four or five recordings, each lasting 20 minutes, at 2-hour intervals, and recording EEG, EOG, and EMG. Daytime hypersomnolence is a very common complaint in the elderly and an overnight PSG is essential for detecting the cause.

Obstructive sleep apnea syndrome is the most common cause of excessive daytime somnolence and there is a high incidence in middle-aged to elderly men (143). It is important to diagnose this condition because there is effective treatment by using continuous positive airway pressure (CPAP), which may prevent serious complications such as congestive cardiac failure and cardiac arrhythmias caused by repeated apneas and hypoxemias at night (144). There are many other causes of daytime hypersomnolence in the elderly, including neurological (145), medical (146), and psychiatric disorders (147). Another indication for PSG in the elderly is male impotence. For this evaluation nocturnal penile tumescence (NPT) is included in the PSG study (148). Penile erections occur during REM sleep. This REM-related penile tumescence shows a linear decrease in percentage from youth to old age (e.g., from 88% at 20–26 years to 64–74% at 60–90 years) (149, 150). To interpret the neurophysiological tests of PSG and MSLT correctly it is important to be aware of the changes in the normal elderly and the limitations of such tests.

1. *Sleep EEG and sleep architectural changes*
   in the elderly

There is an increased incidence of microsleeps (bursts of sleep-like EEG lasting for several seconds) in the elderly (151). An important change in the elderly is a reduction of slow-wave sleep (SWS). It is actually related to the reduction of the amplitude of the delta waves during SWS (152) and, therefore, in the usual Rechtschaffen-Kales (153) scoring technique the amount of SWS decreases. This reduction of the delta amplitude could be related to a reduction of neuronal synchronization in the neocortex, alteration in the skull, and changes in the subarachnoid spaces in the elderly (152,154). There are also a number of changes noted in sleep spindles (155): decreased frequency, amount, and amplitude. The spindles often slow down from 14 to 12 and are poorly formed and poorly developed.

As far as rapid eye movement (REM)–non-REM (NREM) cyclic pattern is concerned, this remains unchanged, but the first cycle may be reduced. Also there is a reduction of REM density (number of eye movement bursts per minute of REM sleep) and a slight reduction of total REM sleep, but the percentage of REM in relation to the total sleep time remains unaltered (154,156–158). There is also sleep fragmentation due to frequent interruptions at night. In addition, there are frequent sleep stage shifts and awakenings. It is often stated that the total sleep time of the elders is shorter than the total sleep time of younger adults, but this may be incorrect because the elderly subjects often take daytime naps and hence 24-hour sleep time remains the same as that in young adults (156). Carskadon (159,160), Kales (161), Feinberg (162), and coworkers summarized the following important changes in sleep of the elderly: frequent stage shifts and state changes, reduction of slow-wave sleep, reduction of the amplitude of the delta waves, increased stage I sleep, frequent arousals, decreased total nocturnal sleep, and a reduction of the total REM sleep time, but normal REM percentage in relation to the total sleep time. Similar findings have also been noted by Williams and colleagues (163) as well as by Prinz and Vitiello (164). In a longitudinal polysomnogrphaic and diary-based study considered to be the first by Hoch et al. (165a), sleep efficiency but not other sleep measures deteriorated over a 2-year period in a group of 23 healthy "old old" subjects (>75 years) as contrasted with a group of 27 "young old" subjects (60–74 yrs).

There are circadian rhythm changes noted in the elderly subjects (156,165). The monophasic circadian rhythm of young adults gives rise to a polyphasic ultradian rhythm of old age. There are frequent awakenings at night with reduction of wakefulness, causing increased daytime naps. There is also a phase advance in the elderly with a tendency to go to sleep early and awake early. These alterations may be related to age-related changes in the core body temperature rhythm (166,167). The physiological changes in the circadian rhythm may be related to the structural alterations seen in the suprachiasmatic nucleus and brainstem hypnogenic neurons in experimental studies in several species of animals (156). Compared with the young adults the elderly subjects show respiratory changes with an increased incidence of periodic breathing with some periods of apneas and increased snoring at night (156).

Weitzman (154) suggested that the sleep disturbances in the elderly may be related to the morphological alterations in the central nervous system, such as cell loss in the locus ceruleus, pontine and midbrain reticular formation, selective hypothalamic regions, and suprachiasmatic neurons, as well as accumulation of neurofibrillary tangles and abnormal pigment in the hypothalamus.

In the MSLT study the average daily sleep latency is shorter in the elderly than in younger individuals (142). In MSLT studies by Levine et al. (168) and Roehrs et al. (169), subjects aged 21–35 years had an average daily sleep latency of 10 minutes, whereas adults aged 30–49 years had average latencies of 11–12 minutes and those 50–59 years old had an average latency of 9 minutes. In MSLT scoring an average latency of 5 minutes or less is considered pathological, a latency of 5–10 minutes is borderline, and a latency of 10 minutes and above is considered normal.

Another important finding in the PSG of the elderly is an increasing incidence of periodic limb movements (170) in sleep (PLMS), and in some studies these PLMS were found in 50% of the elderly subjects. However, PLMS is an important physiological finding in patients with restless legs syndrome (170); therefore, the diagnosis should be based on the history and the PSG study. It should be finally noted that the age-related sleep changes of the normal elderly individuals may be aggravated and compounded by the superimposed neurological, medical, or psychiatric disorders and those secondary to the use of medications for such illnesses.

E. Autonomic Neurophysiology in the Elderly

Simple noninvasive tests to evaluate functions of the autonomic nervous system should be available in every neurophysiology laboratory of an academic department. Such tests may include the following (171–173): testing for orthostatic variation of blood pressure and heart rate in supine and standing positions or on a tilt table (this tests the integrity of both the sympathetic and vagal functions); heart rate variation with deep breathing (this tests cardiovagal function); 30:15 ratio (ratio of 30th heartbeat to 15th heartbeat immediately after standing); cold pressor and mental arithmetic tests to evaluate the integrity of the sympathetic efferent function; Valsalva maneuver and Valsalva ratio (these test both the sympathetic and parasympathetic functions); sympathetic skin response measured in the EMG laboratory (this tests sympathetic efferent function); and quantitative sudomotor axon reflex test (QSART), which is a sensitive test for postganglionic sympathetic sudomotor function. All of these tests are age dependent and, therefore, the sensitivity (e.g., an abnormal test in a patient with autonomic failure) and specificity (e.g., a normal test in a disease-free individual) must take into consideration several factors, including age. It should also be noted that in autonomic testing variability is more frequently noted than in peripheral nerve conduction testing, so that a larger number of controls will be needed for deriving a percentile response (173). It is important to incorporate autonomic testing in the

clinical neurophysiology laboratory because the elderly subjects suffer from a number of autonomic disorders for which
testing is required. Some examples of these disorders are
neurodegenerative diseases, such as multiple system atrophy
with progressive autonomic failure (Shy-Drager syndrome)
and Parkinson's disease with autonomic dysfunction, diabetic
autonomic neuropathies, and distal small-fiber neuropathy. In
addition, prolonged bed rest and inactivity in old age may be
associated with orthostatic hypotension and orthostatic dizziness. Impotence in elderly men may in some cases be due to
autonomic dysfunction.

1.   *Age-related changes in the autonomic nervous system*

Many of the autonomic functions decline in old age, but some
may show hyperactivity. For example, there may be evidence
of hyperadrenalism in old age (174) as manifested by higher
supine plasma norepinephrine levels in older subjects and
increased muscle sympathetic discharges as shown by microneurographic recordings. Thus the ANS undergoes a variety
of physiologic changes in advancing age. Low (175) summarized the alterations in old age of the autonomic functions
pertaining to the heart, circulation, pupils, thermoregulation,
baroreflexes, and peripheral sympathetic functions and suggested that the pathogenetic mechanisms of changes in the
ANS in old age are of multifactorial origin.

2.   *Orthostatic hypotension and old age*

Mild or asymptomatic OH in old age (176–179), particularly
in those over 70, has been reported by several authors, whereas others did not find an age-dependent reduction in orthostatic BP (175,180). In contrast, OH in the elderly may occur
under conditions of stress (e.g., postprandial stress, prolonged
bed rest, volume depletion, and intercurrent illness). OH in
old age may be related to a combination of factors: age-related
reduction of the preganglionic sympathetic neurons in the intermediolateral column of the spinal cord; reduced sensitivity
of the alpha- and beta-adrenoreceptors; and impairment of the
baroreflex mechanism (181–183).

3. Cardiac sympathetic and parasympathetic functions

Cardiac sympathetic and parasympathetic functions are impaired in old age. Degree of increase of heart rate with exercise and isoproterenol is impaired. This reduced sympathetic drive is due to reduced beta-adrenoreceptor sensitivity. Also atropine-induced tachycardia (an index of vagal activity) decreases with old age (175,184). Sympathetic dysfunction may be related to the age-related reduction of preganglionic sympathetic neurons in the intermediolateral column of the spinal cord and preganglionic ventral roots (181,185,186) as well as reduction of postganglionic neurons in the superior cervical ganglion (187). Howell (188) clearly showed slowing of the resting heart rate in old age. Resting heart rate is controlled by both sympathetic and parasympathetic divisions. In contrast, the intrinsic heart rate controlled by the sinoatrial node also is reduced with aging.

4. Valsalva maneuver

Contradictory results have been obtained regarding Valsalva ratio in advancing age: some found no change (189) whereas others noted clear change (190–194).

5. Baroreceptor reflex changes

Baroreflex sensitivity decreases with age (195). Age-related changes (axonal degeneration) in the afferent (e.g., sinus and aortic nerves) and efferent fibers (e.g., vagus nerves) of the baroreceptor reflex arc may be responsible for depression of baroreflexes in old age (196–198).

6. Beat-to-beat heart rate variation

The beat-to-beat heart rate variation shows a decline in old age that is dependent on a reduced parasympathetic tone as evidenced by the action of atropine administration (184,199). Sinus arrhythmia (heart rate response to deep breathing: HR_{DB}) is reduced with increasing age (175,191,200,201). Low et al. also confirmed this finding in a study involving 122 subjects aged 10 to 83 years (191).

7. *30:15 ratio*

The ratio of the maximum R–R interval (around the 30th beat) and the minimum R–R interval (around the 15th beat) is altered in old age. Thus, cardiovagal function is markedly affected by age and there is a linear relationship between the age and the HR_{DB}, 30:15 HR ratio as well as Valsalva ratio. Low et al. (191) found a linear regression of heart rate range against age, showing a slope of 0.36 × age in years. Thus, in all these procedures, using a normal range without any consideration of the age and the conditions of testing will be fallacious.

8. *Plasma norepinephrine levels*

There is a linear increase of supine plasma norepinephrine levels with increasing age (202), but no such relationship was found with epinephrine. On standing and during cold pressor, and mental arithmetic tests, plasma norepinephrine levels show a higher rise in older than in younger subjects (203). The increased supine plasma norepinephrine levels in old age correlate with the microneurographic findings of increased sympathetic muscle nerve activity in older subjects (204).

9. *Thermoregulatory responses*

These responses are impaired in old age as evidenced by impairment of shivering during cooling and sweating during warming in many normal elderly subjects (205).

10. *Sudomotor function*

Sweat gland density decreases with increasing age, particularly in the lower limbs and after age 60. In addition, there are morphological changes in the unmyelinating axons supplying the sweat glands. Low (175) and investigators found on QSART testing that the axon reflex–mediated sweat response declined with age in the lower extremities.

11. *Pupillary changes*

Autonomic innervation to the pupil (sympathetic pupillodilator and parasympathetic pupilloconstrictor fibers) is impaired with increasing age, which may explain the miosis of old age and a decrement of the dark adaptation of pupil diameter (206, 207).

F. Physiologic Tests to Detect Dysfunction of Gait and Balance in the Elderly

Posture and balance depend on smooth functioning of the afferent stimuli from the visual, vestibular, and somatosensory systems; central integration involving the cerebellum, thalamus, and cerbral cortex; and efferent responses (motor control mechanism) (208–212). Dysfunction in any of these mechanisms may result in abnormal posture and gait, causing disequilibrium, and false sensations of unsteadiness and dizziness. Significant changes occur in balance in the elderly, causing postural instability, impairment of balance, and falls. Electronystagmography, static and dynamic position tests, rotational and caloric tests, and computerized dynamic platform posturography are some of the important tests to diagnose balance disorders (208–210). Age-specific data are needed to differentiate between benign falls and gait problems of the elderly, and the pathological conditions causing such balance disorders.

As stated above, normal postural control consists of motor and sensory components (208–212). Motor components include coordination, motor learning, scaling the postural response, latency to postural response, and biomechanics. Sensory components consist of detection of peripheral sensory stimuli, sensory motor intergration, and central selection.

Static balance is defined as an ability to minimize the vertical and support stance over a normal or narrowed base of support (e.g., standing on one leg). Between the ages of 60 and 69, the individual begins to deteriorate in terms of maintaining static balance (208–212).

The limits of sway include the zones of stability in anteroposterior and lateral planes with feet in the normal bipedal position. Beginning at about 60 years this function begins to deteriorate and significant decrease is noted in the 80s and 90s.

Sensory organization is defined as the ability to integrate sensory inputs into motor response. This can be expressed in terms of sway and loss of balance. Sensory input could be visual, vestibular, or somatosensory. There are measurement techniques available for all of these. Sway limits can be measured and actual sways can be measured by computerized scores. With rotating sway referenced platform (i.e., false visual input) the performance in the elderly declines, but with normal visual and vestibular inputs no decline is seen. With false visual input (i.e., eyes closed) and proprioceptive input, sways decline and the incidence of falls increases.

Dynamic balance tests the motor function and is defined as the ability to respond to destabilizing force. This can be expressed in terms of sway or loss of balance and can be measured by surface EMG and computerized scores. Surface EMG can be obtained from the paraspinal, abdominal, hamstrings, gastrocnemius, quadriceps, and tibialis anterior muscles. The pattern of EMG activation is found to be abnormal in old age.

During rotation of the platform about 50% of the elderly will lose balance during the first trial (208–212). Only about 5% of the younger subjects may lose balance initially. Balance improves in the elderly with repetition, but in younger subjects virtually no loss of balance is seen on repeating the test. It should be noted that women have a higher tendency to fall, particularly during the first trial test.

In summary, the elderly demonstrate a resticted limit of sway and diminished ability to control a narrowed base of support. Their balance thus differs from younger individuals under changing conditions (e.g., limiting the sensory input and difficult motor task). All these factors cause falls in the elderly. The relatively modest age-related change is a factor in the increased incidence of falls in the elderly, especially in older women. It should, however, be noted that balance of older individuals is flexible and effective under most conditions. Finally, this impairment of balance disorder in normal elderly individuals is the foundation of gait disorder in normal as well as abnormal conditions (e.g., CNS diseases) (212).

G. Neurophysiologic Tests to Detect Dysfunction of the Voluntary Movements in the Elderly

The cerebral cortex controls voluntary movements by interacting with the basal ganglia and the cerebellum through the cortical and subcortical circuits (213,214). The cerebellum and basal ganglia have two-way connections with various regions of the cerebral cortex. The cerebellum also has direct connections with the brainstem and indirectly connects with the spinal cord, and these subcortical inputs greatly influence the cerebral cortex in the control of voluntary movements. The cerebellum participates in the initiation and coordination of the movements; the basal ganglia helps influence the direction, force, and amplitude of the movements; and the cerebral cortex, via the supplementary motor area, plans and programs the movements. The corticospinal system then commands and executes the movements, and the spinal segmental motor apparatus finalizes these movements. A breakdown in any of these circuits may cause impairment of the voluntary movements. These circuits may be impaired in basal ganglia, cerebellar, and corticospinal disorders.

In normal elderly individuals voluntary movements are often clumsy and impaired as evidenced by the slowing of walking, grip strength, and a lack of physical agility. Some of these functions can be tested by computerized platform posturography (see above) and by studying ballistic movements and reaction time. In normal individuals ballistic movement (e.g., rapid flexion or extension of the elbow) is associated with a triphasic response: an initial agonist (AG), followed by an antagonist (AN), and the final agonist muscle bursts recorded from the AG and AN muscles by surface EMG recordings simultaneously (214–216). The burst duration is between 50 and 150 milliseconds and the AN burst has the longest duration. Such a study of the ballistic movement comparing young and old individuals has not been performed in a comprehensive manner. The most likely finding is either normal (217) or minimal prolongation of the burst duration in the elderly as compared to the younger individuals. Reaction times (RTs), including both simple and choice, involve cognition in execution of these movements, and have been found to be impaired in Parkinson's disease (218). RT is also slowed in the elderly and therefore neurophysiologic data based on well-executed techniques must be obtained in the young and the old to make a meaningful conclusion.

H. Neurophysiologic Tests to Characterize Abnormal (Involuntary) Movements in the Elderly

A variety of abnormal movements may be seen in the elderly. None of these adventitious movements should be considered normal phenomena except perhaps tremulousness (3) or so-called senile tremor. This may represent an enhanced physiologic tremor or a late manifestation of essential familial tremor. Tests may be performed in a standard clinical neurophysiology laboratory to characterize and differentiate different involuntary movements (214,219,220). In this section I will discuss briefly the tests to identify different types of involuntary movements, such as tremor, myoclonus, and dystonia. Such tests may also be used to characterize chorea, tics, tardive dyskinesia, and restless legs syndrome. In some of these tests (e.g., SER, Bereitschaftspotential, reciprocal inhibition, and blink reflex excitability) what is considered normal in the elderly may be abnormal in a young individual and, therefore, interpretation should be made cautiously.

The following tests may be performed to analyze the involuntary movement disorders (214,219): (1) multiple-muscle EMGs using surface electrodes over both the AG and AN muscles of the limbs bilaterally and over various cranial muscles; (2) somatosensory evoked potential study; (3) electroencephalogram; (4) jerk-locked back averaging technique; (5) accelerometric study with spectral analysis of the average epochs to quantitate tremors; (6) reflex studies, such as long-loop or transcortical or C reflex, H reflex to study reciprocal inhibition and motor neuron excitability, and blink reflex excitability test; (7) polygraphic and polysomnographic tests.

1. *Tremor (214,219,221)*

Rest tremor, characteristically seen in Parkinson's disease, has a frequency of 3–5 Hz, and EMG shows alternating AG and AN bursts.

Physiologic tremor, including enhanced physiologic tremor, has a frequency in the range of 8–12 Hz and the EMG bursts are generally synchronous in AG-AN muscles.

Essential tremor is characterized by a frequency faster than the rest but slower than the physiologic tremor and is in the range of 5–8 Hz. EMG bursts are most commonly synchronous, but sometimes can be alternating.

Intention tremor, characteristically seen in cerebellar disorder, shows rhythmic alternating EMG bursts as the target is approached and the frequency is generally in the range of 4–6 Hz.

Neuropathic tremor, seen in patients with polyneuropathies, shows both synchronous and alternating activities in the AG-AN muscles at a frequency of 6–8 Hz.

Hysterical tremor mostly resembles action tremors with alternating AG-AN EMG activities with varying tremor frequency.

2. *Myoclonus (214,216,219,220,222,223)*

The four most important tests to characterize myoclonus consist of polymyography, jerk-locked back-averaging, transcortical reflex, and measurement of somatosensory evoked potential amplitude following median, peroneal, or tibial nerve stimulation. Startle reflex (224,225) study may also be helpful in audiogenic stimulus-sensitive myoclonus. Based on these tests myoclonus can be characterized according to the site of origin of the discharge as cortical myoclonus, brainstem or subcortical myoclonus, and segmental myoclonus. In addition, there is a special type of propriospinal myoclonus (226,227), which is a variant of spinal myoclonus.

Cortical myoclonus (214,228–230) generally shows the following physiological characteristics: (1) The jerks are focal or multifocal and more distal than proximal. (2) The order of activation is in the rostral-caudal direction with the cranial nerve muscles firing in descending order before the limb muscles. (3) EMG burst duration is brief (e.g., 10–100 milliseconds). (4) Jerk-locked back-averaging shows EEG-EMG time-locked event and an EEG positive or negative transient precedes myoclonus jerks by about 15–30 milliseconds in the arms and 20–40 milliseconds in the legs. (5) SEP amplitude (e.g., N20, P25 components of the median nerve SEP) is very high. (6) The transcortical reflex is often hyperactive.

Brainstem or subcortical myoclonus (214,229,231) shows the following physiological properties: (1) The jerks are generalized and more proximal than distal. (2) The activation order is up the brainstem and down the spinal cord. (3) EMG burst duration is longer (e.g., 100–150 milliseconds). (4) Back-averaging does not show EEG-EMG time-locked event. (5) The SEP amplitude is normal. (6) The reflex is not hyperactive except in reticular reflex myoclonus.

Segmental myoclonus (229) is characterized by the following physiological properties: (1) The jerks are focal or bilateral and often rhythmic. These are noted predominantly in the flexor muscles and are often limited to the affected segments of the spinal cord or brainstem. (2) The burst duration is the longest (e.g., 150–250 milliseconds or even longer). (3) Cortical EEG-EMG correlate is absent. (4) Cortical SEP amplitude is normal. (5) The C reflex is normal. (6) In propriospinal myoclonus the order of activation may be from the midthoracic up the spinal cord toward the cervical region and down the spinal cord toward the lumbosacral region.

3. *Dystonia*

EMG characteristics of the abnormal movements in dystonia may show the following three patterns (214,232,233): (1) continuous EMG activities lasting from 2 to 30 seconds followed by brief silence; (2) rhythmic co-contractions lasting from 1 to 2 seconds followed by relative EMG silence of 1 to 2 seconds (myorhythmia); (3) brief muscle jerks similar to myoclonic bursts (with a duration of 50–100 milliseconds).

EMG of the voluntary movements (214,232,233) shows the following properties: (1) normal reciprocal activation of AG-AN muscles during rapid flexion-extension movements; (2) excessive co-contraction of the AG-AN muscles with overflow to other muscles and prolonged duration of muscle bursts; (3) the first AG bursts in the ballistic movement study are sometimes prolonged.

Long-loop reflex study may show hyperactive C reflex, but this may be due to an inability of the patient to relax the muscle. Median SEP study shows no high-amplitude cortical potentials. EEG-EMG correlate is absent from back-averaging technique.

Reciprocal inhibition between AG and AN muscles in patients with both focal and generalized dystonia shows impairment as shown by the technique of H-reflex study (214, 232,234,235). This may be the reason for co-contraction between AG and AN muscles. Briefly, this technique consists of applying radial nerve "conditioning" stimuli in the spiral group before, during, and after delivery of the median nerve "test" stimuli at the elbow and recording the H-reflex amplitude in the flexor carpi radialis muscle. The H-reflex amplitude is expressed as a percentage of the control amplitude before applying the conditioning shocks. Day et al. (234) found three periods of inhibition at 0, 10, and 75 millisecond intervals between the "conditioning" and "test" stimuli while studying reciprocal inhibition between AG and AN muscles of the forearm in normal human subjects. In dystonic patients there is impairment of all three periods of inhibition.

Blink reflex excitability study (236,237) shows hyper-excitability of R2 component of the blink reflex as shown by the application of the "conditioning" and "test" stimuli at different interstimulus intervals during blink reflex study in patients with spasmodic torticollis, blepharospasm, and oromanibular dystonia. These findings suggest increased excitability of brainstem interneurons that may have resulted from a faulty drive from the basal ganglia upon these interneurons.

IV. CONCLUSION

Neurophysiologic tests are important components of the essential laboratory tests for the practice of gerontologic neurology. With advancing years, reference values for a variety of these tests change and, therefore, it is important to obtain age-related normative data for these tests. Without a clear understanding of these pitfalls, many of the neurophysiologic tests may be misinterpreted and hence misclassifications and misdiagnoses may be made. An understanding of the various changes in the dynamic functions of the body in the elderly is clearly a prerequisite for proper interpretation of clinical neurophysiologic tests in the geriatric population. It is hoped that this brief review of test interpretation involving different physiologic functions of the nervous system will make the students and the practitioners of gerontologic neurology realize that clinical neurophysiology is really an extension of clinical neurology.

REFERENCES

1. Stalberg E, Young RR. What is clinical neurophysiology? In: Stalberg E, Young RR (eds.), Clinical Neurophysiology. Boston: Butterworths, 1981; 1–3.
2. Monjan AA. Sleep disorders of older people: Report of a Consensus Conference. Hosp Commun Psychiatry 1990; 41: 743–744.
3. Adams RD, Victor M. Principles of Neurology, 5th ed. New York: McGraw-Hill, 1993.

4. Behnke JA, Finch CE, Momoent BG, eds. The Biology of Aging. New York: Plenum Press, 1978.

5. Comfort A. The Biology of Senescence, 3rd ed. New York: Elsevier, 1979.

6. Critchley M. The neurology of old age. Lancet 1931; 2:1119–1127, 1222–1230.

7. Critchley M. Neurologic changes in the aged. J Chronic Dis 1956; 3:459–477.

8. Katzman R, Terry R. Normal aging of the nervous system. In: Katzman R, Terry R (eds.), The Neurology of Aging. Philadelphia: FA Davis, 1983; 15–50.

9. Benassi G, D'Alessandro R, Gallassi R, et al. Neurological examination in subjects over 65 years: An epidemiological survey. Neuroepidemiology 1990; 9:27–38.

10. Jenkyn LR, Reeves AG. Neurologic signs in uncomplicated aging (senescence). Semin Neurol 1981; 1:21–30.

11. Potvin AR, Syndulko K, Tourtellotte WW, et al. Human neurologic function and the aging process. J Am Geriatr Soc 1980; 28:1.

12. Potvin AR, Syndulko K, Tourtellotte W, et al. Quantitative evaluation of normal age related changes in neurologic function. In: Pirozzolo FJ, Maletta GJ (eds.), Advances in Neurogerontology, vol 2. New York: Praeger, 1981; 13–57.

13. Jorgensen L, Torvik A. Ischaemic cerebrovascular diseases in an autopsy series. Part I. Prevalence, location, and predisposing factors in verified thrombo-embolic occlusions, and their significance in the pathogenesis of cerebral infarction. J Neurol Sci 1966; 3:490–509.

14. Krall VA. Senescent forgetfulness: Benign and malignant. Can Med Assoc J 1962; 86:257–260.

15. Crook T, Bartus RT, Ferris SH, et al. Age-associated memory impairment: Proposed diagnostic criteria and measures of clinical change-report of a National Institute of Mental Health Work Group. Dev Neuropsychol 1986; 2:261–276.

16. Hazzard WR, Bierman EL. Old Age. In: Smith D, Bierman EL (eds.), Biological Ages of Man from Conception Through Old Age, 2nd ed. Philadelphia: WB Saunders, 1978; 229.

17. Cowley M. The View from 80. New York: Viking Press, 1976; 1.

18. Kimura J. Electrodiagnosis in Diseases of Nerve and Muscle:

Principles and Practice, 2nd ed. Philadelphia: FA Davis, 1989.

19. Robinson LR. Interpreting electrophysiologic data in the elderly. In: Aging: Neuromuscular Function and Disease, 1994 AAEM Plenary Session I. Rochester, MN: AAEM Publication, 1994; 25–29.

20. Robinson LR, Rubner DE. Statistical considerations for the development and use of reference values as applied to nerve conduction studies. In: Kraft GH (ed.), Physical Medicine and Rehabilitation Clinics of North America. Philadelphia: WB Saunders, 1994; 531–540.

21. Robinson LR, Temkin NR, Fujimoto WY, Stolov WC. Impact of statistical methodology on normal limits in nerve conduction studies. Muscle Nerve 1991; 14:1084–1090.

22. Rivner MH, Swift TR, Crout BO, Rhodes KP. Toward more rational nerve conduction interpretations: The effect of height. Muscle Nerve 1990; 13:232–239.

23. Trojaborg WT, Moon A, Andersen BB, Trojaborg NS. Sural nerve conduction parameters in normal subjects related to age, gender, temperature and height: A reappraisal. Muscle Nerve 1992; 15:666–671.

24. Denys EH. AAEM minimonograph #14: The influence of temperature in clinical neurophysiology. Muscle Nerve 1991; 14:795–811.

25. MacDonnell RAL, Shahani BT. Clinical electrophysiology in the elderly. In: Albert ML, Knoefel JE (eds.), Clinical Neurology of Aging, 2nd ed. New York: Oxford University Press, 1994; 266–273.

26. Buchthal F, Pinelli P, Rosenfalk P. Action potential parameters in normal human muscle and their physiological determinants. Acta Physiol Scand 1954; 32:219–229.

27. Feinstein B, Patle RE, Weddel CT. Metabolic factors affecting fibrillation in denervated muscle. J Neurol Neurosurg Psychiatry 1945; 8:1–16.

28. Borenstein S, Desmedt JE. New diagnostic procedures in myasthenia gravis. In: Desmedt JE (ed.), New Developments in Electromyography and Clinical Neurophysiology, vol. 1. Basel: Karger, 1973; 350–374.

29. Wilbourn A. Diabetic Neuropathies. In: Brown WF, Bolton CF (eds.), Clinical Electromyography, 2nd ed. Boston: Butterworth-Heinemann, 1993; 477–515.

30. Oh SJ. Clinical Electromyography: Nerve Conduction Studies, 2nd ed. Baltimore: Williams and Wilkins, 1993.

31. LaFratta CW. A comparison of sensory and motor NCV as related with age. Arch Phys Med Rehab 1966; 47:286–290.

32. Downie AW, Newell DJ. Sensory nerve conduction in patients with diabetes mellitus and controls. Neurology 1961; 11:876–882.

33. Ludin HP. Electromyography in Practice. New York: Thieme-Stratton, 1980.

34. Gregerson G. Diabetic neuropathy: Influence of age, sex, metabolic control, and duration of diabetes on motor conduction velocity. Neurology 1967; 17:972–980.

35. Oh SJ, Kim HS, Ahmad BK. Electrophysiological diagnosis of the interdigital neuropathy of the foot. Muscle Nerve 1982; 5:566–567.

36. Wagman IH, Lesse H. Maximum conduction velocities of motor fibers of ulnar nerve in human subjects of various ages and sexes. J Neurophysiol 1952; 15:235–244.

37. Taylor PK. Non-linear effects of age on nerve conduction in adults. J Neurol Sci 1984; 66:223–234.

38. Buchthal F, Rosenfalck A. Evoked action potentials and conduction velocity in human sensory nerves. Brain Res 1966; 3:1–122.

39. Lascelles RG, Thomas PK. Changes due to age in internodal length in the sural nerve in man. J Neurol Neurosurg Psychiatry 1966; 29:40–44.

40. Troghi H, Tsukagoshi H, Toyokura Y. Quantitative changes with age in normal sural nerves. Acta Neuropath 1977; 38:213–220.

41. Kimura J. Electromyography and Nerve Stimulation Techniques: Clinical Applications (Japanese). Tokyo: Egakushoin, 1989.

42. Cruz Martinez A, Barrio M, Perez Conde MC, Ferrer MT. Electrophysiological aspects of sensory conduction velocity in healthy adults. I. Conduction velocity from digit to palm, from palm to wrist, and across the elbow, as a function of age. J Neurol Neurosurg Psychiat 1978; 41:1092–1096.

43. Wagman IH, Lesse H. Maximum conduction velocities of motor fibers of ulnar nerve in human subjects of various ages and sizes. J Neurophysiol 1952; 15:235–242.

44. Norris AH, Shock NW, Wagman IH. Age changes in the maximum conduction velocity of motor fibers of human ulnar nerves. J Appl Physiol 1953; 5:589–593.

45. Mayer RF. Nerve conduction studies in man. Neurology 1963; 13:1021–1030.

46. Horwitz SH, Krarup C. Conduction studies of the normal sural nerve. Muscle Nerve 1992; 15:374–383.

47. Stetson DS, Albers JW, Silverstein BA, Wolfe RA. Effects of age, sex, and anthropometric factors on nerve conduction measures. Muscle Nerve 1992; 15:1095–1104.

48. Buchthal F, Rosenfalck A, Trojaborg W. Electrophysiological findings in entrapment of the median nerve at wrist and elbow. J Neurol Neurosurg Psychiatry 1974; 37:340–360.

49. Tackmann W, Keaser HE, Magun HG. Comparison of orthodromic and antidromic sensory nerve conduction velocity measurements in the carpal tunnel syndrome. J Neurol 1981; 224:257–266.

50. Litchy WJ, Wibbens LM, Lehamn KA, Hokanson JL, Dyck PJ. Normal values of nerve conduction attributes: The Rochester Random Population Study (Abstract). Peripheral Nerve Society Program, Saint Paul, Minnesota, June 1994.

51. Buchthal F. Electromyography in the evaluation of muscle diseases. Neurol Clin 1985; 3:573–598.

52. Bischoff C, Machetanz J, Conrad B. Is there an age dependent continuous increase in the duration of the motor unit action potential? Electroencephalogr Clin Neurophysiol 1991; 81:304–311.

53. Brown WF. Neurophysiologic changes in aging. In: Aging: Neuromuscular Function and Disease, 1994 AAEM Plenary Session I. Rochester, MN: AAEM Publication, 1994; 17–23.

54. Doherty TJ, Vandervoort AA, Brown WF. Effects of aging on the motor unit: A brief review. Can J Appl Physiol 1993; 18:331–358.

55. Brown WF. A method for estimating the number of motor units in thenar muscles and the change in motor unit count with aging. J Neurol Neurosurg Psychiatry 1972; 35:845–852.

56. Brown WF, Strong MJ, Snow RS. Methods for estimating numbers of motor units in biceps-brachialis muscles and losses of motor units with aging. Muscle Nerve 1988; 11:423–432.

57. Stalberg E, Fawcett PRW. Marco EMG in healthy subjects of different ages. J Neurol Neurosurg Psychiatry 1982; 45:870–878.

58. Davies CTM, White MJ. The contractile properties of elderly human triceps surae. Gerontology 1983; 29:19–23.

59. Davies CTM, Thomas DO, White MJ. Mechanical properties of young and elderly human muscle. Acta Med Scand 1986; 711(suppl):219–226.

60. McDonagh MJN, White MJ, Davies CTM. Different effects of aging on the mechanical properties of human arm and leg muscles. Gerontology 1984; 30:49–54.

61. Stalberg E, Trontelj JV. Single fiber electromyography, 2nd ed. Old Woking, Surrey, England: Mirvalle Press, 1994.

62. Howard JE, McGill KC, Dorfman L. Age effects on properties of motor unit action potentials: ADEMG analysis. Ann Neurol 1988; 24:207–213.

63. Dice JF. Cellular and molecular mechanisms of aging. Physiol Rev 1993; 73:149–159.

64. Chiappa KH. Evoked Potentials in Clinical Medicine, 2nd ed. New York: Raven Press, 1990.

65. Barrett G. Advanced data capture and analysis techniques for clinical evoked potentials. In: Halliday AM (ed.), Evoked Potentials in Clinical Testing. New York: Churchill Livingstone, 1982; 483–505.

66. Goodin DS, Squires KC, Starr A. Long latency event-related components of the auditory evoked potentials in demenita. Brain 1978; 101:635–648.

67. Goodin DS, Aminoff MJ. Electrophysiological differences between subtypes of dementia. Brain 1986; 109:1103–1113.

68. Goodin DS, Squires KC, Henderson BH, Starr A. Age-related variations in evoked potentials to auditory stimuli in normal human subjects. Electroencephalogr Clin Neurophysiol 1978; 44:447–458.

69. Dorfman LJ, Bosley TM. Age related changes in peripheral and central nerve conduction in man. Neurology 1979; 29:38–44.

70. Hume AL, Cant BR, Shaw NA, Cowan JC. Central somatosensory time from 10–79 years. Electroencephalogr Clin Neurophysiol 1982; 54:49–54.

71. Allison T, Hume AL, Wood CC, Goff WR. Development

and aging changes in somatosenory, auditory and visual evoked potentials. Electroencephalogr Clin Neurophysiol 1984; 58:14-24.

72. Desmedt JE, Cheron G. Somatosensory evoked potential to finger stimulation in healthy octogenarians and in young adults: Waveforms, scalp topography and transit times of parietal and frontal components. Electroencephalogr Clin Neuorphysiol 1980; 50:404-425.

73. Lueders H. The effects of aging on the waveform of the somatosensory cortical evoked potential. Electroencephalogr Clin Neurophysiol 1970; 29:450-460.

74. Stockard JJ, Stockard JE, Sharbrough FW. Nonpathologic factors influencing brainstem auditory evoked potentials. Am J Electroencephalogr Technol 1978; 18:177-209.

75. Rowe MJ. Normal variability of the brainstem auditory evoked response in young and old adult subjects. Electroencephalogr Clin Neurophysiol 1978; 44:459-470.

76. Jerger J, Hall J. Effects of age and sex on auditory brainstem response. Arch Otolaryngol 1980; 106:387-391.

77. Rosenthal U, Bjorkman G, Pedersen K, Kal A. Brain-stem auditory evoked potentials in different age groups. Electroencephalogr Clin Neurophysiol 1985; 62:426-430.

78. Bodis-Wollner I, Yahr MD. Measurement of visual evoked potentials in Parkinson's disease. Brain 1978; 101:661-671.

79. Onofrj M, Ghilardi MF, Basciani M, Gambi D. Visual evoked potentials in parkinsonism and dopamine blockade reveal a stimulus-dependent dopamine function in humans. J Neurol Neurosurg Psychiatry 1986; 49:1150-1159.

80. Moody ED, Chokroverty S, Tzanakou E. Frequency domain analysis of visual evoked potentials in Alzheimer's disease. J Clin Neurophysiol 1987; 4:549-552.

81. Coben LA, Danziger WL, Hughes CP. Visual evoked potentials in mild senile dementia of the Alzheimer type. Electroencephalogr Clin Neurophysiol 1983; 55:121-130.

82. Visser SL, Van Tilburg W, Hooijer C, De Rijke W. Visual evoked potentials (VEPs) in senile dementia (Alzheimer type) and in non-organic behavioral disorders in the elderly: Comparison with EEG parameters. Electrencephalogr Clin Neurophysiol 1985; 60:115-121.

83. Smith AT, Early F, Jones GH. Comparison of the effects of

Alzheimer's diseae, normal aging and scopolamine on human transient visual evoked potentials. Psychopharmacology 1990; 102:535–543.

84. Shaw NA, Cant BR. Age-dependent changes in the latency of the pattern visual evoked potential. Electroencephalogr Clin Neurophysiol 1980; 48:237–241.

85. Celesia GG, Daly RF. Visual electroencephalographic computer analysis (VECA). Neurology 1977; 27:637–641.

86. Asselman P, Chadwick DW, Marsden CD. Visual evoked responses in the diagnosis and management of patients suspected of multiple sclerosis. Brain 1975; 98:261–282.

87. Hennerici M, Wenzel D, Freund H-J. The comparison of small-size rectangle and checker-board stimulation for the evaluation of delayed visual evoked responses in patients suspected of multiple sclerosis. Brain 1977; 100:119–136.

88. Allison T, Goff WR, Wood CC. Auditory, somatosensory and visual evoked potentials in the diagnosis of neuropathology: Recording considerations and normative data. In: Lehman D, Callaway E (eds.), Human Evoked Potentials: Applications and Problems. London: Plenum Press, 1979; 1–16.

89. Stockard JJ, Hughes JR, Sharbrough FW. Visually evoked potentials to electronic pattern reversal: Latency variations with gender, age and technical factors. Am J EEG Technol 1979; 19:171–204.

90. Sokol S, Moskowitz A, Towle VL. Age-related changes in the latency of the visual evoked potential: Influence of check size. Electroencephalogr Clin Neurophysiol 1981; 51:559–562.

91. Celesia GG, Kaufman D, Cone S. Effects of age and sex on pattern electroretinograms and visual evoked potentials. Electroencephalogr Clin Neurophysiol 1987; 68:161–171.

92. Halliday AM, McDonald WI, Mushin J. Visual evoked responses in the diagnosis of multiple sclerosis. Br Med J 1973; 4:661–664.

93. Faust V, Heintel H, Hoek R. Altersabhangigkeit der P2-Latenz-zeiten schachbrettmusterevozierter Potentiale. Z EEG-EMG 1978; 9:219–221.

94. Halliday AM, Barrett G, Carroll WM, Kriss A. Problems in defining the normal limits of the VEP. In: Courjon J,

Mauguiere F, Revol M (eds.), Clinical Applications of Evoked Potentials in Neurolgoy. New York: Raven Press, 1982; 1–9.

95. Halliday AM. The visual evoked potential in healthy subjects. In: Halliday AM (ed.), Evoked Potentials in Clinical Testing. New York: Churchill Livingstone, 1982; 71–120.

96. Tobimatsu S, Kurita-Tashima S, Nakayama-Hiromatsu M, Akazawa K, Kato Motohiro. Age-related changes in pattern visual evoked potentials: Differential effects of luminance, contrast and check size. Electroencephalogr Clin Neurophysiol 1993; 88:12–19.

97. Dustman RE, Beck EC. The effects of maturation and aging on the waveform of visually evoked potentials. Electroencephalogr Clin Neurophysiol 1969; 26:2–11.

98. Oken BS. Endogenous event-related potentials. In: Chiappa KH (ed.), Evoked Potentials in Clinical Medicine, 2nd ed. New York: Raven Press, 1990; 563–592.

99. Goodin DS. Event-related potentials. In: Aminoff MJ (ed.), Electrodiagnosis in Clinical Neurology, 3rd ed. New York: Churchill Livingstone, 1992; 627–648.

100. Chokroverty S. Magnetic Stimulation in Clinical Neurophysiolgoy. Boston: Butterworth-Heinemann, 1990.

101. King PJL, Chiappa KH. Motor evoked potentials. In: Chiappa KH (ed.), Evoked Potentials in Clinical Medicine, 2nd ed. New York: Raven Press, 1990; 509–561.

102. Eisen AA, Shtybel W. AAEM Minimonograph #35: Clinical experience with transcranial magnetic stimulation. Muscle Nerve 1990; 13:995–1011.

103. Chokroverty S, Picone MA, Chokorverty M. Percutaneous magnetic coil stimulation of human cervical vertebral column: Site of stimulation and clinical application. Electroencephalogr Clin Neurophysiol 1991; 81:359–365.

104. Chokroverty S, Chokorverty M. Clinical applications of magnetic stimulation in radiculopathy and plexopathy. In: Lissens M (ed.), Clinical Applications of Magnetic Transcranial Stimulation. Leuven, Belgium: Peeters Press, 1992; 107–125.

105. Chokroverty S, Flynn D, Picone MA, Chokroverty M, Belsh J. Magnetic coil stimulation of the human lumbosacral vertebral column: Site of stimulation and clinical applications. Electroencephalogr Clin Neurophysiol 1993; 89:54–60.

106. Eisen A, Siejka S, Schulzer M, Calne D. Age-dependent decline in motor evoked potential (MEP) amplitude: With a comment on changes in Parkinson's disease. Electroencephalogr Clin Neurophysiol 1991; 81:209–215.

107. Rossini P, Desiato MT, Caramia MD. Age-related changes of motor evoked potentials in healthy humans: Non-invasive evaluation of central and peripheral motor tract excitability and conductivity. Brain Res 1992; 593:14–19.

108. Delwaide PJ. Are there modifications in spinal cord functions of parkinsonian patients? In: Delwaide PJ, Agnoli A (eds.), Clinical Neurophysiology in Parkinsonism. Amsterdam: Elsevier, 1985; 19–32.

109. Prout AJ, Eisen AA. The cortical silent period and amyotrophic lateral sclerosis. Muscle Nerve 1994; 17:217–223.

110. Priori A, Inghilleri M, Berardelli A. Transcranial brain stimulation in basal ganglia diseases. In: Lissens MA (ed.), Clinical Applications of Magnetic Stimulation. Leuven, Belgium: Peeters Press, 1992; 175–184.

111. Chokroverty S. The Role of EEG in Epilepsy. In: Chokroverty S (ed.), Newton, MA: Butterworth-Heinemann (to be published).

112. Hauser WA, Kurland LT. The epidemiology of epilepsy in Rochester, Minnesota, 1935 through 1967. Epilepsia 1975; 16:1–66.

113. Blass JP, Plum F. Metabolic encephalopathies in older adults. In: Katzman R, Terry RD (eds.), The Neurology of Aging. Philadelphia: FA Davis, 1983; 189–220.

114. Evans WJ, Starr A. Electroencephalography and evoked potentials in the elderly. In: Albert ML, Knoefel JE (eds.), Clinical Neurology of Aging. New York: Oxford University Press, 1994; 235–265.

115. Katz RI, Horowitz GR. The septuagenarian EEG: Normative EEG studies in a selected normal ambulatory geriatric population (abstract). Electroencephalogr Clin Neurophysiol 1981; 551:35–36.

116. Obrist WD. Problems of aging. In: Remond A (ed.), Handbook of Electroencephalography and Clinical Neurophysiolgy, vol 6A. Amsterdam: Elsevier, 1976; 275–292.

117. Obrist WD, Henry CE, Justiss WA. Longitudinal changes in the senescent EEG: A 15-year study. In: Proceedings of the

7th International Congress of Gerontology. Vienna: International Association of Gerontology, 1966; 35–38.

118. Duffy FH, Albert MS, McAnulty TG, et al. Age-related differences in brain electrical activity of healthy subjects. Ann Neurol 1984; 16:430–438.

119. Giaquinto S, Nolfe G. The EEG in the normal elderly: A contribution to the interpretation of aging and dementia. Electroencephalogr Clin Neurophysiol 1986; 63:540–546.

120. Oken BS, Kaye JA. Electrophysiologic function in the healthy, extremely old. Neurology 1992; 42:519–526.

121. Niedermeyer E. EEG and old age. In: Niedermeyer E, Lopes da Silva F (eds.), Electroencephalography. Baltimore: Urban & Schwarzenberg, 1987; 301–308.

122. Kelley J, Reilly P, Bellar S. Photic driving and psychogeriatric diagnosis. Clin Electroencephalogr 1983; 14:78–81.

123. Torres A, Faoro A, Loewenson R, et al. The electroencephalogram of elderly subjects revisited. Electroencephalogr Clin Neurophysiol 1983; 56:391–398.

124. Arenas AM, Brennar RP, Reynolds CF III. Temporal slowing in the elderly revisited. Am J EEG Technol 1986; 26: 105–114.

125. Katz RI, Horowitz GR. Electroencephalogram in the septuagenarian: Studies in a normal geriatric population. J Am Geriatr Soc 1982; 3:273–275.

126. Hughes JR, Cayafa JJ. The EEG in patients at different ages without organic cerebral disease. Electroencephalogr Clin Neurophysiol 1977; 42:776–784.

127. Visser SL, Hooijer C, Jonker C, et al. Anterior temporal focal abnormalities in EEG in normal aged subjects: Correlations with psychopathological and CT brain scan findings. Electroencephalogr Clin Neurophysiol 1987; 66:1–7.

128. Wang HS, Obrist WD, Busse EW. Neurophysiological correlates of the intellectual function. Am J Psychiatr 1970; 126:1205–1212.

129. Rice DM, Buchsbaum MS, Starr A, et al. Abnormal EEG slow activity in left temporal areas in senile dementia of the Alzheimer type. J Gerontol 1990; 45:M145–151.

130. Drachman DA, Hughes JR. Memory and the hippocampal complexes. III. Aging and temporal EEG abnormalities. Neurology 1971; 21:1–14.

131. Breslau J, Starr A, Sicotte N, et al. Topographic EEG changes with normal aging and DAT. Electroencephalogr Clin Neurophysiol 1989; 72:281–289.

132. Streletz LJ, et al. Computer analysis of EEG activity in dementia of the Alzheimer's type and Huntington's disease. Neurobiol Aging 1990; 11:15–20.

133. Miller JD, de Leon MJ, Ferris SH, et al. Abnormal temporal lobe response in Alzheimer's disease during cognitive processes as measured by ^{11}C-2-deoxy-D-glucose and PET. J Cereb Blood Flow Metab 1987; 7:248–251.

134. Busse EW, Obrist WD. Pre-senescent electroencephalographic changes in normal subjects. J Gerontol 1065; 20:315–320.

135. Kugler J. Fast EEG activity in normal people of advanced age (abstract). Electroencephalogr Clin Neurophysiol 1983; 56:67.

136. Katz RI, Horowitz GR. Sleep-onset frontal rhythmic slowing in a normal geriatric population (abstract). Electroencephalogr Clin Neurophysiol 1983; 56:27.

137. Libow LS, Obrist WD, Sokoloff L. Cerebral circulatory and electoencephalographic changes in elderly men. In: Granick S. Patterson RD (eds.), Human Aging, II. DHEW Publication (HSM) 71-9037, 1971. Rockville, MD: U.S. Dept. of Health, Education and Welfare.

138. Obrist WD, Sokoloff L, Lassen NA, et al. Relation of EEG to cerebral blood flow and metabolism in old age. Electroencephalogr Clin Neurophysiol 1963; 15:610–619.

139. A Report of the National Commission on Sleep Disorders Research. Wake Up America: A National Sleep Alert. January, 1993.

140. Keenan SA. Polysmonographic technique: An overview. In: Chokroverty S (ed.), Sleep Disorders Medicine: Basic Science, Technical Considerations and Clinical Aspects. Boston: Butterworth-Heinemann, 1994; 79–94.

141. Carskadon MA, Dement WC, Mitler M, et al. Guidelines for the Multiple Sleep Latency Test (MSLT): A standard measure of sleepiness. Sleep 1986; 9:519–524.

142. Roth T, Roehrs T, Rosenthal L. Measurement of sleepiness/ alertness: Multiple sleep latency test. In Chokroverty S (ed.), Sleep Disorders Medicine: Basic Science, Technical Considerations and Clinical Aspects. Boston: Butterworth-Heinemann, 1994; 133–139.

143. Cetel MB, Guilleminault C. Obstructive sleep apnea syndrome. In: Chokroverty S. Sleep Disorders Medicine: Basic Science, Technical Considerations and Clinical Aspects. Boston: Butterworth-Heinemann, 1994; 199–217.

144. Sanders M, Stiller RA. Positive airway pressure in the treatment of sleep-related breathing disorders. In: Chokroverty S. Sleep Disorders Medicine: Basic Science, Technical Considerations and Clinical Aspects. Boston: Butterworth-Heinemann, 1994; 455–471.

145. Chokroverty S. Sleep, breathing and neurological disorders. In: Chokroverty S. Sleep Disorders Medicine: Basic Science, Technical Considerations and Clinical Aspects. Boston: Butterworth-Heinemann, 1994; 295–335.

146. Chokroverty S. Sleep and other medical disorders. In: Chokroverty S. Sleep Disorders Medicine: Basic Science, Technical Considerations and Clinical Aspects. Boston: Butterworth-Heinemann, 1994; 349–368.

147. Wooten V. Sleep disorders in psychiatric illness. In: Chokroverty S. Sleep Disorders Medicine: Basic Science, Technical Considerations and Clinical Aspects. Boston: Butterworth-Heinemann, 1994; 337–347.

148. Hirshkowitz M, Karacan I. Techniques for the assessment of sleep-related erections. In: Chokroverty S (ed.), Sleep Disorders Medicine: Basic Science, Technical Considerations and Clinical Aspects. Boston: Butterworth-Heinemann, 1994; 165–178.

149. Karacan I, Hursch C, Williams R. Some characteristics of nocturnal penile tumescence in elderly males. J Gerontol 1972; 27:39–45.

150. Kahn E, Fisher C. REM sleep and sexuality in the aged. J Geriatr Psychiatry 1969; 2:181.

151. Liberson WT. Functional electroencephalography in mental disorders. Dis Nerv Syst 1945; 5:357–364.

152. Feinberg I, Hibi S, Carlson V. Changes in EEG amplitude during sleep with age. In: Nandy K, Sherwin I (eds.), The Aging Brain and Senile Dementia, vol. 23. New York: Plenum, 1977; 85.

153. Rechtschaffen A, Kales A. A Manual of Standardized Terminology: Techniques and Scoring Stages of Human Subjects. Los Angeles: UCLA Brain Information Service/Brain Research Institute, 1968.

154. Weitzman ED. Sleep and aging. In: Katzman R, Terry RD (eds.), The Neurology of Aging. Philadelphia: FA Davis, 1983; 167–188.

155. Williams R, Karacan I, Hursch C (eds.), Electroencephalography of Human Sleep: Clinical Applications. New York: John Wiley & Sons, 1977; 49.

156. Chokroverty S. Sleep disorders in elderly persons. In: Chokroverty S. Sleep Disorders Medicine: Basic Science, Technical Considerations and Clinical Aspects. Boston: Butterworth-Heinemann, 1994; 401–415.

157. Miles LE, Dement WC. Sleep and aging. Sleep 1980; 3:119–220.

158. Kales A, Wilson T, Kales J. Measurements of all night sleep in normal elderly persons. J Am Geriatr Soc 1967; 15:405–414.

159. Carskadon M, Brown E, Dement W. Sleep fragmentation in the elderly: Relationship to daytime sleep tendency. Neurobiol Aging 1982; 33:321–327.

160. Carskadon MA, Dement WC. Sleep loss in elderly volunteers. Sleep 1985; 8:207–221.

161. Kales A, Kales J, Jacobson A, et al. All night EEG studies: Children and elderly. Electroencephalogr Clin Neurophysiol 1966; 21:415–420.

162. Feinberg I, Koresko R, Heller N. EEG sleep patterns as a function of normal and pathological aging in man. J Psychiatr Res 1967; 5:107–144.

163. Williams DE, Vitiello MV, Ries RK, et al. Successful recruitment of elderly, community dwelling subjects for Alzheimer's disease research: Cognitively impaired, major depressive disorder, and normal control groups. J Gerontol 1988; 43:69–74.

164. Prinz PN, Vitiello M. Sleep in Alzheimer's dementia and in healthy not-complaining seniors. In: Program and Abstracts of NIH Consensus Development Conference on the Treatment of Sleep Disorders in Older People. Bethesda, MD: National Institutes of Health, 1990; 41–42.

165. Bliwise DL. Sleep in normal aging and dementia: Review. Sleep 1993; 16:40–81.

165a. Hoch CC, Dew MA, Reynolds III CT, et al. A longitudinal study of laboratory- and diary-based sleep measures in healthy "old old" and "young old" volunteers. Sleep 1994; 17(6): 489–496.

166. Vitiello MV, Smallwood RG, Avery DH, et al. Circadian temperature rhythms in young and aged men. Neurobiol Aging 1986; 72:97–100.

167. Weitzman ED, Molin ML, Czeisler CA, et al. Chronobiology of aging: Temperature, sleep/wake rhythms and entrainment. Neurobiol Aging 1982; 3:299–309.

168. Levine B, Roehrs T, Zorick F, et al. Daytime sleepiness in young adults. Sleep 1988; 11:39–46.

169. Roehrs T, Zorick F, McLeaghan A, et al. Sleep and MSLT norms for middle adults. Sleep Res 1984; 13:87.

170. Hening WA, Walters AS, Chokroverty S. Motor functions and dysfunctions of sleep. In: Chokroverty S (ed.), Sleep Disorders Medicine: Basic Science, Technical Considerations and Clinical Aspects. Boston: Butterworth-Heinemann, 1994; 255–293.

171. Chokroverty S. The Shy-Drager syndrome. Neurology Neurosurgery Update 1986; 7:1–8.

172. Low PA. Laboratory evaluation of autonomic failure. In: Low PA (ed.), Clinical Autonomic Disorders. Boston: Little, Brown and Company, 1993; 169–195.

173. Low PA, Pfeifer MA. Standardization of clinical tests for practice and clinical trials. In: Low PA (ed.), Clinical Autonomic Disorders. Boston: Little, Brown and Company, 1993: 287–296.

174. Rowe JW, Troen BR. Sympathetic nervous system and aging in man. Endocr Rev 1980; 1:167–179.

175. Low PA. The effect of aging on the autonomic nervous system. In: Low PA (ed.), Clinical Autonomic Disorders. Boston: Little, Brown and Company, 1993; 685–700.

176. Dambrink JHA, Wieling W. Circulatory responses to postural change in healthy male subjects in relation to age. Clin Sci 1987; 72:335–341.

177. Johnson RH. Effect of posture on blood pressure in elderly patients. Lancet 1965; 1:731–733.

178. Robinson BJ, et al. Do elderly patients with an excessive fall in blood pressure on standing have evidence of autonomic failure? Clin Sci 1983; 64:587–591.

179. Carried FI, Andrews DR, Kennedy RD. Effect of postural blood pressure in the elderly. Br Ht J 1973; 35:527–530.

180. Imholz BPM, et al. Noninvasive continuous finger blood pres-

sure measurement during orthostatic stress compared to intra-arterial pressure. Cardiovasc Res 1990; 24:214–221.

181. Low PA, Okazaki H, Dyck PJ. Splanchnic preganglionic neurons in man. I. Morphometry of preganglionic cytons. Acta Neuropathol 1977; 40:55–61.

182. Elliot HL, et al. Effect of age on the responsiveness of vascular alpha-adrenoceptors in man. J Cardiovasc Pharmacol 1982; 4:388–392.

183. Thomas PK, Ochoa J. Microscopic anatomy of peripheral nerve fibers. In: Dyck, PJ, et al. (eds.), Peripheral Neuropathy. Philadelphia: WB Saunders, 1984; 39–96.

184. Dauchot B, Garvenstin JS. Effects of atropine on electrocardiogram in different age groups. Clin Pharmacol Ther 1971; 12:224–280.

185. Low PA, Dyck PJ. Splanchnic preganglionic neurons in man: II. Preganglionic ventral root fibers. Acta Neuropathol 1977; 40:219–226.

186. Low PA, Dyck PJ. Splanchnic preganglionic neurons in man: III. Morphometry of myelinated fibers of rami communicantes. J Neuropathol Exp Neurol 1978; 37:734–740.

187. Takahashi K. A clinicopathologic study of the peripheral nervous system of the aged. Geriatrics 1966; 21:123–133.

188. Howell TH. The pulse rate in old age. J Gerontol 1948; 3:272–275.

189. Christensen NJ. Sympathetic nervous system activity and age. Eur J Clin Invest 1982; 12:91–92.

190. Clark CV, Mapstone R. Age-adjusted normal tolerance limits for cardiovascular autonomic function assessment in the elderly. Age Ageing 1986; 15:221–229.

191. Low PA, et al. The effect of aging on cardiac autonomic and postganglionic sudomotor function. Muscle Nerve 1990; 13:152–157.

192. O'Brien IAD, O'Hare P, Corrall RJM. Heart rate variability in healthy subjects: Effect of age and the derivation of normal ranges for tests of autonomic function. Br Ht J 1986; 55:348–354.

193. Persson A, Solders G. R-R variations, a test of autonomic dysfunction. Acta Neurol Scand 1983; 67:285–293.

194. Gross N. Circulatory reflexes and cerebral ischemia involving different vascular territories. Clin Sci 1970; 88:491–585.

195. Gervin B, Pickering TG, Sleight T, Pego R. Effect of age and high blood pressure and baroreflex sensitivity in man. Cir Res 1971; 29:424–431.
196. Duke PC, et al. The effects of age on baroreceptor reflex function in man. Can Anaesth Soc J 1976; 23:111–124.
197. Gribbin B, et al. Effect of age and high blood pressure on baroreflex sensitivity in man. Circ Res 1971; 29:424–431.
198. Shimada K, et al. Age-related changes of baroreflex function, plasma norepinephrine and blood pressure. Hypertension 1985; 7:113–117.
199. Vita G, et al. Cardiovascular reflex tests. Assessment of age-adjusted normal range. J Neurol Sci 1986; 75:263–274.
200. Ingall TJ, McLeod JG, O'Brien PC. The effect of ageing on autonomic nervous system function. Aust N Z J Med 1990; 20:570–577.
201. Clark CV, Mapstone R. Age-adjusted normal tolerance limits for cardiovascular autonomic function assessment in the elderly. Age Ageing 1986; 15:221–229.
202. Pfeifer MA, et al. Differential changes of autonomic nervous system function with age in man. Am J Med 1983; 75: 249–258.
203. Roberts J, Turner N. Age-related chagnes in autonomic function of catecholamines. In: Rothstein M (ed.), Review of Biological Research in Aging, vol. 3. New York: Allen R. Liss, 1987; 257–298.
204. Wallin BG, et al. Plasma noradrenaline correlates to sympathetic muscle nerve activity in normotensive man. Acta Physiol Scand 1981; 111:69–73.
205. Fox RH, Woodward BA, Exton-Smith AN, et al. Body temperatures in the elderly: A national study of physiological, social and environmental conditions. Br Med Ed J 1973; i:200–206.
206. Korczyn AD, Laor N, Nemet P. Sympathetic pupillary tone in old age. Arch Ophthalmol 1976; 94:1905–1906.
207. Pfeifer MA, et al. Quantitative evaluation of sympathetic and parasympathetic control of iris function. Diabetes Care 1982; 5:518–528.
208. Cyr DG. Electronystagmography and posturography. In: Aminoff MJ (ed.), Electrodiagnosis in Clinical Neurology. New York: Churchill Livingstone, 1992; 683–709.

209. Shepard NT. The clinical use of dynamic posturography in the elderly. Ear Nose Throat J 1989; 68:940.

210. Voorhees RL. Dynamic posturography findings in central nervous system disorders. Otolaryngol Head Neck Surg 1990; 103:96–101.

211. Barclay L, Wolfson L. Differential diagnosis of gait disorders and falls. In: Barclay L (ed.), Clinical Geriatric Neurology. Philadelphia: Lea & Febiger, 1993; 145–154.

212. Parker SW. Minisymposium: Disorders of balance: etiology, diagnosis, treatment. Program Book of the ninth annual meeting of the American Academy of Clinical Neurophysiology, Boston, July 14–16, 1994.

213. Alexander GE, DeLong MR. Organization of supraspinal motor systems. In: Asbury AK, McKhann GM, McDonald WI (eds.), Diseases of the Nervous System, vol. 1. Philadelphia: WB Saunders, 1986; 352–369.

214. Chokroverty S. An approach to a patient with diosrders of voluntary movements. In: Chokroverty S (ed.), Movement Disorders. Costa Mesa, CA: PMA Publishing, 1990; 1–43.

215. Hallett M, Shahani BT, Young RR. EMG analysis of stereotyped voluntary movements in man. J Neurol Neurosurg Psychiat 1975; 38:1154–1162.

216. Hallett M. Analysis of abnormal voluntary and involuntary movements with surface electromyography. Adv Neurol 1983; 39:907–914.

217. Hallett M, Khoshbin S. A physiological mechanism of bradykinesia. Brain 1980; 103:301–314.

218. Jahanshahi M, Brown RG, Marsden CD. Simple and choice reaction time and the use of advance information for motor preparation in Parkinson's disease. Brain 1992; 115:539–564.

219. Hallett M. Electrophysiologic evaluation of movement disorders. In: Aminoff MJ (ed.), Electrodiagnosis in Clinical Neurology. New York: Churchill Livingstone, 1992; 403–419.

220. Chokroverty S, Manocha M, Duvoisin RC. A physiologic and pharmacologic study in anticholinergic-responsive essential myoclonus. Neurology 1987; 37:608–615.

221. Gresty NA, Findley LJ. Definition, analysis and genesis of tremor. In: Findley LJ, Capildeo R (eds.), Movement Disorders: Tremor. London: Macmillan, 1984; 15–26.

222. Shibasaki H, Kuroiwa Y. Electroencephalographic correlates

of myoclonus. Electroencephalogr Clin Neurophysiol 1975; 39:455–463.

223. Shubasaki H, Yamashita Y, Dobimatsu S, Neshige R. Electroencephalographic correlates of myoclonus. Adv Neurol 1986; 43:357–372.

224. Chokroverty S, Walczak T, Hening W. Human startle reflex: Technique and criteria for abnormal response. Electroencephalogr Clin Neurophys 1992; 85:236–242.

225. Wilkins D, Hallet M, Wess MM. The audiogenic startle reflex of man and its relationshiop to startle syndrome. Brain 1986; 109:561–573.

226. Brown P, Thompson PD, Rothwell JC, et al. Axial myoclonus of propriospinal origin. Brain 1991; 114:197–214.

227. Chokroverty S, Walters A, Zimmerman T, Picone M. Propriospinal myoclonus: A neurophysiologic analysis. Neurology 1992; 42:1591–1595.

228. Hallett M, Chadwick D, Marsden CD. Cortical reflex myoclonus. Neurology 1979; 29:1107–1125.

229. Marsden CD, Hallett M, Fahn S. The nosology and pathophysiology of myoclonus. In: Marsden CD, Fahn S (eds.), Movement Disorders. London: Butterworths, 1982; 196–248.

230. Obeso JA, Rothwell JC, Marsden CD. The spectrum of cortical myoclonus. Brain 1985; 108:193–224.

231. Hallett M. Chadwick D, Adam J, Marsden CD. Reticular reflex myoclonus: A physiological type of human posthypoxic myoclonus. J Neurol Neurosurg Psychiatry 1978; 40:253–264.

232. Rothwell JC, Obeso JA, Day BC, Marsden CD. Pathophysiology of dystonia. In: Desmedt J (ed.), Advances in Neurology, vol 39: Motor Control Mechanisms in Health and Disease. New York: Raven Press, 1983; 851–864.

233. Marsden CD. The pathophysiology of movement disorders. Neurol Clin 1984; 2:435–459.

234. Day BL, Marsden CD, Obeso JA, Rothwell JC. Reciprocal inhibition between the muscles of the human forearm. J Physiol 1984; 349:519–534.

235. Baldisseri F, Campodelli P, Cavalleri P. Inhibition from radial group Ia afferents of H-reflex in wrist flexors. Electromyogr Clin Neurophysiol 1983; 23:187–193.

236.   Cohen LG, Hallett M, Panizza M. Dystonia. AAEE Course
       D: Clinical neurophysiology of movement disorders. AAEE
       11th Annual Continuing Education Course, Oct. 1988.
237.   Berardelli A, Rothwell JC, Day BO, Marsden CD. Patho-
       physiology of blepharospasm and oromandibular dystonia.
       Brain 1985; 108:593–608.

12

Social and Legal Issues in Geriatric Neurology

H. Richard Beresford

University of Rochester School of Medicine, Rochester, and
Cornell Law School, Ithaca, New York

I. INTRODUCTION

Rising life expectancies among Americans have profound
medical and social implications. The 1990 population of
elders included 31 million persons over 65 years of age, 7
million of whom were over 80. If current trends hold, the proportion of the population over 65 will increase over the next
several years and, by some estimates, elders over 80 will
comprise 20 million or more in 2040 (1). This will happen
even if no major scientific developments occur that further
extend life expectancies.

As a group today's elders probably enjoy better health
and less disability than their counterparts in past decades. Yet
because of overall growth in the elder population, the total
number requiring medical and social services can be expected
to rise. Among them will be many with limiting frailty and
physical impairments, dementias, age-related depressions and
other psychiatric disorders, and inadequate financial or other
resources essential to subsistence. Some will have family or
friends to serve and protect them. Others, however, will depend upon health care providers, social welfare institutions,
and various strangers to meet their most urgent needs, all at
considerable cost to them or the public. Indeed aging of the

population may result in health care and related costs occupying an even higher share of GDP (gross domestic product) than now, despite determined efforts at cost containment and reform of the health care system.

These medical and social consequences of an aging population generate certain legal concerns. Foremost is concern about the capacity of the legal system to protect fundamental rights and interests of increasingly numerous vulnerable elders. A second concern is the law's ability to abet just allocation of stressed medical resources. A third is the need to improve the legal framework for resolving hard questions about care of elders with overwhelmingly severe permanent impairments. This chapter will address these concerns, emphasizing situations of elders with debilitating neurological disorders.

II. PROTECTING VULNERABLE ELDERS

A. Participants

Protecting vulnerable elders may engage all levels of government, the judicial system, and various other participants ranging from physicians and families to friends and neighbors. Legal rules that guide these different actors may take the form of beneficently oriented legislation, bureaucratic (in the nonpejorative sense) regulations and procedures, judicial rulings, and contractual obligations. In the best-case scenario, a network of public officials and private citizens would implement these rules and collectively assure that vulnerable elders receive at least minimally adequate sustenance, shelter, and health care. Even now, however, many vulnerable elders do not enjoy this level of comfort, and their number could grow substantially unless society responds with generosity and foresight. Thus, it is appropriate to consider roles the various actors now play and how these roles might evolve.

1. *Government*

Federal, state, and local governments may all engage in protecting vulnerable elders. But activities of state and local government tend to predominate, and state and local laws are thus the most pertinent. Under these laws, governments exercise two types of power: police power and so-called parens patriae power (under which a state assumes a protective power analogous to that of a parent with respect to a child). Asserting police power entails regulating conduct that threatens public harm. Examples are laws that criminalize elder abuse or bar impaired older persons from driving motor vehicles. The exercise of paternalistic power may be expressed in guardianship laws for incompetent elders or in laws that enable involuntary commitment of mentally ill elders who are endangered or urgently in need of treatment. The principle that guides these laws is that the highest duty of the state is to promote the well-being of its citizens, either by protecting them from harm or by securing their access to necessary human services.

State power in these respects is not unlimited. The legally protectable liberty interests of individuals may greatly constrain actions of state and local governments. Indeed much constitutional jurisprudence centers on tensions between declaredly beneficent exercises of state power and the constitutional rights of individuals. In the case of vulnerable elders, some may lack capacity to assert their own rights because of severe debility or cognitive impairment that produces incompetence in the legal sense. Where this occurs, family members or other proxies must speak on their behalf in challenging state actions that seem overly intrusive or that seem to ignore the elders' best interests.

Federal participation in care for the vulnerable aged lies mainly in the realm of financing. Under the Medicare law, the federal government oversees and substantially funds a national single-payer entitlement program that provides medical care for social security beneficiaries who are over 65 or are disabled (2). Through the joint federal-state Medicaid program, the federal government sets many substantive standards and pays somewhat more than one-half the costs of short-term care for the aged poor (3). In addition, it funds long-term care for an increasing number of aged persons who have "spent down" to levels of Medicaid eligibility. Also, recent legislation has expanded the role of the federal government in regulating nursing homes beyond mere attention to physical plant and now prescribes standards that address quality of the health services offered there (4). This legislation responded to documented failures of many state governments to design or implement effective regulatory programs (5). Some current health care reform proposals contemplate a much greater role for the federal government in financing long-term care than it now plays, but the depth of public support for this very costly expansion of federal obligations is quite uncertain.

2. *Judicial system*

Courts may resolve a wide range of issues and disputes concerning the vulnerable aged. They may, for example, appoint guardians, determine competency, oversee tranfers of property by will or inheritance, order commitment of mentally ill aged who require it in order to protect selves or others, adjudicate disputes over insurance coverage for short- or long-term care, respond to requests to authorize withholding or withdrawing life-sustaining care, and enforce laws against abuse, discrimination, fraud, or malpractice with respect to the aged.

Much of this litigation occurs in specialized courts, such as probate, surrogate, or family courts. Proceedings are often relatively speedy and informal when compared to proceedings in other civil courts. This is especially true where parties do not take strongly adversarial positions on requested orders or rulings (e.g., guardianship orders, determinations of incompetency) or where financial or personal consequences of rulings are modest.

3. *Individuals*

An array of private parties may participate in protective legal proceedings for vulnerable elders, such as guardianship hearings. Families are often the initiators of these proceedings, but most state and local laws permit physicians, friends, social workers, hospital administrators, or others to step in where families are unavailable or fail to act. Although the need for protective proceedings may seem obvious in many cases, potential initiators may be affected by ambivalence, self-interest, concerns about legal expenses, and ignorance about what the proceedings can accomplish.

Physicians, in particular, may find themselves in ethically sensitive situations when deciding on proper management for their aging patients. For example, suppose a physician concludes that her patient could be equally well cared for by his spouse at home or in a nursing home, but that the burden of care on the spouse threatens her health. If the patient adamantly opposes nursing home placement, the physician's obligation to respect his autonomy may collide with her concern for the well-being of the spouse—who is not her patient. If she pressures her patient to accept nursing home placement, she arguably violates an ethical duty to assign primacy to his interests even though her motives are altruistic and he may benefit more in the long run from having a healthy spouse than from receiving care at home.

On occasion individuals may be targets rather than orginators of legal proceedings with respect to elders. Allegations against them might include, for example, physical or psychological abuse, fraud or other financial exploitations, or medical malpractice. In this last respect, an important legal question may be whether an allegedly vulnerable elder was competent to consent to an action that would have been lawful had consent been properly obtained. For example, suppose an elder sustains an incapacitating hemispheric stroke after a carotid endarterectomy to which he had consented after his surgeon informed him that major stroke was one of its significant risks. Assuming the endarterectomy was skillfully performed and no expert medical witness could be found to testify that it was not medically indicated, the central remaining question in any ensuing litigation would be whether the elder was competent to consent to the surgery. If he was, the surgeon will prevail. But if he was not competent to weigh the potential benefit of endarterectomy against the risk of stroke, his consent to endarterectomy was legally meaningless. The surgeon would then be open to liability for battery for non-consensual surgery or negligent failure to obtain an adequately informed consent to a procedure that could lead to a stroke.

B. Protective Legal Proceedings

1. *Guardianship*

The purpose of guardianship proceedings for vulnerable elders is to appoint a fiduciary to protect their property and personal interests. The evolving law of guardianship favors appointments that confine restrictions on the rights of wards to what is essential for their basic welfare (6). The goal is to encourage courts to give wards as much freedom as feasible while assuring that guardians take responsibility for conserving wards' resources or for decisions about health or personal welfare that wards cannot safely make. Although guardianship laws in various states differ in their details, they generally share a commitment to flexibility and minimally sufficient constraints. Thus, a hypothetical guardianship order might empower a guardian to veto purchases that would severely deplete a ward's resources or to determine whether the ward should undergo high-risk medical or surgical treatments. But the order would allow the ward to make small purchases (even if objectively foolish) or to consent to routine or unconventional but harmless medical care.

For a court to tailor the most appropriate guardianship order, it may require information that physicians are best able to provide. A court may, for example, need to know if a ward has adequate vision, hearing, motor skills or cognition for driving, or if the ward has enough intelligence or judgment to make decisions about living arrangements or health care. Ordinarily the opinions of physicians on these issues will carry great weight. However, opinions that fail to elucidate practical consequences of identified physical or mental impairments may not be useful to a court. Merely stating that an elder has "early Alzheimer disease" or "multi-infarct dementia" does not communicate the impact of these disorders on an elder's ability to carry out various activities of daily life. The dire overtones of these unadorned diagnoses could lead a court to issue an inappropriately restrictive guardianship order or could delay issue of an order until clarifying data are provided. Accordingly, an opinion that spells out as precisely as possible what an elder can and cannot do or decide enhances the efficiency of guardianship proceedings and improves prospects that a guardianship order will not be unduly restrictive.

Few guardianship proceedings require personal appearances of physicians or involve contests over medical evidence. Written reports or affidavits usually suffice, provided they meet the simple criteria of usefulness noted above. Occasionally, however, courts will order physicians to testify in person, especially where a potential ward vigorously objects to guardianship or where the guardian is seeking authority to make major health-related decisions (e.g., authorizing a do-not-rescucitate order). Here the court might wish to question a physician in some detail about the clinical basis of an opinion that an elder requires comprehensive guardianship or has an untreatable fatal illness.

The formalities of guardianship proceedings depend on applicable state laws and rules of court. These vary enough that little purpose would be served in cataloguing them here. In general, they specify who can initiate proceedings, establish elements of procedural due process, allow for expedited hearings without rigid adherence to traditional evidentiary rules, give judges considerable discretion in fashioning protective orders, and provide mechanisms for continuing supervision and termination of guardianships.

Guardians themselves are held to fiduciary standards. This implies that they must give primacy to needs of their wards in situations of potential conflict or interest, and that they can be punished for contempt of court if they violate terms of guardianship orders or otherwise neglect their duties.

2. *Determining competency*

Issues of competency often arise in the course of guardianship proceedings, and courts may include a determination of incompetency as part of their guardianship order. However, determinations about competency may be made independently and in other contexts. A court may, for example, be asked to decide if an elder is competent to exhaust his life savings to buy a yacht, was competent when she made the will by which she left her large estate to a friend instead of her children, or is capable of assisting in a defense against criminal charges. Or it may be asked to decide if an elder is competent to consent to high-risk neurosurgery for a brain tumor, to consent to the writing of a do-not-rescucitate order, or to refuse medically indicated treatment for a life-threatening condition. One consequence of a determination of incompetency in these various scenarios may be that a court will appoint a guardian for the elder. But the trigger for judicial scrutiny is often a question about the elder's capacity in a highly specific context.

As the above examples suggest, some incompetency proceedings may be adversarial. Disputes may arise over interpretations of medical data, and physicians who have offered testimony may find their opinions attacked through cross-examination or the testimony of other physicians. This emphasizes the heavy legal connotations of the concept of "competency," the contours of which are in any event rather elastic (7). For example, what is competency for making a will is not necessarily the same as competency for authorizing a DNR order. To execute a lawful will one need appreciate only what one owns and whom one intends to give it to. But to authorize a DNR order, one presumably needs to understand the nature and prognosis of one's medical condition and to be able to deliberate over whether one is willing to renounce the possibility of continued existence. Very different degrees of comprehension and understanding are at play in these contrasting examples. Accordingly, a court might conclude that an elder with, say, multi-infarct dementia is competent to make a will but is not competent to engage in deliberation about a DNR order.

There exists a general presumption in law that adults are competent to make decisions for themselves. The effect of this presumption is that the burden of proving incompetency in a legal proceeding rests on those who challenge competency, not on the alleged incompetent. What it takes to satisfy this burden depends on applicable state law. The burden may be high where a finding of incompetency has major consequences. For example, state courts have held that proof of incompetency due to brain disease must be "clear and convincing" before proxies will be permitted to make major therapeutic decisions for the afflicted persons (8). This is a higher standard than the "more probable than not" standard that prevails in most civil litigation. Moreover, courts are reluctant to adjudicate incompetency merely because a particular choice or action appears foolish or differs from widely held societal norms. Thus, they have upheld the rights of adults to refuse treatments that could clearly sustain their lives or reverse life-threatening conditions over contentions that the refusals bespoke major depressions or other incapacitating mental illness (9,10).

Overcoming a presumption of competency may therefore require marshalling of observational and behavioral data. In many instances, a carefully performed bedside or office-based mental status examination furnishes enough information about cognitive abilities to support a finding of legal incompetency. But in contested cases, detailed accounts of inability to manage work, household, hygiene, and finances and accounts of self-endangering conduct may be needed to buttress abnormal findings on mental status examination. Data from neuroimaging studies may help confirm the presence of severe brain disease, and neuropsychological testing may afford concrete illustrations of a person's inability to reason logically or to complete simple performance tasks. While only a few incompetency proceedings will call for extensive presentations of data, potential medical witnesses are well advised to ascertain the stakes in a decision about competency (e.g., lots of money, major therapeutic decision) and what level of contention to expect. If they produce only a cursory appraisal in a situation of great controversy, they risk embarrassment and attacks on the credibility of their observations. They may also do a disservice to the interests of their patients.

Once courts determine that challengers of competency have met their burden of proof, they will make a formal adjudication of incompetency. It may describe the scope of the incompetency by specifying what decisions a person lacks the capacity to make, leaving an opening for the person to act autonomously in some other respects. A court will ordinarily appoint a guardian or other proxy to represent the person in matters he or she is incompetent to handle, and will indicate the scope of the proxy's decisional powers. Family members are usually the preferred proxies but may be excluded if a court believes they cannot adequately represent an incompetent or a conflict of interest is apparent.

3. *Involuntary hospitalization and treatment*

Mentally ill elders may benefit from psychiatric treatment in hospitals or other mental health facilities. If they are not legally incompetent, they may accept treatment on a voluntary basis and without legal intervention. But if they are incompetent to decide about psychiatric treatment or if they resist hospitalization, laws (13) of all states allow for involuntary commitment if specified statutory criteria are met. In most states involuntary detention requires observance of procedural due process and proof that a person is a danger to self or to others. In some states, proof of an urgent need for psychiatric treatment is an additional ground for involuntary commitment. As a result of the recent decision of the U.S. Supreme Court in *Zinermon v. Burch* (11), states will probably be less willing than in the past to allow physicians to circumvent time-consuming involuntary commitment procedures by inducing persons of doubtful competency to "accept" hospitalization on a "voluntary" basis.

The threshhold requirement for involuntary commitment is mental illness, whether or not a person is legally incompetent. Thus, a nondemented but severely depressed elder might qualify for involuntary commitment even if he or she has the capacity to weigh therapeutic options and has rejected hospitalization. In this situation, those seeking involuntary commitment would have the further burden of proving that the depressed elder is suicidal—and thus a danger to self—or urgently requires inpatient treatment to prevent serious psychological deterioration. As with incompetency, standards of proof for danger to self or urgent need for treatment differ among the states. Some state laws require that evidence be "clear and convincing" because deprivation of liberty, even for therapeutic reasons, is a serious intrusion on fundamental rights. Other states hold to a less exacting standard and allow involuntary commitments on proof that it is more probable than not that a person is a danger to self or urgently requires treatment.

Mentally ill elders may also be incompetent to make decisions about their care. In this event, courts are likely to apply the concept of substituted judgment and appoint a proxy or guardian to represent them in commitment proceedings. The obligation of the proxy is to try to identify what choice a mentally ill elder would have made if competent. If that choice is unascertainable, the proxy's obligation shifts to trying to determine what is in the elder's best interests. After the proxy communicates findings to the court, it will weigh these findings together with the relevant psychiatric evidence about danger to self or need for treatment before reaching a decision about commitment.

If a court orders commitment, it may also specify what treatments are permissible. For example, it might include in the commitment order authority for hospital physicians to administer antidepressant drugs over the objections of a suicidal patient, but might require the physicians to seek approval from the court before administering electroshock treatments. If a court does not expressly authorize nonconsensual treatments after admission, the law of some states would require hospital physicians to secure advance judicial approval for such treatments (12). An exception would be where prompt treatment is necessary to prevent major harm to the patient or to others (i.e., a psychiatric emergency). In short, the fact that a person has been involuntarily hospitalized because of mental illness does not automatically entitle a treating physician to override the person's objections to a particular treatment, even if the treatment is medically appropriate.

4. *Restrictions on driving*

By reason of neurological or other impairments, many elders lose the ability to drive safely. This is reflected in data that crash rates per mile driven in persons over 65 are higher than for any group except those under 25 and are double that of middle-aged drivers (13). Yet despite the obvious danger they represent to selves or others, some elders will resist entreaties from families, physicians, and friends that they forego a cherished activity.

Failure to pass a simple vision or hearing test may cause some elders to lose their licenses; others will be disqualified if they develop epilepsy, cardiogenic syncope, or other disorders that interrupt consciousness; and a few will be intercepted after road tests that some states impose as a condition of relicensure for elders or persons with an unfavorable accident record. But this will still leave undetected and licensed an indeterminate number with impaired judgment, visuospatial dysfunction, slowed reactions, and impaired motor skills. While they may be less overtly antisocial than the impulsive adolescent or the chronic alcoholic or cocaine user, their impairments are such that grievous crashes and harms may ensue. For example, persons over 65 are three times more likely to die of crash injuries than those under 25 and sustain the highest rate of fatalities per mile driven of any age group (13). Improving the process for licensing elders is only a partial solution. Undoubtedly more extensive use of road testing or new driving-simulation technologies would identify some elders who pose unacceptable dangers. Yet this strategy would probably also fail to identify some truly dangerous persons and might mischaracterize some prudent drivers as dangerous. Moreover, by singling out elders this strategy would raise issues of unlawful age-based discrimination and invasion of constitutionally protected liberties. On the other hand, a less legally infirm policy that involves the general population might prove prohibitively expensive.

A selective approach nonetheless seems desirable, one that emphasizes the responsibilities of families, physicians, and other caretakers to identify elders who should not drive and to undertake measures to reduce the risk that they will drive. These measures might extend from gentle persuasion all the way to formal determination of incompetency and appointment of a guardian with explicit authority to bar driving. A highly desirable first step is recognition by caretakers that they are the ones best situated to to appreciate if an elder is a dangerous driver and that they have at least a moral obligation to try to reduce the danger by doing something. For family members, this "something" may include simply confronting the elder and insisting he or she stop driving. In the case of a physician, it might include notifying the motor vehicle licensing agency, even if state law has no provisions about reporting neurologically impaired drivers who do not have episodes of impaired consciousness (14). If these approaches fail, the option of initiating a protective proceeding is available. Under guardianship laws that stress minimizing constraints on those subject to protective orders, the outcome of such a proceeding might be a narrow adjudication that an elder is incompetent to drive and that the guardian's authority is limited only to assuring the elder does not drive.

C. Enforcing Protective Laws

1. *Elder abuse*

The extent of elder abuse in the United States is uncertain. One estimate is that as many as 10% of Americans over 65 are subjected to physical or mental abuse, neglect, or financial exploitation, and that as many as 50% have sustained detectable physical harm (15). The prototypic victim is a chronically ill 75-year-old woman who lives with and is dependent on a spouse or child who is in turn mentally ill or a substance abuser and who himself has been a victim of abuse. But the spectrum is much wider than this, and there is evidence that the likelihood of abuse increases as the dependency relationship becomes longer. In any case, whatever the true incidence and prevalence of elder abuse, state legislatures have enacted many protective laws in the past several years, generally adopting the reporting/investigative format of child abuse legislation.

All states now have laws specifically aimed at deterring abuse of elders (16). These laws differ in how they define elder abuse, the procedures they prescribe, and the penalties they impose. As with child abuse laws, most elder abuse laws require particular persons, notably including physicians, to report instances of suspected abuse to state officials; a few states, however, permit voluntary reporting. States that have adopted a voluntary approach can cite evidence that state agencies often lack the resources or will to take effective action on reported elder abuse. Moreover, opponents of mandatory reporting contend that it is overly intrusive, offers a false promise of help, deters caretakers from bringing elders to physicians, and often results in counterproductive institutionalization of elders thought to have been abused. Nevertheless, the overall trend has been toward expanding and strengthening elder abuse laws.

What constitutes elder abuse as a matter of law may be broadly or narrowly defined. A broad concept would encompass all persons over 65 and define abuse to include infliction of physical and mental harms, neglect, financial exploitation, and failure of a caretaker to meet fiduciary obligations. By contrast, a narrow formulation would include only assaultive conduct. As elder abuse laws have evolved, more expansive definitions have been employed so as to cover instances of genuine abuse less overt than direct physical assaults. Thus, in a recent case, a California appellate court decided that the daughter of a bedridden, partially paralyzed elder could be prosecuted for criminal elder abuse where evidence revealed that she did not provide him with food, liquids, or attention to personal hygiene for several days, as a result of which he developed malnutrition, decubiti, and fatal sepsis (18). Moreover, the current California elder abuse statute criminalizes any conduct by a caretaker that willfully endangers the health of a person 65 years of age or older, or that constitutes theft or embezzlement from such a person (19).

As with child abuse laws, enforcement of elder abuse laws has been spotty or nonexistent. Some state adult protective services are underfunded and understaffed, and others may be overwhelmed by the large number of reports they receive under broadly written mandatory reporting statutes. The result is that only what seem the most egregious cases are investigated, and these may be cases that would have attracted attention from the criminal justice system in absence of a reporting law. Also, reporting of suspected abuse may decline when those under a legal obligation to report come to appreciate that most reports are ignored or mishandled (20). Physicians in particular may find that reporting results in their losing whatever opportunity they might have to further help reported patients and that no one takes their place in trying to provide needed care. The state agency may be too busy to investigate, and the patients' guardians or immediate caretakers may thereafter choose to avoid further contacts with physicians for fear this will generate adverse consequences for them.

Even if reporting laws fall far short of achieving their goals, this is not a lawful justification for ignoring them. Physicians who find plausible evidence of physical or other forms of abuse but take no action may not only violate state civil or criminal laws relating to elder abuse, but may also transgress medical licensure laws and become vulnerable to liability for medical malpractice based on their failure to exercise a professional duty to take reasonable steps to prevent forseeable harm to their patients.

Thus, for physicians who care for an appreciable number of elders, an important legal dimension of practice is becoming informed about the problem of elder abuse and about what state laws require with respect to identification and reporting. When it comes to meting out punishment for failure to avert harm to vulnerable elders, physicians are more inviting targets than harassed civil servants of modest means. Also, state officials may be immune from legal attack because of the doctrine of sovereign immunity that shields government employees from liability for discretionary or good faith conduct, even if the conduct in question causes serious harm.

2. *Financial exploitation*

Anecdotal information suggests that elders are particularly susceptible to frauds and other forms of financial exploitation. If so, various factors may be at work. Cognitive impairment is certainly one. An elder may lack the understanding or judgment needed to grasp that a particular purchase is decidedly unwise, or that a clever "financial adviser" will squander entrusted funds on "safe" or "sure thing" investments that are anything but that. Frail and dependent elders may be easily coerced into turning over assets to caretakers who utilize such assets for selfish purposes. Those with poor vision may be unaware that fine print in papers they sign commits them to long-term financial obligations. And those with poor hearing may agree to an oral offer they would not have accepted had they heard it correctly. In any of these circumstances, elders may either lose money outright or find themselves saddled with heavy and unsustainable financial burdens.

Although laws exist that provide protection and remedies with respect to financial exploitation (21), their actual benefit for elders may be limited. Outright frauds may, if detected, result in criminal punishment for perpetrators. But this seldom means that defrauded elders will regain properties they have lost. Various consumer protection laws may in theory allow elders to recover payments made based on misunderstandings or misrepresentations. And exploited elders may invoke doctrines of contract law to undo certain signed agreements or to defend against demands arising from agreements that were obtained through coercion, misrepresentation, or mistake.

To take advantage of these formal legal remedies may require more assertiveness, initiative, and financial resources than many elders possess. They will need advocates such as family, social workers, or public-interest lawyers. Even then, the best outcome may only be release from onerous future obligations; past losses may be beyond recoupment. The most fruitful strategy would therefore seem to be for families, physicians, and other interested persons to identify elders who may be susceptible to financial exploitation and to help them obtain assistance in managing their assets. For some, this may mean seeking a formal guardianship or conservatorship limited to financial matters. For others, it may mean only informal measures such as encouraging a relationship with a bank that offers simple managerial services at affordable prices.

3. *Rights as patients*

Elders may be subject to various forms of neglect or abuse by those entrusted with providing medical care. Neglect may range from subtle reluctance of a physician to expend much effort in caring for a person who is old, infirm, and unlikely to realize objective gains from care to an unsubtle, age-based withholding of care. The latter is clearly unlawful under federal and state antidiscrimination laws (22) and is probably rare. The former is probably more common than physicians and others are ready to admit and may have serious consequences for elders. For example, in an extensive study of iatrogenic harms occurring among hospitalized patients in New York, investigators found that elders were more likely to incur iatrogenic harm than younger patients and were also more likely to be victims of substandard care (23). They were also less likely to bring malpractice suits than younger patients.

Taking age into account in calibrating intensity of care may be an unspoken element of medical practice. But aside from its dubious ethics, such an approach lacks legal justification. A physician or hospital that is defending against a charge of malpractice would be unlikely to find medical experts who would agree to testify that advanced age is an acceptable basis for withholding otherwise medically indicated treatment or excuses substandard technical performance. Age may be relevant to the issue of whether a particular treatment has an acceptable risk:benefit ratio or is particularly likely to result in unavoidable side effects. Neverthless, age alone does not provide an independent legal basis for withholding care or for providing care that does not meet generally accepted standards.

4.   *Rights as research subjects*

Experimentation in humans is largely regulated by detailed federal rules and procedures (24). Several states also regulate human experimentation in ways that complement and expand federal protections. These regulatory programs clearly reduce the chance that elders will become subjects of the sort of research that occurred at the Jewish Chronic Disease Hospital in the early 60s when aged patients were administered "skin tests" consisting of cultured human cancer cells without being told what they were receiving (25). But since human experimentation is essential to the understanding and effective treatment of many diseases of aging, elders can anticipate continuing requests to participate in research. Much of the research will pose little risk, as in studies designed to profile cognitive decline in Alzheimer's disease. Other studies will carry significant or unpredictable risks, such as clinical trials of new agents for treating neurodegenerative disorders.

Where risks of research are more than trivial, troubling issues may arise. Often the threshhold question will be whether an elder is competent to consent to undertake such risks and, if so, whether consent is informed and freely given. If research involves a dementing illness, few potential subjects will possess the capacity to appreciate the nature of the study or to weigh risks of participation. Even if understanding is deemed adequate, the voluntariness of assent to participation may be uncertain, especially if the study involves a method of treating a disorder for which no satisfactory treatment currently exists. In this instance, an intense desire for treatment may overwhelm concerns about real risks of toxicity. Some of these concerns can be alleviated by resort to proxy consents, thereby assuring that legally competent persons perform some form of advance risk:benefit appraisal.

Proxy consents are not a complete solution, however. A few state laws flatly bar more than minimally risky experimentation involving incompetent subjects or require prior judicial approval of such experimentation, whether or not proxy consent has been obtained. Also, proxies may agree to allow others to assume risks they would not take themselves. This would suggest a need for investigators to be quite conservative in their risk:benefit assessments and to adhere scrupulously to the "first do no harm" principle in deciding whether to expose vulnerable elders to risky investigations. Moreover, some experimentation may offer no realistic prospect that elder subjects will benefit from participating. The only "benefit" will be indirect, such as contributing to knowledge about an important disease of elders. For unequivocally competent elders, agreeing to participate in a risky experiment on this basis raises no particular concerns. But where doubts about competency exist, allowing proxy consent to nonbeneficial experimentation is problematic. While a proxy might believe that the potential gain in knowledge from a study is a form of benefit, it is a tenuous benefit for the one who actually assumes the risk. Also, if the proxy is a devoted family member who harbors an unrealistic hope that an experiment may provide a more tangible benefit to the subject, the proxy's consent is further suspect.

When reliance on proxy consents for vulnerable elders raises these sorts of problems, investigators have various options. Assuming an institutional review board–approved protocol and applicable state law permits proxy consents, they may choose to rely on consent of proxies once they are convinced the proxies are adequately informed and are acting in good faith. As an additional safeguard, they may opt for formal review by an intramural ethics committee before proceeding on the basis of proxy consent. If this sort of review is deemed insufficient and the scientific importance of the investigation seems to warrant it, they could seek judicial approval to proceed. This would allow for an intensive weighing of whether the potential value of an experiment is great enough to justify exposing subjects to nontrivial risks they cannot comprehend. In a situation where an experiment offers no promise of direct benefit to elder subjects, it is not easy to envision that it is this valuable.

III. ALLOCATING STRESSED RESOURCES

A. General Considerations

The United States has abundant resources and an array of social programs capable of allocating resources to those in greatest need. Popular support for these programs is uneven, however, and programs that lead to increased taxes or that are perceived as causing too much redistribution of wealth often generate strong opposition, no matter how beneficent their purposes. The result is that millions of citizens, including elders, lack health insurance, decent housing, or minimally adequate nutrition. Although Medicare and Medicaid enable most elders to obtain health care, not all meet eligibility criteria and others are incapable of taking advantage of these entitlement programs. Moreover, having Medicare or Medicaid coverage does not in itself assure access to health care, especially in areas where the supply of medical providers is limited (e.g., inner-city slums, some rural areas) (26). Similarly, while federal and state welfare and old-age assistance programs provide considerable material support for many vulnerable elders, some of these programs are so underfunded or inefficient that they can meet the needs of only a fraction of elders.

Filling the gaps in these programs for elders would undoubtedly require substantial additional public funding, even if administrative inefficiencies are largely corrected. Because the only evident sources of additional funding are new taxes or reallocations of existing public expenditures, prospects for early progress are unpromising. However, as the median age of the population rises and societal awareness of the need for better services for elders grows, public support for needed measures may sharpen. This of course assumes concomitant economic growth adequate to supply the resources to fill the gaps. The particular challenge to the legal system here is to assure just allocation of whatever resources are available. While medical resources are but one concern, what follows will consider only allocational issues in health care.

B. Federal Programs

1. *Impact of health care reform*

Until the shape of health care reform becomes clearer, projecting its effects on health care for elders is difficult. The broadest—and least likely to succeed—proposals would create a national single-payer system for all citizens, thereby assuring elders access to health care. Other proposals would leave Medicare intact as a separate program for qualified elders, although some would open it up to other persons who are unable to obtain private health insurance. Many proposals call for reducing Medicare's share of public funds through increased cost sharing by beneficiaries and largely unspecified administrative efficiencies. Some proposals would, in addition, scale back Medicare payments to medical providers. The fate of Medicaid under various proposals ranges from abolition to expansion, depending in part on whether subsidies are given to those who cannot pay for private health insurance.

A reasonably safe guess is that Medicare will survive in much like its present form, that cost sharing by beneficiaries will increase, and that relatively wealthy beneficiaries will pay higher premiums than they pay now. A shakier guess is that the gap between what Medicare pays providers for particular services and the higher amounts private insurers pay for the same services to nonelders will stabilize or perhaps narrow. The suggestion here is not that Medicare will pay providers more than it does now; it may even pay somewhat less in certain instances. Rather the suggestion is that "managed competition" will constrain the prices that providers can command from private payors, and that this will keep the disparity between what private insurers pay and what Medicare pays for identical services from continuing to widen. In any event, it is probable that Medicare will continue to cover eligible elders for substantially the same services they now receive, whether or not their premiums or cost-sharing obligations rise.

Even if Medicare remains largely intact, the exigencies of cost containment will probably evoke increased scrutiny of the medical necessity for services. This will be buttressed by better analytic tools than existed in past years. Technical assessments are beginning to yield reliable data about outcomes of various treatments, and better information technologies enable faster and surer identification of providers' patterns of practice and how they deviate from relevant norms.

For elders, heightened and more efficient attention to the medical justification for services may have some unpleasant consequences. Most directly bothersome will be denials of reimbursement for certain services that are determined medically unnecessary by reviewers of claims. Less obvious, but perhaps even more troubling, could be the adverse effect of this sort of scrutiny on attitudes of physicians caring for elders. Already many physicians believe they are underpaid for services to beneficiaries of federal programs. Their response to "micromanagement" by Medicare claims reviewers could take the form of scaling back their Medicare practice, reducing time spent with elders during office or hospital visits, or increasing the volume of marginally indicated but well-reimbursed services (e.g., some ultrasound or electrophysiologic studies) in the hope that enough of these services will survive review as to be profitable. Any of these responses by physicians could impair the essential quality of elders' care. Merely because physicians' services are defensible under generally nonstringent legal standards or are reimbursable under existing administrative guidelines does not necessarily mean they are medically or ethically appropriate for particular patients.

Proponents of health care reform at the federal level have largely dodged the issue of long-term care, a matter of great importance to elders. The dauntingly high cost of long-term care best accounts for this evasion. Nearly 5% of persons over 65 are now in nursing homes, although the majority spend less than 90 days there (27). In any case, several million persons who are now alive can anticipate spending at least some time in a nursing home or other chronic care facility during their lifetime. Annual average costs of care in ordinary nursing homes now range from $50/day in low-cost locales up to as much as $200/day in high-cost locales. The costs of care in skilled nursing facilities are proportionally higher. Few persons now have insurance for long-term care, largely because of limited availability and high costs. The result is that many who enter nursing homes exhaust their retirement and other assets and must apply for Medicaid, the major residual source of coverage for long-term care. Those who don't qualify for Medicaid in effect become public wards and must depend on resource-starved state and local welfare bureaucracies to obtain access to chronic care. A sustained political effort will be required to remedy the most unsatisfactory features of long-term care in the United States. But progress in this direction will probably have to await outcome of the current struggle over how to improve access to any form of health care.

2. *Impact of "managed competition"*

Even if new federal legislation does not restructure the health care system, emergence of "managed competition" as a dominant model of delivery in a private system has important implications for elders. Currently many providers who care for both elders and nonelders depend on the relatively higher payments from insurers of nonelders to make up for what they perceive as insufficient payments from Medicare (or in some cases, Medicaid).

a. **Cross-subsidies.** Shifts of funds from private payors to public programs may diminish considerably as managed competition takes hold in the private medical marketplace. As indicated above, this may cause some physicians to alter their practice styles with respect to elders in ways that adversely affect care. It may also encourage physicians to try to contract with elders who can afford such arrangements for care outside of Medicare. Whether physicians can lawfully do this for some elders and not others is currently being litigated. If they can, one could envision that some physicians might condition care of relatively affluent Medicare-eligible elders on their willingness to forego filing claims for reimbursement under Medicare and to agree to pay prices the physicians charge their non-Medicare patients. In a highly competitive practice environment, physicians may not be able to sustain this approach for long. But if they are in great demand or enjoy a sort of "natural monopoly" with respect to the services they offer (as do some specialists), they might succeed—at considerable out-of-pocket cost to their elder patients.

For hospitals caring for elders the implications of managed competition are somewhat different. As with physicians, many hospitals depend to some extent on cross-subsidies from private insurers to make up for perceived losses in caring for Medicare patients (28). In some instances, these subsidies are built into a state system of hospital rate regulation that explicitly permits higher charges to patients covered by private insurance (29). However, hospitals have had a longer experience with regulatory cost containment than physicians and, under pressure of diagnosis-related groups and related reimbursement schemes, have probably improved, however reluctantly, their overall efficiency in caring for patients. This may mean that, as managed competition takes further hold, elders will notice less difference in the quality and intensity of care they receive in hospitals than they do in their physicians' offices. This is by no means certain of course. Many hospitals are in poor financial condition because of excess bed capacity, past profligacy, profiteering by insiders, and flabby oversight by governing boards (especially those of nonprofit hospitals). The attempts of such hospitals to survive in an increasingly competitive environment may take the form of reductions in services and personnel that translate into recognizably lower quality of care for elders and others who are perceived as unprofitable patients because their insurance does not reimburse enough.

    b. Quality of care. If managed competition indeed influences providers to skimp on how they care for elders, law will play a crucial protective role. A particularly potent remedy is the malpractice suit. Here an elder could assert that he or she sustained harm because the treatment a physician or hospital provided fell below minimum accepted standards of care. Proof of malpractice on this basis would not only entitle an elder to compensatory damages, but would also forcefully remind providers that financially driven undertreatment of elders carries significant legal risks.

Some providers may contend that the legal standard of care with respect to patients who cannot pay "full value" for professional services is lower than the customary standard. The argument might run to the effect that if law requires physicians to bear the same legal risks in caring for patients who cannot pay (or cannot pay enough) as for those who can pay, then physicians will simply stop caring for poor payers or will withhold potentially useful treatments that carry some risks of harm (30). The result arguably would be that elders would experience increasing difficulty finding physicians willing to care for them or would not receive an optimal amount of treatment from those they did locate. The proposed remedy to this problem would thus be to set a lower legal standard of care with respect to elders covered only by Medicare or Medicaid. For example, an elder might be required to prove negligence by clear and convincing evidence (approximately 75% probability) rather than by a more probable than not (51%) standard. Or an elder might be required to prove "gross" negligence rather than ordinary negligence in order to recover damages.

Courts have been reluctant to depart from a unitary standard of care in medical malpractice cases (31). One explanation may be that, although there is no well-defined "right" to medical care, it would be unjust to hold as a matter of law that the poor have a lesser entitlement to care of reasonable quality than other citizens. To some extent, however, this explanation ignores the obvious fact that wealth-based disparities in access to medical care are pervasive in the United States. The judicial hesitancy to adopt a sliding-scale standard of care may also stem from the perceived difficulty of engaging in this sort of calibration. In this regard, some courts have taken into account the resources available to a malpractice defendant in determining if the standard of care has been satisfied (32). For example, a physician who fails to diagnose a noncalcified subfrontal meningioma that could have been visualized with a CT scan might be excused from liability for negligence if no CT scan was reasonably accessible and there was no reasonable way to make the diagnosis with accessible modalities. Or if the diagnosis could probably have been made by an appropriate consultant, there would be no liability if such a consultant was not reasonably available. In other words, while the insurance status of an elder is irrelevant to the legal standard of care, the nature of the resources available to a medical provider may very well be.

As managed competition drives more and more physicians into large groups or integrated delivery systems, constraints on physicians' capacity to utilize resources in diagnosis and treatment will grow. These constraints may occasionally result in harms to patients because physicians do not deploy resources that could have averted the harms. In this context, the constraining entities, not the physicians, may be the appropriate defendants in malpractice suits. To date, suits against third-party payors based on allegations that their cost-containing strategies caused physicians to withhold needed treatments have enjoyed little success (31). One explanation is that testimony in these cases disclosed that discretionary conduct of treating physicians was the principal factor in the harms, not the workings of cost-containment programs. However, cases may eventually arise in which injured persons can succeed in showing that, but for a network's or third-party payor's constraints on physicians, they would not have suffered harm.

C. State and Local Programs

1. *Long-term care*

State Medicaid programs play a central role in long-term care for frail and chronically ill elders. Although the federal government provides considerable funding and sets many standards, administrative responsibility largely falls on state governments. Moreover, Medicaid spending is often the most rapidly rising component of state budgets, with long-term-care costs being a major contributor. Many states have therefore established increasingly rigorous cost-containment programs, including managed care, shifts from institutional to home-based care, tight controls on payments to providers, and close scrutiny of fiscal practices of nursing homes and other long-term-care facilities. Greater efficiencies may result from these programs, but some elders are also likely to experience reductions in services and amenities, particularly in states where the stress on Medicaid budgets is greatest.

Independent of the Medicaid program, state governments also have major oversight responsibilities with respect to nursing homes and other long-term-care institutions. Among other regulatory measures, states set standards for accreditation and licensure, establish and monitor fiscal and solvency requirements, and conduct inspections related to safety and quality of care. Because many state governments have been lax or ineffective in their oversight activities, Congress has enacted several laws designed to improve the quality of care in nursing homes and to lever states into taking a stronger role in nursing home regulation (33). These laws set detailed standards that nursing homes must meet before they can be certified to receive payments under federal programs (e.g., Medicare, Medicaid), and they spell out the sorts of inspections that state regulators should make in order to ascertain compliance with these standards. By creating uniform national standards for nursing homes, these federal laws may have reduced some of the wider disparities among nursing homes in the various states. But they do not solve the problems that arise when individual state governments lack the funds or political commitment needed to upgrade care in long-term facilities.

2. *Rationing programs*

The pressure on Medicaid budgets has forced many state governments to consider innovative ways of controlling and directing spending on medical services for the poor (34). One of the most controversial innovations is Oregon's formalized rationing program for Medicaid beneficiaries (35). After input from various experts and from citizens at a series of town meetings throughout the state, the Oregon legislature established a prioritized list of over 700 "condition-treatment pairs." The idea is to rank treatments by urgency and utility such that a treatment for an acute, life-threatening or painful curable illness ranks highly and a treatment for a chronic, invariably fatal nonpainful illness ranks at the bottom. A line is drawn on the list, depending on available funding, such that any condition below the line does not qualify for Medicaid reimbursement. Providers are excused from liability for malpractice if a treatment they withhold is below the funding cutoff line. The projections are that the cost savings from omitting nonbeneficial treatments under this program will allow Oregon to add substantial numbers of needy persons to the pool of Medicaid eligibles. It may also result in withdrawal of treatments from persons who are now receiving them because the particular treatments are below the line.

The Oregon program has attracted praise for rationality and democratic foundation and vilification for conducting utilitarian social experimentation on the vulnerable poor (35). Also, the federal government delayed granting a waiver from Medicaid rules that would have barred the program until it was satisfied that the stratification scheme would not discriminate against persons with existing disabilities in violation of the Americans with Disabilities Act (22). Also noteworthy is that elders on Medicaid are currently excluded from the rationing program. In theory, this could lead to the anomaly of an 80-year-old receiving a treatment that was denied to a 40-year-old. The chance this would happen appears slim, however. Few, if any, nonqualifying treatments would meet the test of medical necessity that governs reimbursability under existing Medicaid rules, and it seems unlikely that elders' physicians, patients, or families would insist on treatments that are widely regarded as useless for younger persons. It would seem more likely that the priority scale will influence the treatment of all Medicaid beneficiaries, regardless of age, and that the formal exception of the aged will have little practical effect. Whether this is a good or bad thing is an issue in the ongoing debate about the ethical acceptability of the Oregon plan.

Other state governments may pay close attention to what happens under the Oregon program. If it meets the goals of proponents and achieves more equitable distribution of scarce Medicaid resources, without wreaking major harms on identifiable individuals, other state governments may be encouraged to try a similar form of rationing. Gaining sufficient popular support may be a problem, no matter how successful the Oregon program appears to be functioning. But if no meaningful health care reform emerges at the national level and state Medicaid budgets continue to escalate at anything like their current rates, some state governments may grow desperate enough to push the "Oregon solution" whatever the opposition.

IV. DECISIONS ABOUT LEVELS OF CARE

A. Context

Many chronically ill elders suffer due to physical or psychological afflictions. At some point, a proportion may conclude
that living is no longer desirable and may resist treatments that
prolong life but do little to achieve a sense of well-being. A
few will even contemplate or attempt suicide, or ask physicians or others to help them end their lives. When elders begin
to think or act in these ways, they can come into conflict with
caretakers who see matters differently or who feel legally or
morally bound to continue life-sustaining treatments. Although
legitimate doubts may exist about the competency of some
elders to make decisions about levels of care, many are clearly
capable of making informed judgments on such matters. Yet
these competent elders may, because of illness or great frailty,
lack the strength or determination needed to end their lives or
to convince others to accede to their wish to stop or reduce
care. In this respect, they may be no better off than the incompetent among them who are utterly dependent on what
proxies decide.

B. Justifications

Decisions to reduce or stop care for disabled or dying elders
can raise difficult ethical and legal questions. The easiest decisions to accept are those which competent elders make for
themselves. The most difficult to justify arise when elders are
incompetent and when genuine uncertainty exists as to what
they would prefer or what choice would be the least harmful.
In what follows, I will consider some justifications for reducing or stopping care for elders and discuss their legal dimensions. An underlying assumption will be that elders are sick
with an illness that cannot be cured or substantially modified
and that will cause death or great disability and suffering.

1. *Autonomy*

Our ethical and legal culture assigns high value to individual
rights and liberties and will countenance diverse acts or words

that offend against the beliefs or sensibilities of a substantial number of citizens. In health care, this tolerance permits competent individuals to refuse measures that others firmly believe are in their best interests, and—though hardly without serious protest—allows women to abort pregnancies before their fetuses are "viable" (36). Indeed the U.S. Supreme Court in its Cruzan decision (37) indicated that the right of an individual to decide whether or not to accept life-saving medical care is a "liberty" protected by the federal constitution against efforts by states to limit that right. The Court also indicated, however, that the interest of society ("the state") in protecting the lives of its citizens permits state legislatures to require clear and convincing proof that a decision to withhold life support from an incompetent person accords with preferences the person had expressed while competent. In other words, if doubt exists about what a person's self-determined or autonomous choice would be, the federal constitution would allow states to err on the side of life, even if this means that a permanently unconscious Nancy Cruzan would be kept alive indefinitely and even if this contravenes the wishes of parents or significant others.

What this implies for chronically ill elders is that their caretakers have lawful justification for relying on their decisions about levels of care, provided the choices are competent in the legal sense. Thus, if a competent elder with motor neuron disease verifiably declines a respirator or demands its removal, a physician could be charged with battery if he or she forcibly applied or continued a respirator without the elder's consent. The fact that an elder is depressed does not excuse ignoring or overriding the elder's wishes unless a caretaker has convincing evidence that the depression impairs cognitive functions (9). A logical corollary is that a physician could not be charged with medical malpractice for removing or withholding a respirator an elder patient had rejected. Moreover, while a state legislature could conceivably enact legislation that criminalizes any act by a physician that intentionally and knowingly causes death, a successful criminal prosecution under such a law would seem unlikely where an elder has an incurable and fatal disease, where the elder has rejected treatment that could do no more than extend life, and where the physician's motive is to respect the elder's wish to avoid further suffering (38).

The high value accorded autonomy may, somewhat paradoxically, limit the freedom of families, physicians, and other caretakers to relieve the suffering of elders who are incompetent or whose competency is in doubt. Thus, if autonomy is viewed as the only moral and legal justification for action that results in an elder's death, then advocates of such an action may be stymied by their failure to establish that it reflects an informed choice by the affected elder (37,39). If they firmly believe that stopping or withholding care is the correct response to the elder's plight, they may seek to justify their actions or omissions in other ways. The most convenient justification would be existence of a formally valid advance directive that the elder prepared when competent and that either clearly indicates that stopping or withholding treatment in the extant circumstances accords with the elder's wishes, or that designates a proxy who is empowered to make a decision of this nature. Although one can debate whether a directive prepared in a time past can truly be said to express an elder's current intentions, it may offer plausible support for the view that a decision to withhold or stop treatment respects the elder's knowable preferences and is thus consistent with the autonomy principle. Absent an advance directive, however, reliance on respect for autonomy as a basis for decision becomes more tenuous.

2. *Substituted judgment*

The legal doctrine of substituted judgment envisions that a designated decision maker knows enough about an incompetent person to permit a reliable approximation of the person's preferences (40). As such, the doctrine derives from the autonomy principle since its intent is to implement supposed preferences of an incompetent person, not those of the actual decision maker. Who qualifies as a decision maker will de-

pend on applicable state and local laws, but may include a
close family member, a guardian, or a court itself. Where a
decision has major import, such as stopping or withholding
life-sustaining care, applicable laws may require some form
of prior judicial authorization or approval for the decision.
This does not mean that a court order is necessary in every
case. But it does suggest that the actual substitute decision
maker, if not a court, should be able to identify some source
of authority for acting, such as an unambiguous advance directive or a guardianship order that clearly contemplates allowing a guardian to make such a decision.

Where judicial approval is sought for a substituted judgment for an incompetent elder, a court may appoint a neutral
party, sometimes called a guardian ad litem, to investigate all
the circumstances of the elder's case and prepare a report
citing grounds for and against stopping or withholding care
(41). The court will then review the report and reach a decision about whether to order the requested action or to authorize a family member or other lawful representative of an
elder to take such action. In some instances, little reliable
information will be available about what an elder's preferences
might be in the particular circumstances. The elder may have
no surviving family members or close friends, or family and
friends may have no recent knowledge of what the elder might
or might not prefer. Where this is the case, deciding on the
basis of "substituted judgment" would be largely guesswork.
Some other justification for a decision would then be necessary if interested parties desire to persist in seeking to stop or
withhold care.

3. *Best interests*

For some elders, it will seem obvious to both caretakers and
disinterested observers that trying to extend their life will only
prolong suffering or do no more than preserve them in a non-
sentient state. Caretakers may then agree that survival offers
no benefits or that its burdens outweigh its benefits. When this
occurs, they may conclude that stopping or withholding life-

sustaining treatment is in an elder's "best interests" and assert this conclusion as a legal and moral justification for a decision to stop or withhold treatment. In some cases, caretakers may be confident enough in the rightness of their conclusions to act without seeking prior legal approval. In other cases, risk aversiveness or institutional rules may cause them to go to court, or at least to seek review by an institutional ethics committee.

If caretakers go to court they could encounter hurdles, especially where they cannot prove that an elder is actually suffering by remaining alive. A guardian ad litem might, for example, cite a generalized societal interest in preserving life as one argument against stopping treatment for an elder who is not demonstrably suffering by remaining alive. That this argument might have some legal force is apparent from the Cruzan litigation in which the Missouri courts rejected efforts by Nancy Cruzan's parents to have her feeding tube removed until the courts were satisfied that Nancy herself would have wanted this (42). The fact that she was in a permanent vegetative state was not in itself viewed as an adequate legal justification for removal. Moreover, as the Conroy litigation (43) in New Jersey reveals, even courts that utilize an unalloyed "best interests" calculus may require proof of intractable physical pain before concluding that a life is burdened enough to allow withdrawal of life-sustaining measures. In other words, proof that an elder has a severe and untreatable dementia with abject dependency may not constitute proof of a cognizable legal burden for purposes of applying a "best interests" analysis. The operative burden is what the elder is experiencing, not the anguish of families or physicians' sense of futility.

4. *Democratic utilitarianism*

One lesson of the Oregon Medicaid experience is that legislative bodies can reach a consensus that some afflictions are not worth treating—or at least not worth the allocation of public funds. Moreover, various national polling data seem to suggest that the public views certain conditions as worse than death, including permanent unconsciousness or severe dementias, and proposals to allow physician-assisted suicide in certain circumstances have attracted considerable popular support. Also, virtually every state allows its citizens to write advance directives that would permit at least some life-sustaining treatments to be withheld or withdrawn in a variety of circumstances. These pieces of information suggest that a substantial portion of the public now believes that physicians should not be morally or legally bound to deploy life-sustaining treatments in all circumstances, and that there are many situations in which physicians are justified in stopping or withholding care.

If this account accurately reflects a societal consensus that there are finite limits on how far physicians should go to sustain life, there would appear to be a basis for democratically arrived at legislation that goes beyond that of advanced directive laws. This legislation might, for example, expressly authorize physicians and lawful representatives of incompetent patients to apply a "best interests" analysis in decisions about life-sustaining care. It might further explicitly permit consideration of mental or emotional suffering in the calculation of benefits and burdens. Still further, it might allow the physical, emotional, and financial stresses on caretakers to be taken into account in calculating burdens of continued treatment.

Any such legislation would of course evoke concerns about the slippery slope to selective nontreatment of those perceived as social burdens (44). As to elders or other vulnerable persons, there are risks associated with formally empowering persons to make decisions about the lives of vulnerable others based on imprecise criteria (45). What is a benefit or burden may vary with the eye of the beholder, and ostensibly objective criteria may mask intensely subjective ones. One who views aphasia or quadriplegia as fates worse than death may be unable to grasp that others may not experience these disabilities in this way. Also, one who has never experienced a neurological impairment may fail to recognize that a seriously disabled person is capable of experiencing pleasure in things that seem insignificant to the nondisabled. Federal and state antidiscrimination laws attempt to protect the disabled against these forms of subjectivity by penalizing differential treatment of the disabled that turns solely on the fact of their disability (22). Indeed any proposals that purport to expand the decisional power of proxies or caretakers with respect to disabled persons may run afoul these laws. This would include a proposal to increase the power of proxies to weigh benefits and burdens in the absence of guidance as to what disabled persons would actually prefer.

C. The Problem of Assisted Dying

The Kevorkian saga has energized public debate about the role of physicians in relieving suffering. At one pole is the view that physicians' highest duty is to relieve suffering, even if this means aiding a person to die (46). At the other pole is the view that physicians' highest duty is to preserve life and that any compromising of this duty will dangerously undermine public confidence in the medical profession (47). Current law favors the latter view, and the majority of states have statutes criminalizing actions designed to assist suicide. Moreover, physicians who aid their patients in dying risk various professional sanctions.

Despite the existing state of the law, anecdotal accounts suggest that many physicians have in various ways responded to requests from their patients for aid in dying. This aid may range from "hypothetical" discussions of the most effective ways to commit suicide (e.g., effective drugs and their dosages) to administration of morphine or other analgesics with full awareness that they might cause fatal respiratory depression. These actions by physicians virtually never eventuate in criminal prosecutions, even where there are no systemic efforts at concealment. One explanation may be that those closest to the action agree that it is morally appropriate behavior that ought not be brought to the attention of law enforcement. Another possible explanation is a disinterest of prosecutors in bringing charges against persons whose intentions are altruistic and are likely to be so viewed by a jury. Also, a state's criminal statutes may not clearly reach such conduct, as had been the case in Michigan before Kevorkian began his campaign there.

A more technical question about assisted-suicide laws is whether they meet constitutional standards. One Michigan appellate court has opined that the new Michigan statute unconstitutionally infringes upon individual liberty by erecting barriers to "rational" suicide (48). And a federal court in the state of Washington recently held that a state law banning physician-assisted suicide is an unconsitutional intrusion on protected liberty (49). These decisions, if upheld by higher courts, could do much to protect physicians who conscientiously determine that assisting their elder patients to die is the best treatment they can offer. They could also lend support to the view that a legitimate part of the physician's professional role is to aid the suicide of elders whose suffering is severe, intractable, and beyond endurance. And they might encourage medical organizations concerned with care of elders to rethink their opposition and to develop guidelines that safeguard interests of elders and instruct physicians in how to respond to requests from competent elders for aid in dying (50).

Even if legal developments legitimize physician-aided dying, many physicians are likely to eschew such a role for reasons of conscience or fear of professional sanction. A nightmare scenario is a scattering of "dying centers" staffed by the few physicians willing to aid dying and a further fragmentation of the care of the chronically ill. Presumably this misfortune will not occur. Still it would seem desirable for physicians to continue dialogues about what is the correct response to elders and others whose suffering exceeds the reach of current treatments.

REFERENCES

1. Randall T. Demographers ponder the aging of the aged and await unprecedented looming elder boom. JAMA 1994;269: 2331–2332
2. Iglehart JK. The American health care system: Medicare. N Eng J Med 1992;327:1467–1472
3. Iglehart JK. The American health care system: Medicaid. N Eng J Med 1993;328:896–900
4. Skolnick AA. After long delay, federal regulations for enforcing nursing home standards may be issued this year. JAMA 1993;269:2348–2353
5. Estate of Smith v. Heckler, 747 F 2d 583 (10th Cir 1984)
6. American Bar Association. Personal and Estate Planning for the Elderly. ABA Satellite Seminar 1989, Washington DC, 147–265
7. Appelbaum PS, Grisso T. Assessing patients' capacities to consent to treatment. N Eng J Med 1988; 319:1635–1638
8. In re Storar, 52 NY 2d 363, 420 NE 2d 64 (1981)
9. Ross v. Hilltop Rehabilitation Hospital, 676 F Supp 1528 (D Ct CO 1987)
10. Satz v. Perlmutter, 362 So 2d 160, affd 379 So 2d 359 (Dist Ct App 3d Dist FL 1980)
11. Zinermon v. Burch, 494 US 13 (1990)
12. Rogers v. Okin, 634 F 2d 650 (1st Cir 1980)
13. Underwood M. The older driver. Arch Int Med 1992; 152: 735–740
14. Beresford HR. Competency and medicolegal issues related to the aging nervous system. In: Albert ML, Knoefel JE (eds.), Clinical Neurology of Aging. New York: Oxford Press, 1994; 679–680
15. Council Report. Elder abuse and neglect. JAMA 1987; 257: 966–971
16. Ehrlich P, Anetzberger G. Survey of State Public Health Departments on Procedures for Reporting Elder Abuse. Public Health Rep 1991; 106:151–154
17. Silva TW. Reporting Elder Abuse: Should It Be Mandatory or Voluntary?. 9 No. 4 HealthSpan 13 (April 1992)
18. People v. Heitzman, 23 CA App 4th 1041, 23 CA Rptr 2d 199 (1993)

19. CA Penal Code 368, West's Ann Cal Penal Code 1993
20. Daniels RS, Clark-Daniels CL, Baumhover LA. Abuse of elders: Physicians are confused. JAMA 1988; 260:3276
21. Lewis LA. District of Columbia Survey: Toward Eliminating the Abuse, Neglect, and Exploitation of Impaired Adults: The District of Columbia Protective Services Act of 1984. Catholic Law Rev 1986; 35:1193–1212
22. Americans with Disabilities Act of 1990, 104 Stat 327 (1990)
23. Brennan TA, Leape LL, Laird NM, et al. Incidence of adverse events and negligence in hospitalized patients. New Eng J Med 1991; 324:370–376
24. Goldner JL. An overview of legal controls on human experimentation and the regulatory implications of taking Professor Katz seriously. St Louis Univ Law J 1993; 38:63–137
25. Hyman v Jewish Chronic Disease Hosp, 248 NYS 2d 245 (NY Sup Ct 1964)
26. Kahn KL, Pearson ML, Harrison ER, et al. Health care for black and poor hospitalized medicare patients. JAMA 1994; 271:1169–1174
27. Cotton P. Bang more of a whimper, health economist avers. JAMA 1993; 269:2333
28. Iglehart JK. The American health care system: Community hospitals. N Engl J Med 1993; 329:372–376
29. United Wire v. Morristown Memorial Hosp, 995 F 2d 1179 (3d Cir 1993)
30. Siliciano J. Wealth, Equity, and the Unitary Standard of Care. Virginia Law Rev 1991; 77:439–484
31. Frankel JJ. Medical malpractice law and health care cost containment: Lessons for reformers from the clash of cultures. Yale Law J 1994; 1297–1331
32. Hall v. Hilbun, 466 So 2d 856 (MS Sup Ct 1985)
33. Annas GJ, Law SA, Rosenblatt RE, Wing KR, American Health Law. Boston: Little Brown, 1989; 516–524
34. Moon J, Holahan J. Can states take the lead in health care reform? JAMA 1992; 268:1588–1594
35. Thomas WJ. The Oregon Medicaid proposal: Ethical paralysis, tragic democracy, and the fate of a utilitarian health care program. Oregon Law Rev 1993; 72:49-156
36. Planned Parenthood v. Casey, 112 S Ct 2791 (1992)
37. Cruzan v. Director, 110 S Ct 2841 (1990)

38. Barber v. Superior Court, 147 CA App 3d 1006, 195 CA Rptr 414 (1983)
39. In re O'Connor, 72 NY 2d 517 (1988)
40. In re Quinlan, 70 NJ 10, 355 A 2d 647, cert den 429 US 922 (1976)
41. Superintendent of Belchertown State School v. Saikewicz, 373 MA 728, 370 NE 2d 417 (1977)
42. Cruzan v. Harmon, 760 SW 2d 408 (MO Sup Ct 1988)
43. In re Conroy, 98 NJ 321, 486 A 2d 1209 (1985)
44. Beresford HR. Legal aspects of termination of treatment decisions. Neurol Clin 1989; 7:775–787
45. Herr SS, Hopkins BL. Health care decision making for persons with disabilities. JAMA 1994; 271:1017–1022
46. Quill TE, Cassel CK, Meier DE. Care of the hopelessly ill. N Eng J Med 1991; 327:1380–1384
47. Kamisar Y. When is there a constitutional "right to die"? When is there no constitutional "right to live"? Georgia Law Rev 1991; 25:1203–1242
48. Michigan v. Kevorkian, 1993 WL 603212 (MI Cir Ct 12/13/93)
49. Egan T. Federal judge says ban on suicide aid is unconstitutional. New York Times 5/5/94:A1
50. Miller FG, Quill TE, Brody H, et al. Regulating physician-assisted death. N Eng J Med 1994; 331:119–123

Index

Index

Index